Wondrously Wounded

SRTD
STUDIES IN RELIGION, THEOLOGY, AND DISABILITY

SERIES EDITORS

Sarah J. Melcher
Xavier University, Cincinnati, Ohio

and

Amos Yong
Fuller Theological Seminary, Pasadena, California

Wondrously Wounded

Theology, Disability, and the Body of Christ

Brian Brock

BAYLOR UNIVERSITY PRESS

Cover Design by Savanah N. Landerholm
Cover image: Kendall Cox, *In a Green Light*, acrylic on canvas, 2018
Book Design by Diane Smith

The Library of Congress has cataloged this book under ISBN 978-1-4813-1012-3.

Printed in the United States of America on acid-free paper with a minimum of 30 percent post-consumer waste recycled content.

For Stephanie

This is my movie. This is my life. Be cool.

For I am poor and needy,
and my heart is wounded within me.

Series Introduction

Studies in Religion, Theology, and Disability brings newly established and emerging scholars together to explore issues at the intersection of religion, theology, and disability. The series editors encourage theoretical engagement with secular disability studies while supporting the reexamination of established religious doctrine and practice. The series fosters research that takes account of the voices of people with disabilities and the voices of their family and friends.

The volumes in the series address issues and concerns of the global religious studies/theological studies academy. Authors come from a variety of religious traditions with diverse perspectives to reflect on the intersection of the study of religion/theology and the human experience of disability. This series is intentional about seeking out and publishing books that engage with disability in dialogue with Jewish, Christian, Buddhist, or other religious and philosophical perspectives.

Themes explored include religious life, ethics, doctrine, proclamation, liturgical practices, physical space, spirituality, or the interpretation of sacred texts through the lens of disability. Authors in the series are aware of conversation in the field of disability studies and bring that discussion to bear methodologically and theoretically in their analyses at the intersection of religion and disability.

Studies in Religion, Theology, and Disability reflects the following developments in the field: First, the emergence of disability studies as an interdisciplinary endeavor that has impacted theological studies, broadly defined. More and more scholars are deploying disability perspectives in their work, and this applies also to those working in the theological academy. Second, there is a growing need for critical reflection on disability in world religions. While books from a Christian standpoint have dominated the discussion at the interface of religion and disability so far, Jewish, Muslim, Buddhist, and Hindu scholars, among those from other religious traditions, have begun to resource their own religious traditions to rethink disability in the twenty-first century. Third, passage of the Americans with Disabilities Act in the U.S.A. has raised the consciousness of the general public about the importance of critical reflection on disability in religious communities. General and intelligent lay readers are looking for scholarly discussions of religion and disability as these bring together and address two of the most important existential aspects of human lives. Fourth, the work of activists in the disability rights movement has mandated fresh critical reflection by religious practitioners and theologians. Persons with disabilities remain the most disaffected group from religious organizations. Fifth, government representatives in several countries have prioritized the greater social inclusion of persons with disabilities. Disability policy often proceeds based on core cultural and worldview assumptions that are religiously informed. Work at the interface of religion and disability thus could have much broader purchase—that is, in social, economic, political, and legal domains.

Under the general topic of thoughtful reflection on the religious understanding of disability, Studies in Religion, Theology, and Disability includes shorter, crisply argued volumes that articulate a bold vision within a field; longer scholarly monographs, more fully developed and meticulously documented, with the same goal of engaging wider conversations; textbooks that provide a state of the discussion at this intersection and chart constructive ways forward; and select edited volumes that achieve one or more of the preceding goals.

Contents

Preface

> Now I only inquire when I find myself *inquired of*. Inquired of, that is, by people, rather than by scholars. There is a human being in each scholar, who inquires and stands in need of answers. I am anxious to answer the scholar *qua* human being, but not the representative of a certain discipline, that insatiable, ever inquisitive phantom which like a vampire drains the one whom it possesses of humanity. I hate that phantom as I do all phantoms. Its questions are meaningless to me. On the other hand, the questions asked by human beings have become increasingly important to me.[1]

Most people would consider my son Adam profoundly intellectually disabled. One of Adam's many gifts to me is to make the terms "profound" and "disabled" feel painfully misleading. Far from pointing toward an entity with crisply defined boundaries, the term "disability" points into a complex terrain populated by remarkably diverse conditions and crisscrossed by highly charged political disputes. Adam's life is tangled in that jungle. Should Adam emerge in these pages as a person, citizen, and churchman in his own right I will have succeeded in one of my main goals: to offer readers a sense of the ways common distinctions like able and disabled, high functioning and the profoundly disabled can obscure the lives that are so much more than the labels.

Living with Adam has meant doing theology under the pressure of those who *ask*. People ask about Adam—serious and probing questions that admit of no easy answers. Even to attempt to answer them demands revisiting widespread assumptions about God and the world in which we both must live: industrialized, consumerist, secular Western democracies.[2] The process has surfaced substantial questions about some of the sterile boundaries imposed in much academic theology. As an academic theologian trained in medical ethics, I was being given a good shakedown by Adam, unsettling the very foundations of my understanding of what it means to *do* theology. He even forced me to the realization that much that goes under the heading of disability theology still takes too many common assumptions for granted, is still insufficiently shaped by the realities to which Christians commit themselves when they confess themselves to be followers of Jesus Christ.

A central presumption of this book is that our lives with God, neighbor, and world cannot be understood independently of one another. Though what we call disability is never a purely individual experience, it is one that can only be lived out by individuals.[3] The term "disability" points to a "deep" phenomenon, a rupture not just in conceptual categories but in people's lives, much more than a phenomenon unfortunately afflicting "some people." The term "disability" is first and foremost a sign hanging over a doorway that opens into existentially dangerous territory, an unexpected portal into an apparently alternative reality. Nobody goes through that door willingly. And nobody who goes through it is unchanged.

This book is held together by a life lived under the label disability, that of Adam Brock. Adam's body and mental world are vastly different from anything I have personally lived. To know Adam at all demands letting him tell me what his life is, and aligning myself with what he reveals. Devoid of any power of projection, he nevertheless articulates profound things with wide-ranging implications. His quiet voice has called me through the door of disability and emboldened me to embrace the suffering of finding the right words to let you hear it too. My hope is to give you a sense of the wondrous beauty of Adam's form of life. It has been a privilege to have a front-row seat on the work of a healer in a church founded as a hospital for fallen humanity.[4]

The chapters in this book broadly track the various stages of Adam's life. As my reflections on his life unfolded over many years, the book was bound to end up the story of a conversion—mine. Conversion stories are notoriously hard to tell, as the slow transformation of the author's view of the world must be tangibly depicted. The various fractures and shifts of viewpoint in this book are unified by an underlying story about how living with Adam has overturned my narrative of my own life, my fears and hopes, as well as my views of God and the church. Through it all I am constantly puzzling through what it could possibly mean to call him disabled.[5]

If Adam is going to appear before you in his own right, there are limits to what I can and should tell about him. Only one of us has the power to define both our lives by telling our story, and this imbalance comes with real dangers. The first is to tell his story as a way of proving my credentials to speak on this topic, a gesture that has become so familiar in disability theology circles.[6] Telling stories always engages an audience and builds powerful ethical momentum. Stories can easily overwhelm theoretical discussions and draw undue attention to the storyteller. It is for me a matter of the ethics of discourse to forgo the deployment of stories to convey my credentials as a credible authority on this topic. I will therefore strictly limit myself to only telling stories that advance the reader's understanding of the sort of actions in the world that I am trying to describe in more theoretical terms. Every story is an interpretation. I will tell stories as occasions to display the *theological hermeneutics of experience* that I understand to be my main contribution to the scholarly discussion of disability. The stories I present are the ones necessary to understand the theoretical discussions that most often precede them. In this book, *narratives* and arguments are interpreting each other. Telling stories in this way may validate my credentials to speak, but this is an effect, not the aim, of my telling them.

My aim will be to write his life as we have lived it: *together*. To tell his story at all risks obscuring important aspects of lives like his, as narrative conventions enforce their own rules of coherence and closure. It would be easy for these narrative conventions to sanitize his story by masking what is unsettling and different about him—his pain, shame, and frustration. Ultimately none of us will know whether my stories about Adam map onto *his* perception of our shared experiences. I am not certain, for instance, that Adam's experience of the world has a narrative structure with a past, future, and present. He may inhabit the world in something like a perpetual present tense not easily fit into conventional narrative forms. Such difficulties of talking well about Adam's life must not be obscured or evaded if his own personality is to emerge. Honoring his uniqueness thus demands *dramatizing* the difficulties of narrating his life, making them *more* palpable. One of the most important gains of not using stories to establish my credentials as an author is that I am empowered to depict my bewilderment, my lack of understanding of given situations, and so to let his certainties emerge as genuinely other than mine. To be true to Adam's life on his own terms demands working to push myself as the storyteller into the background, a task in palpable tension with relating the story of the conversion he has catalyzed in me. Such tensions must not, and indeed ultimately cannot, be evaded.[7]

If I can tell our story in ways that rob Adam of his own (nonverbal) voice, the problem recurs in relation to the many other people who are part of his story. Disability happens in the gloriously repetitive stuff of the day-to-day, and the day-to-day of Adam's life is highly social, woven together with the lives of his family, his school, and his local and national governments as well as his church. I hope to offer some glimpses of what this dailiness entails in all its joys and difficulties. Yet to articulate my own difficulties in living day to day with someone who is genuinely different from me implicates other people and social orders, exposing the frictions between them. My wife, Stephanie, has her own views of many of the events that will be narrated in this book, as do our other children, Caleb and Agnes. Their stories would be subtly but importantly different from the ones I will tell.[8] Though it will be my voice you will hear in these pages, it is one I hope has been shaped by these other voices and the ways they tell our story, as well as by voices of the saints through the ages, from whom I have learned the story of all our lives together with God.

Approaching a theological treatment of disability as a reflection on my life with Adam has the advantage of concretizing my discussion and limiting its scope. It will also foreground the questions raised by cognitive disability, as well as the particular set of theological questions raised by congenital conditions.[9] Loving Adam in all his concreteness is thus a good place to start to talk about disability but can also foreshorten the discussion. Both conditions exacerbate the problems of representation just outlined. Concentrating analysis on a young man with intellectual challenges may also buffer the *political* challenge of his life, since it is easy for parents to infantilize people like Adam by assuming they will never grow up and out of their households. I will need to find ways to keep my relation to him as his father from sequestering him in the private zone of the family. His parents are not the only ones responsible to Adam. As threatening as it feels to relinquish him to others, this is a constant responsibility of a parent. It includes letting his vulnerability be visible to readers who need to be challenged by *his* predicament as a citizen of a developed democratic society, and as a church member.[10]

Why tell all these stories without a shred of evidence that Adam cares whether his story is told or not? I tell Adam's story as a witness to his witness. It is a confession, a testimony. I seek to listen to and join in with *his* song of praise. To put the matter this way is to be released from the worry that I am illegitimately "using" or "operationalizing" Adam to score theological points or gain territory in a culture war. Much like the early Christian parents who did not shirk martyrdom because it would deprive their children of parents, our hope is only that Adam will not be disadvantaged by our amplification of what we have heard from him about the church and society in which we live.[11]

By daring publicly to amplify the quiet joy of Adam's witness I hope to explode some of the layers of uncomfortable avoidance and outright censorship that surround disability in churches, in public discussion of social care policy, and in medical contexts. In each of these contexts most people assume they know what disability is. In fact their views are often skewed by unacknowledged fears of disability as a dark thundercloud threatening to destroy lives and eject people into a desolate life of social isolation, grinding practical difficulties, and unbearable expense. It is difficult for any of us to eradicate the fear evoked by the term "disability," which threatens at the very least an unbearable diminishment of the life choices available to us. This fear points to an enslavement to the desire to control others, to make them into our images, and to make ourselves into an image of perfection. It is an enslavement that renders our lives, and our societies, frightfully two dimensional—efficient, homogenous, and so unsurprising.[12]

One way of summarizing the Christian gospel is as an empowerment to risk living as the vulnerable beings we in fact are, to make peace with our limits and blemishes and to delight in the unexpected. Human redemption consists in the recovery of the joy and freedom that come with being content to be creatures rather than aspiring to be gods. The central theological task of this book is to give theological density as well as contemporary tangibility to this claim. In short, I hope to convey as richly as I am capable that what Christians should hear in the term "disability" is the rumble of something approaching that is much bigger than our fears and dreams, and forces from us an enlarged capacity to love, wonder, and praise.

None of this is meant to suggest that pain and suffering are not part of the human experiences typically labeled disabilities. The title *Wondrously Wounded* highlights the entanglement of blessing and suffering at the heart of the story of God's people. Jacob is on the run from his brother Esau, whose birthright blessing he has deceitfully stolen from their old and blind father Isaac (Gen 27). Jacob's nomadic life on the run is upended by a rude attack of an unknown man in the middle of the night at the ford of Jabbok (Gen 32:22-32). In the course of that extended wrestling match Jacob realizes he is wrestling with God and demands a blessing. Dawn arrives to find Jacob exhausted but exultant, the desired blessing secured. With the blessing has come the gift of a new name commemorating for all generations such wrestling as the very essence of faith.[13] An unwelcome attack has been transformed into the discovery of Jacob's true place in God's story. But the process has not been easy, the wrestling so violent that Jacob is left with a permanent bodily impairment and a very visible limp. The unexpected attack, the bravery of clinging to God instead of running, the pain, the permanent wound, the social marker of a funny walk—come together in a transformation of Jacob so deep that he now sees literally everything differently: himself, his feud with his brother, God, and his place in the created realm. In time the whole people of God come to identify themselves with this wrestling.[14]

Human eyes can see the wrestling with society, with the medical establishment, and with the church that disability so often provokes. But wrestling with the human experiences labeled disability is ultimately to wrestle with God. These are experiences that bring human beings face-to-face with creaturely limits and personal brokenness. In them reality tears through the paper-thin beliefs about human life that are characteristic of modernity, shattering the individual hopes built on them. Precisely in the shattering of superficial hopes does disability become a crucible for the radical remaking of hope. With this remaking comes new awareness of the blessings and responsibilities that are ours alone. Letting my own wrestling at times appear will hint at how, for Christians, this wrestling is understood as the interruption of a Christ who graciously attacks the constricting expectations that blind us to others.[15]

The subtitle, "Theology, Disability, and the Body of Christ," alludes to my ambition in this book to offer a *theological reconstitution* of the very idea of disability. The body of Christ is the result of God's gracious attack on the antihuman certainties that keep each fallen human generation estranged from one another. Throughout this book I will regularly use the language of "people who carry the label disabled" to highlight the contemporary relevance of this divine attack on contemporary assumptions about disability. It is the experience of one's self as "able" in comparison to others that is fundamentally problematic for the Christian. It tends to entrap both those who believe themselves "able" and those they believe are not within patterns of relating that blind them to what the Spirit of Jesus Christ has for the church and the world in and through each human life.

To name disability as the site of struggle with God is to insist on the primacy of theological description. For me, writing is an extended attempt to discover the words from the biblical traditions that illuminate my life with Adam. I say "attempt" because far more than any before, this book has been constructed in fits and starts, in first stabs at stories and analyses, some of which were initially published elsewhere.[16] Passages from those first attempts appear here interspersed with much new material and in what I hope is a more developed, clear, and readable form. Re-presenting some of this earlier material often lends older descriptions quite different colors, yet another reminder that the struggle is not an abstract one, but an ongoing quest to find the words for the life I live with the living person of Adam Brock. A kaleidoscopic treatment results, in which each chapter picks out one facet of this lived life. Eventually a set of central theological themes was to emerge—the revelatory role of the human experiences currently labeled disabilities, the importance of the body, with its embedding in social and linguistic structures, as well as the counterintuitive nature of health and wholeness when viewed within the fullness of redeemed community. These points of clarity were achieved by means of a classic theological approach; using biblical texts, and traditional readings of them, to find my way into the coherence of my own story. This required holding rather loosely to the usual academic divisions of theology from the Bible, the Bible from historical analysis, historical analysis from appeals to experience, and experience from cultural criticism. Points needed to be found where typically very discrete discourses—literary, philosophical, political, and theological—meet and even fuse to open unexpected ways of perceiving and living in our world. The central problem is to accurately formulate what might be reasonably hoped for all of us in the middle of the world we *already* inhabit. It all must be in play in order to speak with any thought about the redeeming work of Jesus Christ, and the life of the community of faith in the contemporary world.

Disability is so much more than a medically diagnosed impairment, a social stigma, or political activism engaged in the fight against manifest injustice: it is an existential struggle. Foregrounding this personal struggle is theologically important because most people do *not* find disability disturbing in this deeper and more personal way. Most assume disability is a sad departure from what human beings were meant by God to be that befalls an unfortunate few. Ironically, the most severely intellectually disabled also do not struggle with disability, being wondrously free from pondering what others suppose them to lack. I write then for those who have for some reason found themselves forced genuinely to wrestle with disability. With any luck what we will together discover are truths hidden by the illusions of the great majority. That majority continues, mistakenly, to labor under the greatest illusion of all—that disability is a marginal note to the human condition.

Acknowledgments

Writing is revision, making generous and critical readers indispensable. Amos Yong pushed me to produce this book, Martin Wendte to keep the stories in, and Carey C. Newman to trim the fat. Students in the 2017 Theological Ethics and Practical Theology Research Seminar in Aberdeen pointed out the tricks I'd missed, and I'm especially grateful for the engagement of my colleagues John Swinton, Grant Macaskill, and Leon van Ommen. I benefited from a trial run of some of the material at the Summer Institute on Theology and Disability at Azusa Pacific University in 2017, where I received especially insightful feedback from Brian Lugioyo, Helen Ree, and Paul Shrier. In the last leg of revisions, the hospitality of the monks of Pluscardin Abbey was a lifesaver (yet again!), as was the feedback I received from those who read near-final drafts: Amos Yong, Sarah Melcher, John Swinton, Tom Greggs, Susan Parsons, Jake Rollison, Julie Lamb, Kevin O'Farrell, Tony Stiff, Alex Mason, Steve Hickey, and Topher Endress, to whom I am doubly grateful for preparing the index.

Introduction
Disability as a Matter of the Heart

Practitioners of disability theology and the churches of the developed West are at a crossroad. Virtually every public building, including churches, has been modified for accessibility, and the importance of making the lives of people with some disabilities a little bit more livable is now widely fixed in the public consciousness. Yes, most will admit, there is more to be done—perhaps much more—but at least the peoples of the developed West can be proud of having accomplished the task of including people with disabilities in the collective life. Down this self-congratulatory road we can already see public attention turning to supposedly more pressing social issues. And that is the rub. Accessibility modifications have made everyone's lives easier without demanding more substantive change.[1] They may even have stalled progress in increasing the hospitality of secular society by generating the illusion that interpersonal change is less important than infrastructural improvement.[2]

Facing the possibility that the accessibility movement has hardened problematic views of disability is to confront the central problematic of a theological account of disability: the resistance of the human heart to being claimed and reshaped by genuine difference. As the wellspring of affective personal attachment, the human heart is the origin of a person's basic orientation in the world as well as the place where people genuinely meet one another, the locus of interpersonal union. A deeper resistance to having one's sense of what counts as a "normal" human life can fester in human hearts. To admit that this resistance is widespread is to be forced to consider that Western society may not have achieved as much for people labeled disabled as it would be comforting to assume. With this admission another, harder, road becomes visible, that winds down into the badlands of the human heart, where inner resistance to finding joy in the disabled other persists.[3]

The main aim of this book is to beckon readers down this harder road. It will not be all darkness. When the genuine breadth of human life lodges in human hearts, it profoundly reshaped the way people look on the world. Conversely, all the ramps and lifts in the world are a poor substitute for open hearts, as hearts hardened to otherness radiate rejection and resistance even in physically accessible public places. This contrast will need to arise before the reader in vivid detail. As the painter's task is to bring to canvas the beauty and ugliness she sees in the material world, this book must display the ugliness our self-image as members of the enlightened and humane modern world so desperately wishes to hide. Facing the ugly rejection and marginalization still suffered by people with disabilities is only tolerable in the light of a gospel with the power to reveal its alternative: the community of open human hearts.[4]

Human hearts take shape in specifically configured cultural contexts. The term "disability" is always a label that attempts to capture several types of liminal conditions within ever shifting webs of human relations. Gaining any substantive purchase on disability will therefore demand historical and genealogical work. In an up-to-date definition of disability that would be difficult to improve, Rosemarie Garland-Thomson captures the vast semantic range of contemporary deployments of the label "disability."

> Disability is in an overarching and in some ways artificial category that encompasses congenital and acquired physical differences, mental illness and retardation, chronic and acute illnesses, fatal and progressive diseases, temporary and permanent injuries, and a wide range of bodily characteristics considered disfiguring, such as scars, birthmarks, unusual proportions, or obesity. Even though the prototypical disabled person posited in cultural representations never leaves a wheelchair, is totally blind or profoundly deaf, most of the approximately forty million Americans with disabilities have a much more ambiguous relationship to the label . . . . Disability, then, can be painful, comfortable, familiar, alienating, bonding, isolating, disturbing, endearing, challenging, infuriating, or ordinary. Embedded in the complexity of actual human relations, it is always more than the disabled figure can signify.[5]

The highly complex and contradictory meanings inherent in contemporary usage of the term "disability" offer little more than a starting point for a theological treatment of the various life experiences to which that label points.

COMPLEXIFYING THE WORD "I": SELF-KNOWLEDGE BETWEEN GOD AND NEIGHBOR

Writing stories and novels was Franz Kafka's way of seeking an abundant life. As a Jew living in the Austro-Hungarian empire, a functionary in a large insurance agency reaching ever greater heights of bureaucratic complexity, an unmarried first son of an overbearing and socially aspirant father seeking family advantage through his marriage, and then a man of soldiering age kept home from the gruesome trenches of the First World War, he needed to find a way to articulate the tensions and dilemmas of his existence to avoid being psychologically dismembered by the forces at work in and upon him. As he constructed fictional characters who were themselves sufferers and resisters of inhumane forces, Kafka patiently searched for coherences within his own life narrative. These fictional characters would somehow, by way of hints and gestures, uncover more promising ways of living to an author who was himself also a sufferer and resister. His writing was his wrestling, and his resistance.[6]

In writing novels and stories Kafka was attempting to gain purchase on his "I" without falling into one of the fundamental paradoxes of modern identity: the habit of thinking of ourselves as discrete beings whose identities are essentially self-determined. Kafka knew that if he was to have an "I" at all, it would have to be laboriously wrested from the illegitimate moral demands assumed by most people in his time and place.

The fourth-century African Christian Augustine of Hippo also wrote his life, offering his own life to the reading public instead of a fictional doppelganger, as did Kafka. Neither could say exactly where their own faults ended and the cruelties of the societies in which they lived began. Augustine's main concern was to praise God for having rescued him out of this confusing predicament, offering his own life as testimony that Jesus Christ is still at work even today. What is so memorable about the stance Augustine strikes in the *Confessions* is that he never makes claims *about* God that are not set within prayerful speech *to* God. His search for the narrative coherence of his life is part of a deeper and wider conversation with God.

Confessing himself a Christian has committed Augustine to an account of himself as a character who has been set on a path toward the *discovery* of his true "I"—one constituted within a set of relationships that precede him, with God, creation and the neighbor. If Augustine's life has any unity, he confesses, it has been given to him from beyond himself. It will take active work to receive it, the claim of Jesus Christ having radically decentered his former self-identifications.[7]

The task before him is to come to terms with what Scripture and the Christian community say about who he is. He starts over at the beginning, the beginning of his own story in the works of the God who has created him and claimed him for life with the people of God. He discovers that there are three stories that encapsulate his origin, and so his true identity. The first is the story of having been captured, against his will, for the plans and programs of the Lord of history. Confession commits him to witnessing having seen the action of Jesus Christ afoot in world affairs. But this story of the origin of his own faith is not intelligible without locating the points where his particular story interweaves with the story of the origin of creation and of the church within it. His story of conversion, of the origin of the world, and of the saving work that births the redeemed community are all necessary parts of knowing his identity in its enfoldment within the greater story of God's ways with the world.

No one has full possession of their own story, because everyone is ultimately called into existence by the story of Jesus and incorporated into this story by the Holy Spirit. *The vulnerability intrinsic to reliance on the Spirit reveals vulnerability as ultimately not a threat, but the condition of relation, and indeed, its very promise*. Augustine's own point of greatest vulnerability was his relations to two people, his pre-Christian mistress and their son he named Adeodatus ("gift of God").[8] To tell the story of his vulnerable relationship with God meant telling of the vulnerability he experienced in his relations with other human beings.

Theological writers like Augustine levy a crucial challenge to contemporary theologians: to refuse to let discussions of theological concepts drift free of a more basic confession of relational intimacy with a living God, what Martin Luther was later to call the "for me" aspect of the Christian confession.[9] What is being claimed when a Christian doctrine is invoked gains substantial traction when readers can see how the author believes such a doctrine orients people in the world in which they live.

The examples of Augustine and Kafka highlight why it is impossible for me to imagine talking in any serious way about disability and health, Christ the healer, Christian theology, or myself without reference to Adam. Whoever "I" am is also and irrevocably Adam's father. His characteristic round face and vaguely Asiatic eyes makes him instantly recognizable as a bearer of the medical label Down syndrome. Fewer will recognize his lack of speech and characteristic arm flapping gestures as signs of his autism. Adam is now a teenager, a fact that I cannot but contemplate with genuine wonder. This book is an apparatus for discerning how to live with integrity with him and the God from whom he has come in the modern, developed West.[10]

WRITING DISABILITY AS COMING TO TERMS WITH CREATURELY VULNERABILITY

"My soul was wounded, and my life as it were torn to pieces, since my life and hers had become a single thing."[11] So Augustine described the death of his faithful Christian mother, Monica. Human beings are constituted by their ties with others, ties so tight that when they are severed our "I" can go missing. The terms "I" and "you" are in the end only names for aspects of a relation composed neither by "I" nor "you." Human beings must constantly puzzle through and laboriously differentiate where "I" begins and "you" ends. "Let's face it. We're undone by each other. And if we are not, we're missing something."[12]

The language of disability is almost inextricably bound up with distinctions between us and them—with the ones doing the talking assuming themselves to be the "us" and the people being talked about the "them." I have chosen to explore my life with Adam in the public forum of an academic monograph because it allows me constantly to unsettle these deep-seated linguistic habits.[13] Human beings estranged from their Creator have not found suitable words to express all that needs to be said about those currently called disabled. To escape becoming entangled in this us-them thinking, I want to begin differently: from the wonder at the heart of the creaturely life human beings live. I write as a prayer for God to transform misshapen fears and repulsions into joy and delight.

I also write to digest events and gazes that have left an unsettled and finely textured sediment in my soul. I write in response first to averted gazes, confused and repulsed gazes, mocking and annoyed gazes, and more powerfully by gazes and gestures of joy and delight. Behind every word of this book is a wall of gazes; not gazes on its author, but toward the one he gazes at in love—a gaze itself provoked and consoled by the gaze of the One who created us both as we are. I have been made part of that community sensitized by gestures of disdain and dismissal that fundamentally challenge the politics of Christian love.

Perhaps more powerfully than anything else, the gaze and the gesture produce the feeling of threat in modern societies within which those bearing the label "disabled" must live their lives. As a man of fighting age kept home from the front by his role as a "war-indispensable" insurance company employee, Kafka felt intensely the barrage of disapproving gazes trained on him by the citizens of Prague as he walked the streets of his home town. The war directly impacted all he thought and felt, but at an emotional level. He experienced himself a victim of constant personal attacks prosecuted through sneers and glares. Before the rise of the surveillance society he described how the weight of a gaze lingers long after the act of gazing has passed, how approval and disapproval burrow into the soul of those looked upon.[14]

It is notoriously difficult to read gazes, a problem further complicated by the ambiguity and essentially contested nature of disability ascriptions.[15] It may then be one absurdity too far for someone whose body and mind locate him right at the center of the Western ideal form of humanity to claim any real experience of disability—a healthy white male, articulate and in the prime of life, and a card-carrying member of the aggressively competitive and hypercognitive world of the academy to boot. Yet Adam has come to live in me. Were Adam to die, he would live on in me, since I can forget neither his face nor the faces the world has turned toward him—nor that through him God has confronted me.[16] This has rendered the person I point to as "I" sensitive to the slights, glares, and curiosity of the general public. The realization that something has changed comes in moments of noticing oneself internally bracing to weather the field of gazes that crisscross public space or assuming a defensive crouch at curious stares. Along with such winces comes wondrous surprise at discovering a sense of kinship or affection passing in a glance with someone in a wheelchair, or with an autistic teen and her harried loved one. Having been disabled in this manner means, above all, becoming acutely aware that some human beings are never invisible in a crowd.

Just as people with bodily impairments can experience being "abled" by intimate and supportive relations with others, so too can loving someone lead to a vicarious internalization of their (largely social) disablement.[17] To say that "Adam has disabled me" is to confess having been drawn into his world, with its time and its politics. Modern political philosophy struggles to account for the passion and grief and rage that draw people out of themselves and binds them to others, overspilling the vocabulary and ontology available to secular liberal rights holders.[18] Christians, in contrast, have a ready vocabulary for this process of *being made members of one another*.

It is finally from Adam then, not Kafka, that I learned the power of gesture and gaze. The process has been accelerated because Adam withholds his speech. To know him at all has demanded expanding my grasp of the richly communicative rhythms of his various forms of bodily communication. The power of disability to expand communicative bandwidth is prodigious. Laying paralyzed and unable to communicate as a sufferer of locked-in syndrome, Martin Pistorius gained special insight into the ubiquity of communicative signaling.

> People revealed themselves . . . in a touch that was gentle and caring or rough and unthinking; in feet that shuffled with fatigue when they walked into a room. If someone was impatient, they would sigh as they washed or fed me; if they were angry, they would pull off my clothes just a little more roughly than usual. Happiness fizzed off of them like a small electric pulse, while anxiety had a thousand telltale signs from the nails people bit to the hair they pushed behind their ears again and again to try to contain their worry.[19]

In the end, everyone wears their heart on their sleeve. Becoming attuned to finer-grained modes of communication allows glimpses of a more subtle and gentle politics tuned in to the happiness that fizzles off people's bodies "like a small electric pulse" and can respond with gentle empathy to pains too deep for words. At the same time, it is also to be sensitized to the blundering, blind violence of our age and the cloak of words behind which it hides.

To say "Adam has disabled me" is ultimately to draw attention to the hard work that goes into mediating between him with his limits and capacities as he negotiates a world in which it is assumed that he lacks the basic capacities of "normal" citizens. The suffering that goes with this hard work for Stephanie and me, as his parents, relates to the diminishment of our ability to live the lives we have been led to expect people with our levels of education and privilege deserve. Thankfully, this is a diminishment that Adam himself does not suffer. It is equally true to say that Adam has empowered me—as is the slave in Hegel's master-slave dialectic—by liberating me from the illusion of all masters: that they live without the help and support of others. Adam makes the need for networks of supportive human relationships for a flourishing human life palpable. My use of the utterance "Adam has disabled me" thus represents a ruthless exploitation of the ambiguity of the term "disability," so that the *theological* reality hidden within aspects of the secular term "disability" can be exposed.

Kafka offers a final provocation. The tuberculosis that eventually killed him did not proceed quickly. The metamorphosis of his body was decisively altering all his relationships and rendering him a foreigner to his own society. As the horizon of death loomed ever larger in his body, he sensed himself slipping into a rival time, one very different from that inhabited by the citizens of the general public. In such a situation, he mused, "what else can happen but that the two worlds split apart, or at least tear away at each other in a fearful manner."[20] He penned his greatest works as he slipped ever deeper into what has come to be called "crip time." The rending of time by a disabling condition proved the crucial catalyst for crystallizing his deepest insights into the everyday challenges facing nonstandard human lives in modernity.

One of the founding documents of contemporary disability theology was born out of a not dissimilar experience of a broken body, written—that of Nancy Eiesland. Her writing, too, was a living engagement with the everyday reality of Christian faith in a modern world not often fully welcoming of people with disabilities. In the tearing away of the time of her disablement from the public time of modernity, she was able to see more clearly the most problematic political, material, and anthropological implications of much modern Christian theology.[21] Adam's existence, his experience of illness, as well as his very active engagement with his church and the general public has likewise alienated me from the common sense of our age, making this book, too, part of the tradition of suffering writers like Eiesland and Kafka, and others, such as Flannery O'Connor and Franz Rosenzweig.[22]

Eiesland was finally a political insurrectionist. Insurrection, being an assault on the great inertia of modern common sense, demands great discipline, at once intellectual, linguistic, and practical. Passion is insurrection's fuel.[23] First comes seeing the systematic ways in which the status quo disadvantages and slights some, the least able to defend themselves, while making life as easy as possible for others, the most able. I have been disabled because Adam rubs my face in the barbarisms of our civilized world. Not so long ago people like Adam were routinely hidden away, not offered education or a place in their own family—and today the vast majority of people like him are killed before being allowed to assume their rights as citizens of modern Western democracies. I dream of exposing and demolishing the configurations of words and ideas that make that barbarism seem reasonable. Yet raw outrage is sterile or simply destructive if not focused to yield constructive proposals about how Christians might go on with any integrity in a society that condemns some people to die because they cannot speak, or because their lives are considered too divergent from common pictures of the good life.

This book will at many points burn with angry protest at certain gazes and gestures, as well as the unexpected joy and comfort that beams from faces suffused with love. The anger cannot and must not be an end in itself. *If*—and here the conditional is emphatic—the anger at the way our world is arranged that burns through some of what follows is theologically defensible, it can only be as *lament and protest at the habitual disdain of God's good gifts. That* really is worth protesting.

THE SHAPE OF THINGS TO COME

Focusing on the architecture of the gaze and gesture provides an initial access point into the dynamics that shape the lives of those labeled disabled in the various scenes of modern life. In this book I will develop and deploy a doxological hermeneutic to indicate how these cultural scenes and domains might be negotiated in a faithfully Christian manner. The language of doxology and anti-doxology emphasize the inescapability of the activity of praise for human beings as emotive and communicative beings. What and how we praise has wide-ranging epistemic implications. Within a doxological hermeneutic, to speak about the phenomenon that is normally called disability is to understand it as a creaturely phenomenon strung between creation and the final judgment. At the center of this history is Jesus Christ, who, as creation's Origin and Redeemer, is the active opponent of all sinful and so destructive human gazes.[24]

The book is organized into five sections. Interested readers can grasp the general thrust of the book by reading the codas to the five sections, especially the coda to part 4, which summarizes the first half of the book and points to the aims of the second. Part 1 positions modern presumptions about disability against the horizon of patristic Christianity. A theological approach to disability is introduced by way of an extended investigation of the hermeneutics of anomalous births. Very early on, Christians began to develop countercultural attitudes to the socially marginalized, especially abandoned children. Where citizens of the ancient world saw an anomalous birth as a threatening sign, Christians saw a much more positive divine creative work (chapter 1). The modern period sees the ancient division of anomalous births into either curses or wonders joined by a third option, the anomalous birth as a biological accident. The severing of human birth from the realm of divine action has not only affected how moderns see their own children, but how they understand their own acts of compassion. Chapter 2 draws attention to the ways in which Jesus' very physical attunement to the presence and need of others in all their contingent particularity both taught and modeled the importance of understanding human acts of compassion as fundamentally resting on divine mercy. Theologically speaking, human mercy and works of compassion are best understood as responses to divine mercy. A genuinely theological account of the various phenomena grouped under the label disability depends on reconnecting these conditions to God's working in the world.

Part 2 puts this discussion of the hermeneutics of anomalous births alongside contemporary prenatal screening practices. Chapter 3 offers Adam's origin story to reveal some of complex tensions and implications that have come with the new world of diagnostic genetic testing. The moral, technical, and social mechanisms characteristic of the modern medical establishment are exposed as assuming some people to be expendable. The claim that prenatal testing is not a judgment on disabled lives becomes difficult to sustain in light of such testing practices. Chapter 4 goes deeper into the conflicts and tensions appearing in the story told in chapter 3. A doxological cultural hermeneutic is developed as an analytical tool for spotting the false hopes and fears that drive violence against people labeled disabled. Language rooted in fear can be distinguished from that which arises from praise, and both take flesh in socially elaborated routines. Drawing on social scientific studies of prenatal testing, it reveals how the fear of negative outcomes has come to play an architectonic role in organizing modern screening practices. This fear can be theologically narrated as a form of misdirected praise, a living, articulate, and institutionalized embodiment of fear that is the opposite of the praise of a good Creator.

Part 3 investigates how the fear-praise polarity shapes contemporary practice in schools, churches, and the political realm. The remarkable silence of mainstream medical ethicists on issues of disability is the focus of chapter 5, which outlines the role of the discipline of medical ethics in establishing and sustaining the current status quo. Furthermore, and just as troublingly, it also shows how the work of academic practitioners of medical ethics has, in effect, politically disempowered medical professionals. A recent damning report on the healthcare outcomes for people with learning difficulties in England is the focus of chapter 6, and raises questions about why people with disabilities, especially intellectual disabilities, seem not to receive the same health care that most people in society are afforded. Paradoxically, the creaturely concreteness and particularity of people labeled disabled have become increasingly difficult to accommodate in modern healthcare systems. On closer examination it appears that many of the problems people with disabilities experience in modern healthcare contexts are not different in kind to those they can expect to face in other sectors of modern Western societies. To have a unique mind or body, and especially to be unable to speak, renders one a painfully bad fit in all these domains. A communication gap has opened that is best understood as an artifact of creation being fallen, of human beings having been rendered insensate and unresponsive by sin. Sin causes human beings to strain against their limits as contingent creatures and so to devalue the givenness of others. This overlaying of false images of wholeness onto others is compounded by medical systems that minimize the time and importance of listening to them.

Part 4 begins to flesh out a constructive account of how the lives labeled disabled today might be received as a divine judgment and invitation to renewal. The most important work of divine mercy is to liberate human beings from their sinful desires and misshapen hopes. Divine mercy does its liberating work in the mundane spaces of daily life. The term "disability" must be extracted from its etymological linkage with lack and brokenness by weaving it into an account of creaturely flourishing that is not only bodily but admits that human beings were created for a temporally extended engagement with God. Chapter 7 opens this constructive account by interrogating the theological assumptions embedded in modern views of health. Chapter 8 furthers this theological account of health by asking what health looks like in the case of autism. Answering this question takes the discussion into questions about the role of eschatology in a theology of disability. Because autism is primarily a nonstandard way of living as a social being, it proves an especially fruitful condition for highlighting the mundane differences between sinful and redeemed social orders.

The final section develops a detailed account of the politics of the Christian community, highlighting how the ways listening and attending to one another decisively determines the social forms that will emerge in a community. Part 5 thus extends and concretizes the contrasts between the grammars of the modern scientific-objective view of all creatures and the church gathered to worship and receive the gifts of the Holy Spirit. Chapter 9 takes up the theme of inclusion, suggesting that Paul's depiction of the social order that is church leaps far beyond the modern aspiration to be more "inclusive." The chapter lays out the book's central constructive proposal: that the body of Christ is a circulator of spiritual gifts. In the body of Christ, the needs associated with the label "disability" can be recognized—at the same time the common sensibility that deficiency and dependency are somehow the sum of what can be expected of people with disabilities is overturned. Chapter 10 makes explicit a theme that has been running through the treatment from the beginning—a narrative of the Christian God as a militant God. The self-absorption and truncated visions of the good life that are characteristic of fallen humanity have a real intergenerational momentum, one not easily interrupted by mere education or infrastructural adjustments. It is out of his passionate love of Jesus Christ for humanity that he actively, even militantly, combats the hardness of heart that sustains the injustices that bedevil the lives of people with disabilities. Real political insurrection, it turns out, demands rooting the dismissal and "othering" from the human hearts out of which it springs. The church is presented as a community within which resistance to the depredations of our world is being learned because in it human beings hear something promising. They have found themselves drawn into worship around the One who is worthy of worship—worthy, not least, for implacably resisting human beings' rejection of one another.

PART I

DISABILITY IN THE CHRISTIAN TRADITION

1

Wonders from Jesus to Augustine

A PASTORAL DILEMMA: WONDER OR MONSTER?

Many strange and wonderful stories come down to us from the first centuries of the Christian era, but few are stranger than the story of Augustine's strange vocations. Early in the fifth century CE, a Christian bishop in a provincial port city on the southern edge of the Mediterranean took up a theme that had never received sustained treatment by Christians: how to understand the birth of an abnormal child. Like everyone else at that time, Augustine of Hippo understood such a birth as a clear departure from the orderly progress of nature. Questions would immediately be swirling about the probity of the child's parents in the bedroom, about the fortunes of the community into which the baby was born, and about whether the baby was in fact even human. By beginning with this last question, Augustine opens questions about the hermeneutics of viewing the body that reverberate down to the present day.[1]

Christians, too, have heard the many stories circulating in pagan culture about "certain monstrous races of men."[2]

> If these tales are to be believed, it may be asked whether such monsters are descended from the sons of Noah, or rather from that one man from whom the sons of Noah themselves have come. Some of these are said to have only one eye, in the middle of their forehead. Others have feet which point backwards, behind their legs. Others combine in themselves the nature of both sexes, having the right breast of a man and the left of a woman, and, when they mate, they take it in turns to beget and conceive.

> Others have no mouths and live only by breathing through their nostrils. Others again are only a cubit high, and these are called Pygmies by the Greeks, after their word for a cubit, *pygme*. . . . It is not, of course, necessary to believe in all the kinds of men which are said to exist. But anyone who is born anywhere as a man (that is, as a rational and mortal animal), no matter how unusual he may be to our bodily senses in shape, colour motion, sound, or in any natural power or part or quality, derives from the original and first-created man; and no believer will doubt this. It is, however, clear what constitutes the natural norm in the majority of cases and what, in itself, is a marvellous rarity.[3]

This being Augustine, the pastoral is intertwined with the exegetical, in this case a question about the repopulation of the earth after the flood. After asking how animals released from the ark could have reached even far flung ocean islands, he has taken up the question of whether, as the myths of the pagans indicate, there might be other races of humanlike beings.[4] His conclusion is unambiguous: human beings are creatures born from other humans, and therefore must be affirmed as rational in kind and in possession of a rational soul. He also insists that *every* human being in existence is good because they are *created by God exactly as they are*.

> For God is the Creator of all things: He Himself knows where and when anything should be, or should have been, created; and He knows how to weave the beauty of the whole out of the similarity and diversity of its parts. The man who cannot view the whole is offended by what he takes to be the deformity of a part; but this is because he does not know how it is to be adapted or related to the whole. We know of men who were born with more than five fingers or five toes. This is a trivial thing and not any great divergence from the norm. God forbid, however, that someone who does not know why the Creator has done what He has done should be foolish enough to suppose that God has in such cases erred in allotting the number of human fingers. So, then, even if a greater divergence should occur, He whose work no one may justly condemn knows what He has done.[5]

Scripture, for Augustine, is never read well without one eye on the material world, and here his earthy empiricism yields the observation that most people seem to be born in a rather predictable configuration. Hence the pastoral question: how should parents whose child seems different, out of the ordinary, perceive this child? After all, as bewildering as it might be for the individuals involved, it is not exactly a rare occurrence.

> Who could call to mind all the human infants who have been born very unlike those who were most certainly their parents? It cannot be denied, however, that these derive their origin from that one man, Adam; and the same is therefore true of all those races which, by reason of their bodily differences, are said to have deviated from the usual pattern of nature exhibited by most—indeed by almost the whole—of mankind. If these races are included in the definition of 'human', that is, if they are rational and mortal animals, then it must be admitted that they trace their lineage from that same one man, the first father of all mankind.[6]

A theological question remains that goes to the heart of Augustine's pastoral response to the parents of an apparently anomalous child. If there are races of different sorts of human beings, they must have been created by God for a reason.

> Perhaps it was so that, when monsters are born of men among us, as they must be, we should not think them the work of an imperfect craftsman: perhaps it was so that we should not suppose that, despite the wisdom with which He fashions the nature of human beings, God has on this occasion erred. In which case, it ought not to seem absurd to us that, just as some monsters occur within the various races of mankind, so there should be certain monstrous races within the human race as a whole. I shall, then, conclude my discussion of the question with a tentative and cautious answer. Either the written accounts which we have of some of these races are completely worthless; or, if such creatures exist, they are not men; or, if they are men, they are descended from Adam.[7]

Augustine's pastoral response offers all Christians a densely layered accounting of the unexpectedly formed human child. A child's body is legible as a work of God in the same way as the myths of fabulous races.[8] While clearly comforting parents confused by the birth of a child who looks very unlike them, Augustine's wider aim is to normalize human diversity as a natural part of God's story with creation.

Even more strikingly, Augustine urges Christians to read this expected appearance of the unexpected not as freakish or repulsive but a special *communicative act* of God. "Not many years ago, within living memory, a person was born in the East who had two heads, two chests, four hands, as though he were two persons, but one stomach, and two feet, as though he were one. And he lived long enough and the case was so well known that many people went to see the wonder."[9] Disability, the divinely communicative "wonder" of a loving Creator. It had not always been thus. This chapter tells the story of the transformation of the ancient world's views of the human that arose with the advent of Jesus Christ. In so doing it sets out some of the fundamental insights necessary for a Christian account of the human phenomena we today label disabilities.

THE POLITICAL POTENCY OF A HEALING JESUS

The roots of the revolutionary understanding of the human that developed in the patristic period lay in the New Testament. The revolutionary nature of the New Testament's view of human life has, however, been masked for many modern readers by the tendency to picture Jesus' healing activity as not unlike that of the modern doctor. Since those labeled disabled often experience modern medicine as aiming for a healing that looks like an attempt to make them "normal," the specter of Jesus being an irresistibly powerful healer has appeared to many as a decidedly threatening prospect.[10] To recover the roots of the creative practices of Christians in the patristic period requires revisiting the Jesus who inspired them.

Modern views of healing rest on very narrowly conceived presumptions about human life. The phrase "deficiency in need of a cure" is shorthand for the convergence of what has come to be called the medical model of disability and the anthropology of political liberalism.[11] These accounts position disability as the biologically rooted incapacity of an individual to achieve mainstream pictures of economic productivity and aesthetic beauty. Given the dominance of medical accounts of health and liberal political philosophies throughout the modern period, it is unsurprising that post-Enlightenment thinkers have often figured Jesus as an otherworldly healer. This Jesus gathers outcasts and sufferers to himself for a cleansing and healing while remaining unsullied by their deficiencies. The Jesus of the transfiguration is taken to present the icon of the resurrected body for which every human being ought to hope.[12] To present Jesus as a precursor of the modern medical project is to annex him as an ally of a violently paternalistic desire to fix every so-called disabled body to make it "normal."[13]

It is both unlikely and anachronistic to assume that the earliest Christians understood Jesus as the great eradicator of disability, a view equally hard to square with the evidence of Scripture. The medicalization of the Messiah is only achievable by overlooking the characteristic insistence of the Old Testament narratives on Israel's identification with the oppressed slaves of Egypt. To erase the defacing bondage of Israel obscures in turn the pride of place the writers of the Synoptic Gospels gave to the vision of the suffering servant of Isaiah 53. The Jesus of the Synoptics is no serene Olympian, but grotesque: "despised, rejected, a man of suffering, acquainted with infirmity, one from whom others hide their faces."[14]

Being predominantly from the underclasses, Christians in the early centuries gravitated to the miracle stories. These stories offered them a healer and liberator who freed people from the disfiguring oppression under which they groaned.[15] The story of the people of God whose bodies had been subjected to the political whims of the rulers of Egypt, Babylon, and now Rome was continuously concerned about slavery of every type—and Jesus' power to bring release from it. When these early Christians heard rumors of Jesus' miracles, what excited them was the destabilization of the powers that ruled their own age that they promised. Jesus had the power to effectively disrupt the prevailing imperial definitions of a worthwhile life.[16] Jesus' healing miracles were claimed by the earliest Christians as a direct challenge to the prescriptive regimes of control by the ruling political powers. This is why, for them, Jesus' miracles were powerfully *hopeful* signs. A more biblically rounded account of Jesus' healing activity understands it as an attack not on the ethical claims characteristic of the Roman status quo, but on the whole ethos that grounded it.

Liberation from bondage is the key term. The New Testament positions Christians as people looking for and living into the liberation offered by Israel's Messiah *now*, a tangible release from the powers that break and maim human life.[17] The potency of early Christian hope that the reign of the lowly servant king would overturn the oppressive rule of the pagan emperors is signaled by a deluge of images in the first Christian centuries of Jesus as a healer and miracle worker.[18] This linkage of Jesus' healing with the breaking of the denuding rule of the powers of the age requires some unpacking to be intelligible in contemporary terms.

The intentionally spectacular and highly martial procession of the Roman emperor on parade was a pageant designed to evoke the fear and awe that renders a population docile and subservient before an irresistible power. Such parades were called in Latin the emperor's "adventus." It was thus a direct challenge to this tradition when the earliest Christians called the triumphal entry of Jesus on Palm Sunday Jesus' advent. A multitude of early pictures and carvings depict Jesus making his advent in the highly biblically symbolic city of Jerusalem not on a gilded horse-drawn chariot of war but riding sidesaddle (as women did) on a lowly donkey made miraculously docile by the power of his touch. In such pictures the marginalized earliest Christians depicted the miraculous healings of Jesus as stronger than military might. Even riding a donkey, this Jesus was overthrowing the merely military might of the very power who crucified him—the imperial rulers. It was their excitement about this power to free and liberate and restore that so energized and emboldened the Christians of the first centuries, and it is likely that these images and the ideas they promulgated ultimately played a pivotal role in the fourth-century triumph of Christianity that drew the patristic era to a close.[19]

This Jesus might have been lowly, but he was also a miracle worker throwing down the politically powerful. The earliest Christians grasped the political explosiveness of this prominent strand of the New Testament. After the miraculous conception of Jesus, Luke depicts Mary as speaking of this trait of the Messiah in its most potent form:

> . . . *his mercy* reaches from age to age for those who fear him . . . .
> *He has pulled down princes from their thrones and exalted the lowly*
> The hungry he has filled with good things, the rich sent empty away.
> He has *come to the help of Israel his servant, mindful of his mercy*
> —*according to the promise* he made to our ancestors—
> *Of his mercy* to Abraham and to his descendants forever. (Luke 1:50-55, New Jerusalem translation)

Though Jesus' healings were associated with political potency, this potency was not the promise to normalize every human body, but to break the power of sin and reopen a relationship with God.[20] The dream of having a "normal" body is one of those sinful dreams, one that has led moderns to fundamentally misunderstand Jesus.

Since doctors and magicians were closely associated in the first Christian centuries, emphasizing Jesus' power to heal also brought him into contest with magic. The hopeless entanglement of medicine and sorcery in the late antique world is signaled by the English translation of the Greek *pharmakeia* in Galatians 5:20 as "witchcraft." The same people made and sold drugs for medicinal purposes alongside abortifacients and magic potions. If Christianity was to succeed in the ancient world, Jesus' power to heal would have to coopt powers claimed by the gods and demons to heal.[21] Magic had the cultural dominance that medical expertise has for modern Westerners. Magic was not just for a show but was considered the normal form of treatment for those needing healing. And like Augustine after them, the earliest Christians did not respond by denying the efficacy of magic. Jesus, they repeated to the point of cultural saturation, transcended the magician (a pejorative term at the time), by being *the* true and efficacious healer.[22] Jesus was not only more powerful than the emperor; he was also more powerful than the magicians, like Moses before him, who had vanquished the magicians of Pharaoh and all the enchanters of the east. And it was different in kind from the magicians—he could *give* life. Early Christian art emphasized this latter point by presenting the three wise men as magicians laying down their potions and magical arts at the feet of the baby Jesus.[23] In Jesus God had given a gift to humanity that had drastically, extravagantly, outdone the gifts any magician could muster.[24]

To emphasize the uniqueness of Jesus as healer these early Christians invented a wholly novel imagery—of Jesus at the very moment of healing. Perhaps because street magicians were outlawed in the ancient world, this moment of healing had never been depicted in Roman or Greek art. Nor was the god most associated with healing, Asclepius, ever shown in the actual act of healing. Even doctors were depicted in paintings and sculptures only as diagnosing, never treating or curing. It therefore must be considered a work of evangelism when early Christian artists consciously styled Jesus in the dress and stance of Asclepius. Jesus was given the fatherly looks and gentle manner of Asclepius and incessantly replicated on objects that people would regularly encounter—on tombs, tableware, and clothing.[25]

In the images of the fourth century, Christ has absorbed the attributes and attitudes of the magician and in a manner wholly unthreatened by imperial authority. Both aspects of this posture are important. Magic was too potent a power base to bypass; it had to be redirected and made to serve Christian purposes. In the venerable tradition of Moses embarrassing Pharaoh's magicians and the infant Jesus outgifting the magi—combined with Daniel and his companions who walked through the fire stoked extra hot by a pagan potentate for their execution—Christ is depicted as the magician who confronts the emperor's representative and pulls his ultimate trick. With perfect equanimity he accepts execution, confident of his resurrection.[26] The resurrection that proved him to be the one true healer exposed all false magicians and in so doing demolished the claims to superiority of all political rulers.

Jesus is more powerful than the pagan protectors of Rome, but his power is different in kind. His was a power to heal, and his political power took forms that were visibly and distinctly pacific, nonmilitary, and nonimperial.[27] Stories emphasizing the difference between Jesus' power from that of the Roman rulers were to be repeated in myriad iterations for centuries to come, many of which were preserved in apocryphal gospel traditions. The legend of Veronica is one such tradition. Veronica presented an image of Jesus' face preserved on a cloth to the emperor Tiberius with the words, "if thy lord will devoutly gaze upon his face, he shall obtain forthwith the benefit of health."[28] The emperor becomes enraged at the scoundrel Pilate who has executed the "innocent doctor Jesus," whose power remains so resplendent that it can still heal an emperor if only he will gaze on a shadow of the man.

"God chose what is low and despised in the world, the things that are not, to reduce to nothing the things that are" (1 Cor 1:28). Jesus came into a world where the martial might of Roman emperors was ceaselessly emphasized by images on coins picturing them magnanimously reaching out to bestow favor on women kneeling in obeisance. The earliest Christians surely knew that the world was being turned upside down by a Jesus whose gentleness and approachability encouraged the woman with the issue of blood to reach out to touch his hem and be healed.[29] He came as one labeled shameful, but in this very social location he overturned the dominant ideals of the socially and politically powerful. The rulers of the age who crushed life out of the lowly were living on borrowed time with the advent of the healer who had vanquished the god of healing.

ANOMALOUS BIRTH FROM GREECE TO AUGUSTINE

Jesus' precedent unleashed an avalanche of creative thinking and countercultural practices among the first Christians. To return to our opening example, Augustine took anomalous births as ontologically dense and revealing phenomena. In the ancient world, conditions today classed as disabilities, especially congenital disabilities, were not viewed as meaningless mistakes in biological processes. In classical Greece and Rome, the dominant cosmological and religious beliefs positioned an anomalous birth as the product of a complex web of natural and supernatural forces. The shape of deformities mattered and upon appearance were immediately perceived through a library of stories, with deformed limbs evoking various half-human, half-animal, half-demonic figures.[30] Disfiguring congenital conditions were assumed to be the work of supernatural powers needing placation and exorcism for the protection of the polis. The responsible thing to do was to protect the household and city against the ill effects associated with such children by leaving them to die of exposure.[31]

Between the ministry of Jesus Christ and the Emperor Constantine's decriminalization of Christianity, those who confessed that every human being was "one for whom Christ died" (1 Cor 8:11) came to refuse such justifications for killing people considered substandard contributors to the household or city. Among Christians a set of global sensibilities about human life converged to form what might be called the *rule of human solidarity*. It was a rule worked out through a myriad of countercultural practices.

During the first to the fourth centuries of the Christian era, the elites of the Roman empire tended to view this minority sect with some suspicion for its tendency to question conventional pieties—the observance of pieties being directly linked to the wellbeing of the community.[32] The Athenians executed

Socrates for the same reasons that the Romans were prone to unleashing spasms of violence against Christians: for subverting the claims of the gods. Roman punishments included execution and being sent to the gladiatorial games. As many of the first Christians were slaves,[33] they were all too aware that their beliefs might render them subject to capital punishment or less draconian disadvantages. Many Christian writers during this period attempted to defend Christians as nonthreatening to the powers that be. Though the violence was spasmodic and locally enacted, it hung over the early generations of Christians as a constant threat.[34] This explains why, as these centuries wore on, the martyrs came to play an ever more central place in Christian self-identification. Those who had joined a movement inaugurated by a God-man, whom the Roman authorities had tried to kill, developed very early on a deep sympathy for all those devalued and oppressed by the powers of Rome.

The threat of martyrdom was important in the formation of early Christian attitudes toward human life in heightening the opponent of the rule of solidarity: the *law of scarcity*.[35] In Greek and Roman antiquity human life had no independent value. A person's value was largely defined in social terms, calibrated according to his or her potential to contribute both materially and through acquired virtues to the good of the family and society. This valuation of social contribution was combined with a deep-seated aesthetic of bodily integrity in Greco-Roman pictures of virtue and rationality. As beings composed of earth and spirit, human beings were expected to stand erect, their spirits rising within them to pull them upright and, in the course of their natural development, even beyond the body into speech and concepts—into philosophy. Greek cities were full of detailed and aesthetically perfect statues of human bodies, and bodily imperfection was frowned upon and seen as a sign of the degeneration of the city. In this aesthetic, being bent toward the earth, to lack speech or the ability to think clearly was to exhibit signs of regression toward the subhuman.[36]

Since Plato (like most of the ancients) understood the body to take its form according to the pattern of the soul, developmental disabilities were inextricably linked with belief in deformity as rooted in defective and incurable souls. Insinuations of moral disability were thus added to the social burden already carried by those with congenital disabilities. The moral disabling did not end there. Since Plato (like almost all other Greek thinkers) considered virtue to be the capacity to contribute to society gracefully and well, in his view only those capable of living normal healthy lives could hope to become truly virtuous.[37] In one infamous passage Plato has Socrates suggest that there is no point for a chronically ill carpenter to receive medical treatment since his life is of little use to him if he cannot fulfill the social role that gives his life structure and allows him to develop in virtue.[38] Plato's views are representative of the wider ancient grounding of human worth in its value to the community combined with a complete inability to imagine any value in a disabled life on its own terms or in supporting people with disabilities.

The heroic deaths of great statesmen and soldiers were the ideal in Greco-Roman societies, and an ethos of nobility and aesthetic harmony defined the ethics of suicide and end of life care. Committing suicide to protect one's honor or being killed in battle were taken as paradigmatically noble acts utterly unrelated to medicine with its interest in healing.[39] Similarly, by the late antique period, the notion of a peaceful death undergone without pain had come to be positioned within the same moral calculus that justified infanticide as a socially meaningful ending demonstrating the cooperative values of the city state.[40] While Christians did occasionally apply the term "good death" (*euthanasia*) to describe martyrdom,[41] they intentionally severed it from Stoic images of rising above pain and strictly ruled out intentionally taking one's own life.[42] Christians might glory in martyrdom, but definitively repudiated seeking it. Human life has been made for service to God and is never at one's own disposal.[43]

Christianity was also born into a world in which a great weight of social expectation bore down on the work of procreation. Lifespans were low, child mortality high, and birth dangerous for mothers. To ensure its survival the ancient city needed couples to direct significant energy and ingenuity toward begetting and raising healthy, legitimate heirs. Girls were recruited young for the task, in their early teens, and needed to bear an average of five children each for the population to remain steady.[44] The family was the site where the body of the newborn was judged worthy of entry into organized society in Greek and Roman antiquity. Mere birth from a woman did not establish a child as a legal person, but the decision of the head of the household to lift the child from the floor. It was wholly legal for the father to kill (by exposure or any other means) both the healthy and the deformed.[45] As this act was not understood as murder but as offering the child back to the gods, it was not considered unseemly to abandon even a healthy child in a public place. If the gods did not reclaim them, they were available for other families, typically to become a slave.[46] Greco-Roman perceptions of the limited value of precarious lives directly determined healthcare ethics of the Roman Empire. According to the most famous medical textbook in antiquity, Soranus' *Gynecology*, the care of defective newborns was not even classed as one of the responsibilities of doctors. Plato depicts Socrates as unapologetically advocating the exposure of defective infants, and Aristotle turns this into an explicit injunction.[47]

The rise of Christianity marked a turning point in late antiquity in holding every human life to have achieved infinite worth in being the object of Christ's love. The radical divergence of this Christian ethos with its rule of human solidarity diverged markedly from the dominant ancient ethos. Christians also attacked the "games," the gladiatorial shows, highlighting the callousness toward human life that was accepted as a normal within the ancient ethos. Around 200 CE in North Africa Tertullian decried the games as repugnant to Christian views of the worth of human life, an argument repeated fifty years later in Rome by Novatian.[48] While some of the New Testament documents were still being written, Christians rewrote the Old Testament Decalogue for gentile converts and glossed the command "thou shalt not commit murder" as a blanket refusal of abortion and infanticide.[49] This refusal had become so widespread and well known among Christians by 200 CE that in an apologetic text Tertullian held the whole Christian community up for public scrutiny as nowhere being guilty of murder, including abortion.[50] The habit of taking in children who had been left to die on the hillsides soon became a widely known practice among Christians, and was a practice that was especially important to Christian communities committed to celibacy that formed in the eastern part of the empire.[51]

Christians and pagans alike understood all these behaviors as rejections of the independent powers of the pantheon of gods and demons. Human life was no longer given its worth by a judgment of authorities in the family or the state about who would be capable of contributing to the community. Thus, a sweeping opposition to the universally held worth calculus of the ancient world solidified among Christians.

Taken as a whole, it is not accurate to claim that Christians in the patristic period were obsessed with perfect bodies.[52] Indeed, at the climax of the patristic period Augustine routinely made precisely the opposite claim: that after the fall human beings are prone to loving the *physically* beautiful and being *repulsed* by the physically deformed—despite the theological reality that they should be attracted to moral beauty and repelled by moral deformity.[53]

> I repeat, the eye with the capacity to appreciate the beauty of righteousness is within you. If there were no beauty in righteousness, how could we love a righteous old man? What bodily charms has he to offer that could delight our eyes? All he has is a bent back, a wrinkled face, white hair, weakness, and bodily complaints throughout his frame. Nothing to please your eyes in this worn-out old man, then. But perhaps there is

> something to delight your ears? His speaking voice? His singing? What are they like? Even if he did sing well as a boy, all such talent has fallen away with age. Is even the sound of his speech pleasant to your ears, when he can scarcely get his words out, having lost his teeth? Yet all the same, if he is a righteous man, if he does not covet other people's property, if from his own possessions he is generous to the needy, if he gives good advice and is a man of sound judgment and honest faith, if he is prepared to sacrifice even shattered limbs in defense of the truth (for many martyrs were elderly)—then, isn't that why we love him? What good do our carnal eyes find in him? None at all. This proves that *righteousness has a beauty of its own, which we perceive with the eyes of the heart, and love, and kindle to, a beauty which people have dearly loved in the martyrs, even when their limbs were being torn by wild beasts*.[54]

Christians had decisively repudiated the Greek idea that only those with good bodies could be virtuous, as well as the Roman idea that only healthy bodies could be beautiful. It is the viewer who has the problem. Those who are repulsed by any human being are in need of repentance and the renewal of their minds.

The sinfulness of the human tendency to pity or shun those considered "monstrous" was a theme regularly preached by Augustine. Believing every human being to have a rational soul led him to the belief that there was hope for this sinful proclivity to be healed.[55] Minds need to be sanctified to be brought into a right relationship to all of God's creatures. This sanctification is necessary because Augustine held it to be blasphemous to disparage any of God's handiworks. In the basis of this claim he develops a substantial critique of (Platonic) physical beauty as a type of idol obscuring the more basic truth that God has created every human being precisely as they are—even if at times he also deploys a Platonizing account of healing that devalues nonstandard human bodies. But his revolutionary thought is that *an observer's shame or embarrassment in the presence of nonstandard human life is an artifact of disunion with his or her Creator, a mark of humanity's common guilt not easily overcome and certainly not by human powers*. People with disabilities thus both reveal human disunion with God and stand as a promise of his resurrecting and sanctifying power over it.[56]

Much, then, of Augustine's account of disability was inherited from the patristic church, specifically, the emphasis on the universality of the human race rooted in the works of a benevolent Creator and the salvific work of Jesus Christ. Augustine's own distinctive contribution was to think through the issues associated with the revelatory and eschatological implications of nonstandard human lives.

As always, Augustine's thinking circled around exegetical questions. His engagement with the theme of the anomalous birth appears in a dispute with non-Christians about the veracity of the Scriptures. Miracles, unbelievers say, disprove the truth of Scripture, since the Bible is full of impossible events. But the existence of the world itself is a miracle, replies Augustine; creation is brimming with the miraculous. Christians will agree with the common wisdom that many natural substances have traits that seem unnatural, he continues, such as rocks capable of being simultaneously wet and dry. Such traits may surprise us, but they are not contrary to nature. At the same time, he suggests, most people do hold *some* beliefs that are not susceptible to rational proof, "yet they will not deign to believe us when we say that Almighty God will perform things which transcend their experience and sensation, even though we do give a rational [i.e., scriptural] explanation."[57] Given the story of God's works recounted in Scripture, Christians do in fact positively expect God at opportune times to do things that people regard as impossible, "because he has foretold that He will; and what He promises He fulfils, so that the unbelieving nations may come to believe the unbelievable."[58]

That fallen human wonder is upside down is indicated by cases like identical twins. Twins evoke wonder for being indistinguishable, and in so doing only highlight the more wondrous (despite more regularly occurring) miracle of every single human being, differing just enough to be distinguishable despite all being members of a single kind.[59] Like the generations of ancient peoples before him, Augustine takes astronomical anomalies as paradigmatic instances of the miracle or wonder, given that the usual laws of the heavens are so unvarying. But, he insists, the wonders that fill the earth are no less marvelous and are there for all to see. What is interesting about the kind "human being" sharing a single set of basic traits, suggests Augustine, is that "it is a consideration of the differences which ought to make us wonder; for similarity seems to be more consistent with our common nature."[60] These subtler wonders should be paradigm cases.

A twofold movement is being proposed by Augustine. On one level Christians should learn to appreciate the diffuse and plenteous mundane wonders characteristic of the diversity of creation. At the same time, they are also to expect the God who created nature sometimes to work outside of its regular course to further God's own purposes.[61] It is here that Augustine locates anomalous births.

Beginning from the assumption that because God has created each human they must be good, he had moved to the belief that some impairments had to be understood positively as divine speech to the world. The consequences he now drew were as bold as they were novel in his context. The ancient language of anomalous births as "portents" and "monsters" would have to be decontaminated. Rather than *dissociating* the anomalous birth from divine revelation, he chose instead to *invert* the Greco-Roman understanding of the revelatory message conveyed by the surprising appearance of nonstandard bodies and minds. No longer were nonstandard physical or mental traits to be understood as forbidding omens: they became, for Augustine, a divine communicative act challenging human expectations of worldly occurrence.

> This is why there has sprung up so great a multitude of those marvels which are called "monsters," "signs," "portents" or "prodigies." If I chose to recall and mention them all, would this work ever come to an end? The word "monster" we are told, clearly comes from "to demonstrate" [*monstrare*], because monsters are signs by which something is demonstrated. 'Sign' [*ostentum*] comes from 'to show' [*ostendere*]; 'portent' from 'to portend', that is 'to show in advance' [*praeostendere*]; and "prodigy" from "to speak of what is far away" [*porro dicere*], that is, to foretell the future. Let those who divine by such means see for themselves how often they draw false conclusions from them. . . . *For our part, however, these things which are called monsters, signs, portents and prodigies ought to demonstrate to us—to show us, to portend to us, to foretell for us—that God will do with the bodies of the dead what He foretold: that there is no difficulty to impede Him, and no law of nature to forbid Him, from so doing.*[62]

The appearance of a wonder displays the will of the Creator to resurrection, the spectacular central claim of the Christian gospel. Augustine's revolutionary thought grows from his insistence that God creates every human being. This thought turns the wonder from an evil omen into a sign of benevolent divine involvement in human affairs.[63]

While insisting that Christians not become obsessed with portents, Augustine nevertheless concluded that there were theologically weighty reasons to attend to anomalous human births as divinely communicative.[64] He did so out of pastoral solicitude for Christians facing the shock of a surprising and unexpected child but also out of a cold realism about the alternative—the strong tendency of fallen humans to pity or shun those considered "monstrous." Jesus Christ had come to eradicate this sinful desire to protect one's self against the "other" through the renewal of the mind.[65] Only a redeemed mind could discern these "strange vocations" in their true light, without pity or fear.[66]

Augustine was not sanguine about the very tangible physical problems associated with some congenital conditions as well as mental and physical illnesses. Over many years Augustine explored a range of speculations, none presented as definitive, about God's reasons for allowing the more problematic human impairments and deviations from what he understood to be the normal human form. He did assume that some suffering and impairments were ultimately an effect of the Fall. Some cases, he also allowed, could be understood as divine interventions serving pedagogical purposes for the individuals involved, while others might best be understood as the effects of the Fall disrupting the normal causal mechanisms of the material world.[67] What is important to note, however, is that he grasped very clearly the injustice against God built into the claim that disabilities are nothing more than signs of the brokenness of creation.

The Fall might have something to do with anomalous bodies, but it is more important for Christians to appreciate the unbelievable diversity of the created realm and to expect God to speak through surprising human differences. Human beings whose bodily and mental form appears to lie at the margins of the familiar should be attended to as having been created as a divine communicative act. From a cosmic perspective, some people's impairments simply cannot be deficits. "Such persons are predestinated and brought into being . . . in order that those who are able should understand that God's grace and the Spirit, 'which bloweth where it listeth' (John 3:8), does not pass over any kind of capacity in the sons of mercy, nor in like manner does it pass over any kind of capacity in the children of Gehenna, so that 'he that glorieth, let him glory in the Lord.'"[68] Augustine finds himself forced to conclude that some cases of impairment happened "so that the work of God might be displayed."[69] He labels these cases "strange vocations," his paradigm case being an individual who is both intellectually impaired and an exemplary Christian.[70] It was this chain of reasoning that protected Augustine from embracing the conclusions to which some of his Neoplatonic assumptions often pushed him, in which physical and intellectual disability is by definition a sad marring of the human visage.

In his willingness to conceive disability as, at least in some cases, evidence of God's having given some people "strange vocations," Augustine effects what is perhaps the most remarkable conceptual reversal of the patristic era. For centuries before him Christians had repudiated the Greco-Roman view of nonstandard newborns as the work of malevolent supernatural powers by rescuing these babies, a politically subversive act tempting the wrath of angry gods and breaching the law of scarcity. Augustine undergirded this clear but inchoate practical insight with a robustly theological account of the anomalous birth.

Augustine's encapsulation of the whole patristic era's sensibilities about anomalous lives and bodies was to determine the development of views of disability in Christendom for centuries to come.[71] This included its strengths and weaknesses. Augustine was not, for instance, able sufficiently to break with the prioritization of the male gaze. The questions of women and slaves had never been worth discussing to the literate men who ruled the ancient world. Educated Greeks and Romans had praised marital concord in glowing terms, but not the griefs, pains, and illnesses that came with marriage and childbirth. Not until the Christian literature defending virginity as superior to the married state arose in the first Christian centuries did people speak in public of the physical realities of the married state for women; the dangers of childbirth, the pain of nursing a child, or the shame associated with infertility.[72] Within this context it is clear that Augustine is in important respects pushing toward the modern world in directing such sustained discussion to the question of the anomalous birth as a pastoral problem—and in a book that begins with an extended address comforting Christian nuns dealing with the aftermath of rape. Augustine may not have been able to see things from a woman's perspective, but he did see women and their problems. In his world, disability was one of those problems.

Augustine's deep engagement with the philosophies of his day led to several problems in his theological positioning of disability. His rationalist anthropology and his speaking in terms of a charity model of care couched in language of "deformity" have decidedly negative rhetorical valences that have been widely noted.[73] At the same time Augustine was also clearly aware of some of the more problematic aspects of his own philosophical presumptions. Though drawing deeply from Neoplatonism, he unambiguously refused its presumption that all disability is a result of humanity's fallen condition. Nor did Augustine unambiguously assert that all human beings should hope to be "normalized" in the resurrection. Sometimes his speculations about the resurrection did point to a hope that God would restore all people to the "normal" human form by healing all physical disproportions as well as sensory and mental deviations.[74] At the same time, he also insisted that there are good theological reasons to hope that the physical marks of the roles each saint played in God's story will endure in the resurrected life.[75] It is a line of speculation that commits Augustine to the intriguing claim that those who had lived out "strange vocations," like the early Christian martyrs, should not expect to lose the proud marks of their witness in life in the healing of the resurrection. Though the sometimes mixed messages of Augustine's thought undoubtedly deserve critical scrutiny, he clearly offered a richly theological reconceptualization of the various phenomena lumped today under the heading "disability." His case also shows why it is best to view with skepticism all blanket charges that patristic theology illegitimately diffused the liberating and healing power the New Testament writers ascribed to Jesus.

PREACHING INVERTED PERCEPTION

A single sermon encapsulates the patristic view of disability.[76] We see in it a working out of this combination of Jesus' redemptive and healing work as a challenge to the political status quo. Exegetical sermons of this type played a pivotal role in breaking down the ethos of the Roman world and forming the ethos of the Christian middle ages.[77] Gregory of Nazianzus first preached it in the cathedral at Caesarea (central Turkey) around 370 CE, in support of his friend Basil's efforts in providing public care for the sick and poor.[78] At the time this sermon was preached, Basil of Caesarea was a bishop engaged in building a large complex just outside Caesarea called the Basiliad, which included a poorhouse, hospice, and hospital, and was a genuine "new city" in the fullest theological sense. Having first been converted to the monastic life as a young and wealthy young man, Basil had a second conversion to the public dimensions of belief in Jesus and was ordained a priest in 365 CE. Within a few years a serious drought, followed by a famine, struck the region. Basil found his interests gravitating toward the plight of the poor and the outsiders in his diocese, expending his considerable family fortune in the process. The Basiliad drew together his various work feeding the starving, reforming thieves and prostitutes, and caring for the ill, all of which he accompanied with public calls for civic officials to fairly administer justice.[79]

In the sermon we see a pastor hard at work planting in his congregation an entirely new vision of human life. Gregory aims to overturn some deep-seated repulsions to human difference in his congregants. To bring them to the surface he forces them to examine their repulsion at the leper. He must show precisely how Christian faith opens a rival counterethos to the aesthetics and politics of the Greco-Roman world. At the same time, he needs to attend to the existential disorientation induced by a direct attack on his congregation's internalized allegiance to that ethos. The sheer rhetorical creativity deployed in the sermon signals Gregory's awareness of the magnitude of the transition to which he is challenging his congregation.

The theme of the sermon is immediately presented, and succinctly states the theological affirmation that united patristic Christianity.

> . . . as I feel pain at the weaknesses of my own flesh and sense my own weakness in the sufferings of others, reason urges me to say this: brothers and sisters, *we must care for what is part of our nature and shares in our slavery*. For even if I lay charges against it . . . still I stand by it as a friend,

> because of the one who bound me in it. And *we must, each of us, care no less for our neighbors' bodies than our own, the bodies both of those who are healthy and of those who are consumed by this disease. "For we are all one in the Lord*, whether rich or poor, whether slave or free" [Gal 3:28], *whether in good health of body or in bad*; and there is one head of all, from whom all things proceed: Christ . . . . *So we must by no means overlook or neglect to care for those who experience our common weakness before we do*, nor should we delight more in the fact that our bodies are in good condition than we grieve that our brothers and sisters are in misery. Rather, we must consider this to be the *single way towards the salvation both of our bodies and our souls: human kindness shown towards them.*[80]

The preacher then deploys the most powerfully evocative imagery at his disposal to evoke empathy in his congregation for the most liminal of human beings: the leper.

> There stands before our eyes a terrible, pitiable sight, unbelievable to anyone who did not know it was true: *human beings both dead and alive*, mutilated in most parts of their body . . . As marks of identification, they call out the names of their fathers and mothers, brothers and sisters and homes: "I am the son of so-and-so, so-and-so is my mother, this is my name, you were once my dear companion!" They do this because *they cannot be recognized by their former shape; they are truncated human beings*, deprived of possessions, family, friends and their very bodies, *distinctive in being able both to pity themselves and hate themselves at once*. . . . For *even the kindest and most humane of neighbors is insensitive to them*; in this instance alone, we forget that we are flesh, clothed in this lowly body, and we are so far from caring for our fellow creatures that we think the safety of our own bodies lies in fleeing from them. *One approaches a body that has been dead for some time, even if it has begun to reek*; one carries about the stinking carcasses of brute animals, and puts up with being full of filth; *yet we avoid these lepers with all our might (what inhumanity!)*, almost taking offence at breathing the same air as they breathe.[81]

The criticism Gregory is developing of the Roman ethos is structurally identical to Tertullian's attack on the gladiatorial games in *aiming to foster a new public consensus organized by a more empathetic gaze toward human lives devalued in that dominant ethos*.

For both thinkers it was not statistics, political pressure groups, or moral arguments that offered Christians purchase on the ethos of their present, but gazes and gestures. The ways people look at the world reveals the particular truth of the specific times, places, and relationships that orient their perception. Gregory, like Tertullian before and Augustine after, views the gaze as the most direct route to understanding the regnant moral order. The emotional tenor of a political community is detectable in the gaze, as revealed by those who, in diverging from the regnant norms, are disapproved of through glares and dismissive looks that they experience much as a physical attack. This is the transmission mechanism allowing patterns of public shared life to be formed by the outward projection of people's inner worlds.[82]

One particularly evocative turn of phrase highlights Gregory's intention to change the way Christians gaze on the leper. He aims at evoking a more empathetic gaze by highlighting the absurd and painful situation of lepers who are "distinctive in being able both to pity themselves and hate themselves at once." Knowing that their condition is degenerative and that they have been culturally positioned as the lowest of the low, their deepest suffering is that "even the kindest and most humane of their neighbors is insensitive to them." Gregory increases the rhetorical potency of this observation with the exclamation "what inhumanity!"—one of the earliest known uses of the term "inhumane" as a term of general moral opprobrium. To accuse the highest ideals of the day of being inhumane is a clear sign that under the light shed in Christ, disability has become the fulcrum by which ancient values are being overturned, the remaking of the heart and the gaze its workshop.

While the voices of people with what we would now call disabilities appear all too rarely in early Christian texts, this example ("I am the son of so-and-so . . .") makes it clear that such voices do fleetingly appear, and indispensably so.[83] Gregory cannot humanize these misshapen bodies without asking each of his congregants to recall their own experiences of these ignored voices. By remembering such suppressions, the individual conscience is implicated in the violence of physical ostracizing. And the immorality of this stance is further compounded by the admission of physical revulsion at the leper's deformed body. With this empathetic focusing of the congregation's attention on the pleas of afflicted people, Gregory drives hard into the existentially sensitive wounds of his congregation to provoke what Nietzsche was later to call a revaluation of values. Should it be effective, the resulting inversion of perception was recognizable as a prime marker of the transforming work of Jesus Christ.

Gregory draws attention to the grief of parents, highlighting how the suffering of a child can sow the seeds of a false and barbarous compassion for those very offspring.

> Who could be more upright than a father? *Who more sympathetic than a mother?* . . . The father looks at his own child, whom he begot

> and raised, whom alone he considered the light of his life, for whom he prayed often and long to God, and now *both grieves over that child and drives him away*—the first willingly, the second under compulsion. The mother recalls the pangs of childbirth and her heart is torn apart: she calls his name wretchedly, and when he stands before her she *laments for her living child as if he were dead*: "Unfortunate child of a miserable mother, bitter disease has come to share you with me! . . ." There have been instances when *people have allowed a murderer to live with them*, have shared not only their roof but their table with an adulterer, have chosen a person guilty of sacrilege as their life's companion . . . ; *but in this person's case suffering, rather than any injury, is handed down as a criminal charge*. So crime has become more profitable than sickness, and we accept inhumanity as fit behavior for a free society, while we look down on compassion as something to be ashamed of.[84]

It is worth noting the preacher's need for the laments of parents of disabled people to call the church to be the church—that is, to see people with the compassion of Jesus Christ. It is also worth reflecting on the fact that the pain of a mother was viewed as no more a fit subject for public discussion in the ancient world that was the suffering of a disabled person. The Christian preacher breaches these taboos against speaking about the dilemmas of women and the disabled because Christ's claim demands it. In a world where even parental kindness is rent for the leper, the mercilessness of the general populace is even more crushing. Deeply entrapped in a malignant social positioning, those stricken with leprosy find their hopes of kindness reduced to the hope that they will not be sent off with a sharp stick.

But even lepers must eat, and despite knowing that they are detested, they find themselves driven back into human company. They even appear at the margins of the great church festivals—not because Christians want them to take part but because Christians refuse to supply their needs. Absolute outsiders, they come only to beg. Gregory draws his sermon to a climax by deploying the witness of the martyrs to devastating effect. Christians have gathered to celebrate the martyrs, "who witnessed to the truth, so that by paying honor to their struggles we might also imitate their piety."[85] But Gregory has introduced a discomforting figure at the margin of the celebration: the hungry, hated, and feared lepers, dying the death of the outcast outside the camp. Christians only truly celebrate the lives of the martyrs, Gregory insists, when they see their broken and hacked bodies not as repulsive, but beautiful. The beauty of lepers' bodies may be denied in Greco-Roman aesthetics but ought not be among those who follow a despised and crucified Savior. Genuinely to love the martyrs with their mangled and disfigured bodies demands a fundamental overturning of the aesthetics and politics of the Greco-Roman ethos.[86]

Paralleling the art of the patristic period, Gregory's sermon articulated the impelling inner core of a broad-spectrum challenge to common understanding of medicine in the Roman world. Impelled by the words, "Insofar as you have done it to the least of these brothers of mine, you have done it unto me" (Matt 26:40), patristic Christians felt their way toward new institutions of care. The rich in the ancient world were tended in their homes by private doctors. Some medical services were available in the temples of Asclepius, but the care was rarely professional and presumed a donation (fee) would be paid. Nor were cases that appeared hopeless welcome, as a death inside the temple constituted a ritual impurity.[87] Some medical care was available to the masses, also for a fee, in storefront practices. But the modern care institutions today called hospitals are a Christian invention. Christians were the first to assume that there *should* be institutions providing beds and meals, as well as round-the-clock care for patients undergoing medical therapies provided by a professional physician without concern for payment. It was the Christians of the patristic era (like Basil) who came up with the idea that health care should be provided in institutions open to patients of all classes and both sexes.[88]

To achieve this new institutional arrangement meant consummating Jesus' cooption of healing from the magicians by making peace with pre-Christian medicinal arts. The pre-Christian institutions in which some healthcare services in the ancient world (such as bathhouses) would also need reconfiguration. What is clear is that over relatively few centuries this Christian reconfiguration of the very conception of health care won the day. The theologians and pastors of the patristic period thus laid the groundwork for the view that was to prevail in Christendom—of the practice of medicine as one of the highest forms of Christian love for the neighbor.[89]

INSIGHTS FOR A THEOLOGY OF DISABILITY

The patristic period offers four important initial insights for any theological account of the human phenomena labeled disability. *It is important to attend to the register or level of Christian social engagement*. This formal or methodological insight is helpfully clarified by introducing a distinction between "ethos" and "ethics." "Ethos" designates the characteristic moral sensibility of any given sociolinguistic community, the "atmosphere" within which all the particular questions and answers about right and wrong behavior are formulated. The ethos of a society is the *condition* of public ethical arguments, as well as for individual moral subjects to formulate their own views of how to act well.[90] What most people think of as "ethics" is the work of delimiting what counts as a legitimate or illegitimate ethical question as well as distinguishing good from bad ethical arguments.[91] By attending to the processes whereby one ethos is challenged and displaced by another, Christians are alerted to the types of response necessary if the problem of disability is to go beyond ethical argumentation to challenge the more fundamental ethos that is positioning these arguments.[92] But to gain any grasp of the ethos characteristic of a time and place demands noticing that *attention to place as well as questions of individual emplacement are irreducible in Christian ethics*.[93] Much like the challenge of opening hearts to lepers Gregory tackled in the patristic era, when people are trapped in a malignant social positioning, the light of Christ exposes the ethos that sustains it as one that Christians must challenge.[94]

What stands out today about ethos characteristic of the patristic period was its grounding in the rule of absolute human solidarity and its embodiment in explicit rejections of all sorts of exclusionary practices and attitudes common at the time. The modern Western solution to the problem of exclusion is inclusion. But to rest content with this conclusion to forego the intellectual work of critical engagement with the question animating the modern ethos: "What should *we* do about *them*?" A power differential is built into the ethos that renders a range of contemporary ethical dilemmas intractable. That contemporary Christians have not recognized how deeply this question is malformed is a humbling reminder of their immersion in the ethos of the modern, secular West.[95] Augustine and Gregory read such a predicament through the biblical language of the need for eyes to be opened, for sinful humans to be *given* a new perception. This language renders the existential breach of the taken-for-granted ethical universe as promising rather than threatening. Only the shaking of a person's ethos allows radically different ethical questions to emerge by bringing alternative ethical problematics into view. That graceful disruption of taken for granted ethical certainties is the most important *theological* feature of the phenomena today called disability.

The formation of this new ethos by Christian laypeople, theologians and pastors was broad based and flowed from a will to explore new and more merciful social arrangements. Looking more closely at patristic responses to anomalous human life suggests further that the general claim that every human life is valuable spontaneously led to explorative practices by individuals, such as the rescue of abandoned newborns, as well as institutional responses, such as the building of institutions of universal care. These practices were in due course to be ensconced in law.[96] Through such practices Christians in this period developed and promulgated moral affirmations that paved the way for later conceptual formulations like "universal human rights" that have become the basic furniture of modern secular morality.

As Christians engaged in these new practices, conceptual descriptions of the reality to which they were responding had to be developed, some from scratch. It is therefore unsurprising that formulations came into use that were later to come under critical scrutiny by disability activists, language like "truncated human beings" and "charity for the needy." The modern criticisms of such language are important. In levying them, however, the reasons for its rise need to be appreciated. When the "charity account" of disability was invented, a gesture was being undertaken by Christians very like the one being undertaken today by thinkers attempting to recover aspects of Greek and Roman views of friendship in order to valorize friendship with the intellectually disabled.[97] Christians today seeking to deploy ancient views of friendship have to remove from it the view that friendship can only be between social equals. Patristic Christians developed the charity model of disability as an attempt to circumvent the common prohibition of generosity to social inferiors, which the ancient Greeks and Romans believed "shall be proportionate to the worthiness of the recipient."[98] The rationalism and aesthetics of Greek and Roman views also often found their way into Christian writings without sufficient critical engagement, sitting uncomfortably with the drive of Christian practice to support the marginalized in ancient society. Decisions like that of Lactantius to incorporate the anthropology of humans as the upright creature jar with the aesthetic rehabilitation of lepers and the aged preached by Gregory and Augustine.[99]

The story of the resistance of the first Christian generations will return in chapters to come. Their example has already provided a warning that failing to attend to broader trends in the sociocultural landscape will leave Christians entrapped in superficial ethical positions and mute in the face of fundamental threats to precarious human lives. If today the "normal" is presumed to be the moral ideal into which the disabled must be included, then the only question is whether people labeled disabled will agree to be healed and included according to the terms of the medical account and the rules of capitalist liberalism. Attending to the ethos of secular modernity suggests that Christians dare not imagine themselves to be on a level playing field when interrogating contemporary practices such as prenatal testing, healthcare allocation, or debates about the legalization of euthanasia for the mentally ill and learning impaired. Christians dare to raise questions about the ethos of their age out of hope in a Jesus whose power to heal challenged the ruling powers and ethos of the first century. Such a Jesus is perfectly capable of breaking into the dominant Western ethos today with its characteristic normalizing medical regimes and ableist stereotypes. And we are his witnesses (Luke 24:48).

2

Wonders from Christendom to Modernity

MERCY'S ADVENTUS

The modern West can rightfully be called the first culture in the world no longer looking for wonders. This state of affairs seems impossible to derive from a Christian tradition founded by a community explicitly yearning to see God's wondrous works.

> Praise the Lord!
> I will give thanks to the Lord with my *whole heart*,
> in the company of the upright, in the congregation.
> Great are the works of the Lord,
> studied by all who delight in them.
> *He has gained renown by his wonderful deeds*;
> the Lord is *gracious* and *merciful*.[1]

The first Christians were certainly witnesses to wonders, and it seemed easy for them to understand themselves as participating in a revolutionary aeon in which a new form of life was taking shape. This certainly became true.

By the time of medieval Christian Europe, it was a matter of course, for instance, for lepers to be found in Christian worship. The fifteenth-century "leper's chapel" of St. Michael's Church in Zwolle, Netherlands, provides architectural proof that sermons like that of Gregory had been received and taken on cultural flesh. One of the transepts of St. Michael's was designed to allow lepers to be present for the mass. What is remarkable is the location of the church in the very heart of the city, its marketplace. Even if those afflicted with leprosy were not allowed to enter the nave with the congregation, they could still see the main altar and receive communion through a barred window. This arrangement indicates that for centuries complex intellectual work had been going on among Christians negotiating prudential concerns about infection without compromising the affirmations about the worth of every human life in Christ, and, as they did so, refusing easy equations of disability with sin.[2]

At the same time the barred windows of the leper's chapel are also a reminder that significant conceptual and practical problems remained. Christians in the medieval period inherited the language of "charity toward the unfortunate" developed by patristic Christians. Disability rights advocates have rightly protested this positioning of disabled people as eternal recipients, a rejection that was fundamental in the founding of the discipline of disability theology. Patristic Christianity bequeathed a problem for modern Christians who care about "disability issues": to escape understanding themselves as those who care *for* disabled people.[3]

It is possible to escape the limits of the charity model by attending to a Christian theological tradition based on the claim that human beings can talk intelligibly about mercy only because God has first been merciful to them. Jesus commands Christians to "be merciful as your father is merciful."[4] Hearing this claim means asking first after the main characteristics of God's works of mercy, and only in a subsequent step investigating what it might mean for humans to attempt acts of mercy in God's name. If the charity model asks, "Where can I find someone who is a deserving recipient of charity?" the mercy tradition offers a different question: "How can God's works of mercy be detected and met by disciples?" In this tradition human acts of mercy never "invent"[5] but only *transmit divine* mercy, at best following God's own breaking into world occurrence on behalf of distressed and vulnerable of human beings.[6] In this tradition all theology is a response to the promise of the God of Scripture continually to uphold and indeed live in and through those fragile lives that everyone else has forgotten.[7]

ANOMALOUS BIRTHS AND THE DIVINE WONDER TRADITION

The task now is to explore from the inside this Christian reasoning about how God's mercy might be perceived and met by disciples desiring to follow Christ's merciful rule. To recap: in pre-Christian Western cultures, anomalous births were taken as threatening portents signifying the wrath of the gods. They therefore evoked terror and demanded the expulsion of the infant and/or repentance among those to whom such children are given as a cosmic warning or rebuke. A second tradition understood such births as marvels eliciting delight and wonder, so increasing the esteem and respect accorded to God and nature. Such births were rarities, yes, but not menacing ones. In the modern age a third perceptual regime with theodical overtones has almost wholly eradicated these two earlier views. As natural errors marring the symmetry of nature, "deformities" might be aesthetically repugnant, but communicate nothing morally. Anomalous births are glitches in highly complex machines, the price of nature's elegant simplicity and regularity which is thrown into sharp relief precisely by these shocking deviations.[8]

It makes all the difference in the world whether we take a surprising birth to be an "unfortunate roll of the dice," a sign of the displeasure of God (or the gods), or a work of God that might plausibly be understood to whisper, somehow, of God's good pleasure in every human life and will to offer abundant life to all. Once this contemporary perceptual frame of anomalous births has been so described, the emotional reactions of shame and disappointment among Christians and non-Christians alike at the advent of supposedly nonstandard human lives makes complete sense.[9] Prereflective perceptions of an anomalous birth have already preconfigured any ethical deliberations that might ensue about how to respond.

The path from Augustine's wonder at the anomalous birth to modern rationalist pathologizing accounts can be quickly sketched. The rationalist strand of Augustine's probably laid the grounds for the loss of the subtle nuances of his legacy among subsequent generations of Christians.[10] By the twelfth century the pre-Christian habit of seeing monstrous births as evil omens had firmly reasserted itself, driven by, and inflaming in turn, the fear of these most vulnerable human beings. This time though, the theologians who specialized in study of the empirical world, the so-called natural philosophers, resisted Augustine's response. Rather than reclaiming threatening omens as divine wonders, they proposed instead to dispel the miraculous entirely, to make wonders cease. In so doing they were to establish modern Western common sense.[11]

The reasons for this transition are complex. The recovery of Aristotle's works in the medieval period catalyzed a revolution in Christian thinking in throwing into question the dominance of more Platonic metaphysical accounts in Christian theology. While famous for having said that wonder is the beginning of philosophy,[12] Aristotle's thought was being taken up in a medieval university increasingly devoted to training professionals, and so having a significant stake in teaching a body of universal truths that could be deployed by students in their subsequent professional careers. Though this shift in the task of theology produced a remarkable body of highly sophisticated work, it also subtly positioned wonder as a passion of the unlearned—the nonphilosopher, the ignorant, the source of old wives' tales. It was in this period that wonder came to be demeaningly associated with ignorance and fear. Believers in wonders reveal themselves ignorant of the natural causes of things. So it is that deeply Aristotelian thinkers like Thomas Aquinas came to hold that wonder, unlike a salutary scientific studiousness, signaled a lack of understanding of both the ways of God and creation.[13] A boundary between nature and supernature was developed in this period that was deeply to shape modern thought when taken up by early modern thinkers. Bacon and Descartes, for example, elaborated this theological separation of nature and grace in the direction of treating nature as a closed system of causes that could be known without reference to faith—and so mastered.[14]

Despite this reduction of the role of wonders among the theologians, there was an explosive reappearance of "wonders" and "portents" in the sixteenth century. Momentous social changes were afoot in this period as feudalism crumbled under the pressure of new mercantilism.[15] In this age of the first great global explorations, the perennial question of disability again became acute: Do these strange races belong to us? Questions of human belonging reignited the hermeneutical problem of anomalous births, and several high-profile "monstrous births" appearing in the nurseries of Christian Europeans became hotly debated portents. Given the cultural energy churning under the discussion of these anomalous births, it was inevitable that these children were to be drawn into that other great upheaval: the Reformation. Both Luther and the Vatican could call for the destruction of deformed infants as a protective measure against the works of the Devil, and Luther in his polemics also all too regularly depicted the papacy as an abominating deformity.[16]

After 1660, with memories of civil and religious disturbances from the Wars of Religion to the French Revolution still vivid, the intellectual, political, and ecclesial elites of the Western world collectively decided to once again make a concerted effort to do away with wonders. Weapons that had fallen into the wrong hands needed to be disarmed. This time around it was not the scientists, but the philosophers and theologians of the Enlightenment who took the lead in attempting to eradicate all belief in the wonderful and miraculous. Philosophers, doctors, and politicians had become wary of wonder as distorting, tempting people to fabricate misleading claims about the material world and in so doing to undermine civil and religious order. During the eighteenth century the assumption that belief in miraculous events led to political upheaval had become so widely held that theologians found themselves needing to defend Jesus against accusations that his association with miracle working was sufficient grounds to reject his claim to be God and to invalidate even his authority as a teacher of respectable moral truths. This snuffing out of belief in wonder and the miraculous might have been politically expedient, but it did create casualties. Simplicity, uniformity, and universality had been decreed the laws of both nature and society, but as a result both God and nature lost the powers of spontaneity capable of shaking the established political order.[17]

This history explains the almost universal belief today that an anomalous birth is a divergence from the statistical norm resulting from an aberrant development in embryonic processes. Such births must be understood as the products of mere chance and causal mechanisms. To see them as anything different is assumed to be the height of ignorance or superstition.[18] In the longer story of Christendom, however, this is only one of three perceptual regimes that have framed anomalous births.

The main issue at stake is not the recovery of miracles. The question is whether Jesus is taken to be willing and able to shake the status quo, and if so, how this comes about. If they think of God at all, inhabitants of secular modernity imagine a deistic Creator of natural laws. Portents and signs are a sideshow. People may still enjoy reports of UFOs and Loch Ness monster sightings, or reading their horoscope, but such pastimes have been rendered politically impotent.[19] In such a landscape it is little wonder that Christians can conceive acts of compassion as, at best, responses to some historically distant creative or redemptive act.

The string of thinkers in Western history who sensed the power of wonder to disrupt the civil order were not wrong. But they were short sighted in assuming that Jesus Christ, and with him Christianity, could only be embraced if the politically disruptive role of the wonder was downplayed or removed. The rise of Christianity *was* politically disruptive, and it was so because it was attractive to people who believed that only a miraculously healing Jesus could threaten the dominating powers that held them captive.

LUTHER ON DIVINE AND HUMAN MERCY

For some, Luther's more infamous comments on disability debar him from any role in a theological account of disability.[20] His contribution to a theology of disability is a theologically sophisticated recovery of Augustine's embrace of "strange wonders"—with its political potency intact. Luther's elaboration of the Augustinian wonder tradition is the road not taken by the contemporary naturalized narrative that so comprehensively positions contemporary perceptions of the anomalous birth. He allows Christians to ask what God might be announcing in and through the wonder of nonstandard human lives.

In Luther's time, theological debates about wonders centered on how God's direct agency was to be related to the workings of secondary causality. One of the prooftexts around which these theological debates were swirling was the story of the sacrifice of Isaac. The problem was how to explain the sudden appearance of the ram in the bush at the precise moment that the angel told Abraham not to sacrifice Isaac.[21]

Luther's preferred theory is that the ram "was brought into existence by the angel's command."[22] Luther allows that both good and bad angels can work wonders. The crucial hermeneutical question is *which* wonders should be attended to and *what* they can reasonably be expected to communicate from God. Luther proposes a clear litmus test: God's wonders conform to the analogy of faith and the promise of God's word. They can thus be expected to yield comfort and joy in those who witness them, not fear.[23]

It is the high status Luther accords the wonderful power of speech, specifically God's word, that leads him to this position. By God's word the world was created and continues to be sustained. Luther concentrates the whole Augustinian wonder tradition in this account of the potency of the word.[24] Because the communicative and creative word of God is the wonder behind all wonders, every other portent is judged by it. Hence the certainty of Luther's assertion that any wonder can be parsed according to the analogy of faith and his allowance that some experiences of portents are "false magic."[25]

Luther's concentration of the Augustinian wonder tradition radicalizes the Christian expectation that God's miraculous activity will be all around and is not confined to events that seem to contravene natural causality. A classic statement of his account of wonder is worth quoting at length. The issue is not God's ubiquity, but the precise form of God's merciful speaking through mediating forms.

> [God] wills to speak, then, namely, when we, almost despairing, decide that He will keep silence forever. But what or in what manner will He speak? Here we must observe the Hebrew way of expression. For when Scripture says that God speaks, it understands a word related to a real thing or action [*verbum reale*], not just a sound, as ours is. For God does not have a mouth or a tongue, since He is a Spirit, though scripture speaks of the mouth and tongue of God: "He spoke, and it came to be" (Ps. 33:9). And when He speaks, the mountains tremble, kingdoms are scattered, then indeed the whole earth is moved. This is a language different from ours. When the sun rises, when the sun sets, God speaks. When the fruits grown in size, when human beings are born, God speaks. Accordingly the words of God are not empty air, but things very great and wonderful, which we see with our eyes and feel

> with our hands. For when, according to Moses (Genesis 1), the Lord said "Let there be a sun, let there be a moon, let the earth bring forth trees," etc., as soon as He said it, it was done. No one heard this voice, but we see the works and the things themselves before our eyes, and we touch them with our hands.[26]

This hermeneutic of divine communication is anchored in the Christian worship service for Luther, specifically, the sermon and the words of institution uttered by the celebrant over the elements of the communion.[27] Precisely in what looks to unbelievers like natural elements, he insists, Christians hear the merciful address of God. Given this location of the miraculous in Christian worship, it is no surprise that his Roman opponents rightly saw him as revivifying the miracle tradition to destabilize the status quo and that wonders so quickly became a central theme in Catholic-Protestant polemics.

If the sacrifice of Isaac was the biblical locus for Luther's recovery of the political potency of wonder, the wider scope of his 1535 commentary on the whole book of Genesis allowed him to elaborate precisely how these continual divine workings of mercy could order human works of mercy. Luther wants to help his students understand the contours of a work of divine mercy so that it is tangible when it appears within their lived experience.

The so-called protoevangelion is the paradigm of divine mercy. God promises to "put enmity between you and the woman, and between your offspring and hers; he will strike your head, and you will strike his heel."[28] This divine promise, eventually to defeat the tempter, is simultaneously a judgment on the serpent and a word of comfort for Adam and Eve in giving them hope that God will defeat the sin that so gravely afflicts them. "Here grace and mercy [*misericordia*] begin to shine forth from the midst of the wrath which sin and disobedience aroused. Here in the midst of most serious threats the Father reveals His heart; this is not a father who is so angry that he would turn out his son because of his sin, but one who points to a deliverance, indeed one who promises victory against the enemy that deceived and conquered human nature."[29] In arresting human rebellion, God displays God's character as concerned both with justice and righteousness yet dominated by the desire to remit punishment. If humans are to find the courage to repent, to change their hearts and turn around, it will come only through internalizing this forgiveness against the visible evidence that they do not deserve it. Therefore, trusting *God's* mercy is for Luther the soul of genuinely *Christian* action.

Luther imagines a chastened Adam and Eve faithfully clinging to this promise and carefully explaining it to their children. Their hope in the promise was so strong that they even expected each new child to be the promised deliverer. The promise of redemption has generated an expectation that events in the creaturely can be tangible acts of divine mercy, good for humans and undeserved. The arrival of a child can be understood as a tangible, wholly concrete divine mercy in that a child is a gift that is undeserved by rebellious humans but is nevertheless given out of God's love and desire to rescue these fallen humans from the clutches of sin.

A much wider range of creaturely occurrences should be understood as divine works of mercy in this way, continues Luther, though they are only known in repentant humility.[30] The language of the three estates, *politia, oeconomia*, and *ecclesia*, concretizes Christian hope in the divine working of quotidian mercies. As a *nation* Israel was God's inheritance. Jerusalem was God's dwelling place, and when Israel became proud and reliant on its own gifts and powers, God withdrew his mercy and bestowed it on other nations as an invitation for them to repent.

> The same thing happens in the family [*oeconomia*]. The purpose for which God gives us good health, wife, children, and property is not that we might offend Him by means of these gifts, but that we might recognize His mercy and give thanks to Him. For this reason He has granted us the enjoyment. . . . But how few there are who do this! Do not almost all of us live in the most shocking abuse of the gifts of God?[31]

The first sacrifice in the fallen world (Gen 4:3) gives Luther an opportunity to round out his explication of the three estates. In accepting sacrifices from the humans expelled from the Garden, God allows a sign of the *ecclesia* to be set up. The cultus of worship is an enacted reminder to all humanity that even fallen humans remain an object of God's concern and regard.

The establishment of these three institutions is itself a work of divine mercy toward fallen humanity. Jumping forward in the biblical narrative, Luther continues:

> This is what God was indicating when He kindled and consumed the sacrifices and offerings with fire from heaven, as we read about the sacrifice of Moses (Lev. 9:24) and of Elijah (1 Kings 18:38). These were true manifestations of the divine mercy [*verae ostensiones divinae misericordiae*] which the wretched people needed in order not to be without some light of the grace of God. In the same way the very Word, Baptism, and the Eucharist are our lightbearers today, toward which we look as dependable tokens of the sun of grace.[32]

God fostered these institutions as an extension of the divine desire to forgive and rescue fallen humans from their idolatrous relations to nation, family, and false religion. The establishment and preservation of the three estates as acts of divine mercy was a central theme for Luther because he understood his own call for reformation of the church to be evidence that the divine promise to judge and preserve the church had not been abandoned.[33] The sheer tangibility of this experience of merciful recovery from idolatrous religion opened his eyes to see God's rescue and care all around him. God "has so richly given us the signs of His grace that we can have them before our doors, yes, even in our houses and in our beds."[34]

The narrative of Cain illustrates the alternative. Cain refuses to receive repentantly and faithfully rely on the divine mercies that rain down on the creaturely realm. He thus lives life blind, careening disorientedly through a disenchanted world. God has no regard for Cain's offering (Gen 4:4-5), comments Luther, because he makes his sacrifice

> without faith, without any confession of sin, without any supplication for grace, without trust in God's mercy, without any prayer for the forgiveness of his sins. He comes in the hope that he will please God by nothing else than that he is the first-born. . . . Abel, on the other hand, acknowledges that he is an unworthy and poor sinner. Therefore he takes refuge in God's mercy and believes that God is gracious and willing to show compassion. . . . [God's different responses to the brother's respective sacrifices shows that] God is not interested in works, not even in those which He Himself has commanded, when they are not done in faith. . . . He is even less interested in the works which have been invented by men without a Word of God; he is interested in faith alone, that is, *the reliance on His mercy through Christ*. Through it people begin to please God, and after that their works also please Him.[35]

While Adam and Eve eventually repent when confronted with their sin by God, Cain remains insolent; he does not understand that "a free confession of sin obtains mercy and overcomes wrath."[36] Those who refuse to look for the rescue of divine mercy are locked into a hermeneutic of refusal toward any signs of divine action in the world. Thus, the heart that refuses to rely on the mercy of God will inevitably become disoriented and homeless.[37]

By tying God's mercy in Genesis so firmly to God's mercy in Christ, Luther is broadening out and existentially thickening his great discovery of God's work of justification.[38] For Luther the grammar of "divine mercy" and "Jesus Christ" are reciprocally defining. The two terms have a messianic logic, since Luther is primarily concerned not with God's character as merciful in the abstract, but with *manifestations* of divine mercy, the capacity of divine mercy to keep human beings part of God's dealings with the world.[39] The faith that God recognizes in Abel is thus not faith that he will go to heaven, but that God will mercifully sustain his life in the day-to-day, that he will "give us our daily bread."

The concreteness of this understanding of God's work in Christ allows Luther to draw all sorts of divine works of deliverance into his account, and paradigmatically, Israel's rescue from Egypt (Exod 3). Jesus constantly reenacts this paradigmatic rescue at the scale of an individual human. Jesus is how divine mercy and rescue look in human form, displaying what it looks like to respond to the command to "be merciful as the Father is merciful" (Luke 6:36). Luther has suggested that Jesus' teaching to his followers to be merciful "as" the Father is merciful is not levying an *ethical* demand, nor proposing Christian acts of *imitative* mercy; humans can only act as those claimed *by* and *for God's* mercy, having been "created in Christ Jesus for good works, which God prepared beforehand to be our way of life."[40]

In short, for Luther the term "mercy" is grounded in the doctrine of God.[41] To speak of mercy is therefore to speak primarily of God and not of Christian ethics. Within the biblical grammar, God's mercy is understood as continually flowing from God to give shape to human lives. Human acts are only merciful by proxy and can only be called merciful as eschatological recognitions of divine blessing: "Blessed are the merciful, for they will be shown mercy" (Matt 5:7). Commenting on this verse in the tradition of Luther, Bonhoeffer insists on the eschatological nature of any ascription of mercy to humans.

> Disciples give away anyone's greatest possession, their own dignity and honor, and show mercy. They know only *one* dignity and honor, the mercy of their Lord, which is their only source of life. He was not ashamed of his disciples. He became a brother to the people; he bore their shame all the way to death on the cross. This is the mercy of Jesus, from which those who follow him wish to live, the mercy of the crucified one. This mercy lets them all forget their own honor and dignity and seek only the company of sinners. If shame now falls on them, they still are blessed. . . . Blessed are the merciful, for they have the merciful one as their Lord.[42]

Luther has provided the key to moving beyond charity models of disability. *Every human being has a place in God's story. To be a Christian is a process of coming to know that place by following God's merciful care for the particular creatures God places before each of us.*[43]

HEARING A WONDER

A defining feature of modernity is the widespread acceptance of a picture of God as having withdrawn to let creation run according to natural laws—should God even exist. In such a deistic (or atheistic) context, recovering a sense of God's engagement with nonstandard lives will demand recovering a sensibility for God's appearance and claim as the act of a *person* who comes to humans as "the Word made flesh."[44] *The tangibility of such personal acts of divine mercy as they appear in the lived spaces of daily life has been undertheorized in modern Christian theology*. If, as we have seen Luther so firmly to believe, God, "has so richly given us the signs of His grace that we can have them before our doors, yes, even in our houses and in our beds,"[45] more attention will need to be given to narrating what it might mean to experience worldly occurrences as "manifestations of mercy."

Such manifestations will have to be in real time, and so "heard" as God's articulate works, to use a prominent Old Testament idiom. Quoting Deuteronomy 8:3, Jesus was keen to emphasize that the human being "does not live by bread alone, but by every word that comes from the mouth of God" (Matt 4:4). To emphasize this biblical theme runs directly counter to the secular-modern sense that "hearing the word of the Lord" is something that no longer happens today, or happens only to prophets on mountains or maybe every once in a while through a sermon or the promptings of conscience.[46]

That hearing is more than the operation of the auditory organs and speaking more than sounds made by the mouth is the basis of the common maxim in special education that "every action is communication." Touch is the basic bodily sensation, physical hearing being one form of the more universal human capacity to touch, and so sense, the world.[47] The grounding of communication in touch makes intelligible the constant intertwining of speech, gesture, and gaze in human communication.[48] Human beings cannot live and move without proprioceptive interactions between their inner depths and their outer surfaces constantly crossing the boundaries of their skin.

These anthropological observations provoke a theological insight. In the parable of the Good Samaritan, Jesus very materially concretizes the descent and advent of divine mercy. The parable of the Good Samaritan pivots on the line, "when he saw him, he was moved in his bowels." The story ends by summarizing the response to this inner movement as a "showing of mercy."[49] The Messiah who has traveled into the far country tells a story of a Samaritan's body reacting immediately and spontaneously to the presence of a suffering human. Jesus is presenting the immanent mercy of God as straining toward the bodily suffering of the neighbor in the way people's stomachs clench and hearts race out of self-concern when approaching a railing above a high precipice. The Hebraism translated into Greek used here, *splanchnizesthai*—"to be deeply moved" as in "deeply in the bowels," appears at several crucial points in the gospels. Jesus is depicted as a being living inside the tent of his skin in a manner that ensures that his outer surfaces are sensitive to the truth of an embodied person. A depth of bodily connection between human beings is powerfully evoked. *Jesus calls everyone to receive this heightened sensitivity*.

Heightened sensitivity is often one of the gifts of physical disability. The loss of certain bodily functions can provoke a greater awareness of the kinesthetic aspect of human bodily existence, what is also called the "kinesis of knowledge."[50] The term "kinesthesia" refers to the aggregate of impressions arising from organic sensations. This aggregate is the basis of one's awareness of body or bodily state, such as an awareness of one's body being vigorous or lethargic. Highlighting this aspect of human communicative sensation, does, however, unsettle Descartes' influential claim that "I" am fundamentally a center of consciousness inside a brain and essentially *other* than my body.[51] Jesus, in contrast, depicts the individual's "I" as possessing a body, and so kinesthetic senses that can be involuntarily drawn outward by the mortal need of a specific, bodily neighbor. Descartes got it right in claiming that the soul touches the body at a particular point, but wrong in locating it in the pineal gland. Jesus looks further south, much nearer the waist, as the place where the "I" is decided and the "soul" is seated.[52]

The redemption Jesus offers fallen humans is of their whole being, and includes restoring them into loving relationship with others.[53] Though Jesus alone fully embodies this congruence of human and divine works of mercy, in his parables he nevertheless insists that human works that are pleasing to God are those that join his works of divine mercy.[54] He models a responsiveness to God embedded in relationships with others and flowing out from the innermost parts of the viscera. Jesus' investment in specific humans in all their concreteness is so central to his being that it erupts from the very fibers of his body.[55] Jesus thus both displays and offers a story that encapsulates the inner dynamics of human life when determinatively shaped as a response to divine mercy. In Jesus Christ we witness a "self," an embodied identity, wholly dedicated to meeting and serving God's mercy toward human beings in need of rescue. The limits and boundaries of the neighbor's body are for Jesus not something that separates people, but the conditions that allow deepening connections with them. In reality this has been God's way since the beginning, God having brought human beings into existence by forming Adam from the dust with his own hands and breathing life into his nostrils with his own lips.[56] Jesus confirms the goodness of God's works of creation in raising up the dying man and restoring his breath of life by giving himself to him through personal presence and touch.

The dis-ease experienced by the Samaritan before the body of the wounded man is presented by Jesus not as a demanding responsibility, but a gift, an invitation to receive our true selves by stepping into the gratuitous love of Christ. From the human side, gratuity needs an occasion and cannot flow out of me unless it is evoked and challenged by you.[57] From the divine side, in Christ, the God who is both over and above the whole of creation, makes human beings part of his story of the world. Human beings are incorporated into God's story when God claims them in the neighbor as participants in his gratuitous acts of liberating, sustaining, and healing mercy. The divine gift is not an opportunity to "do something nice,"[58] to discharge a merit-building act of charity, but a moment when a gratuitous response to God's mercy *to us* is made tangibly available.

Christians respond to the neighbor because in the neighbor the mercy of Christ calls out to them, as emphasized by the passage the Christians of the patristic era took with such deadly seriousness: "Insofar as you have done it to the least of these brothers of mine, you have done it unto me" (Matt 26:40). Whether the one whose need calls out is a good or bad person is irrelevant here, as irrelevant as the past actions of the one who finds themselves drawn to act mercifully. What matters for human beings is to recognize that their own wholeness can only come to them through others. That wholeness is finally their life in Jesus Christ. His presence is the primary relationship that draws people into these secondary relationships. His *humanity* reveals God's love for *all* humanity. And he claims humanity through the humanity of others. As Gregory preached, *the gift of the neighbor, especially the one who makes us uncomfortable, is in Christ a realization that neither they, nor we, are who we once thought.*[59]

Christians love a God who loves justice and whose steadfast love flows throughout the world, but only, the biblical traditions tell us, in and with the neighbor (Ps 33:5; Lev 19). The neighbor with their need activates the bodily compassion that keeps human beings in God's story in specific places and times. Salvation is being made the servants of the bodily survival of other human beings, and in this way to discover the way to each individual's survival as a human being.[60] To *recognize* the reality of our neighbors as subjects of God's merciful love is, for the Christian, a welcoming of divine mercy poured out on creation by becoming attuned to the *physical* concreteness and gift nature of the claim their lives levy. This formed perception must be *repentantly* received and follow up with a *disciplined* response that extends over time.

Disciplined and repentant attention to the concrete bodiliness of the neighbor flowers in the capacity to hear bodily gestures as spoken words. After all, the neighbor in the ditch near unto death would have been unlikely to have raised his voice—the comportment of his body was his only cry. A Christian theology of the gaze and the gesture is rooted here in knowledge-how that grows from so caring for the other as a bodily being, that capacity emerges to read what the body is communicating. Such knowledge is possessed even by those with the most limited cognitive and sensory capacities, who, having bodies themselves, have some awareness of the shape of a face when it smiles, or of the gait of a friend, or of the difference between a caring and an uncaring touch. Attunement to the rhythms of bodily tension and relaxation characteristic of unique individuals grows from concern to know their joy and their pain.[61]

The forms of love and care that are paradigmatic of Israel and the church are ones learned not by grasping the beatific vision of the One, but by grasping that the many vectors of the natural world and the economy of God's action are tangible in *every* unique person and place. Christians do not worship a universal God knowable apart from his presence and action in creaturely locales, supremely in the life and death of Jesus Christ.[62] A genuinely Christian and theological account of mercy turns on formed perceptions that *this* neighbor has been clothed by the divine word of a merciful God. In this Christology and doctrine of creation, things and words are no more antitheses than God and the creature. This is not to claim that every creature is God, but to insist that to know creation at all is to know God in God's word and act, and to know God truly in God's word and act is to know God's mercy—and through it, creation as it truly is.

***

CODA: PART 1

The first four centuries of the Christian era saw Christians discovering a range of fertile, practical, and theoretical links between the work of Jesus Christ and the worth of every human life—links utterly novel within the surrounding ancient cultures. For them, disability was no niche question because the core of the Christian gospel concerns the redemption of every human being. Their example challenges Christians today to find ways to name the variations among human beings that do not introduce divisions and hierarchies and yet retain the capacity to recognize some people as having important bodily and mental differences and legitimate needs for social support. Affixing the label "disability" to some of the differences among human beings is one way to do this, but not the only one, and comes with its own drawbacks. Any serious Christian theology of disability has continuously to interrogate the limits such a label places on modern assumptions about humanness and personhood.[63] Having looked closely at a Christianity deeply committed to vulnerable and ostracized human lives has even revealed much modern disability rights language as rather lacking in ambition and scope.

Tracing the red thread of the wonder tradition has been especially helpful in exposing the modern perceptual frame situating anomalous births. Because in modern secularity wonders have ceased, it is almost inevitable that people who have been labeled disabled will feel condemned to having their whole lives framed by a narrative in which the biological or historical lottery has dealt them a losing hand. Their bodies and personalities are viewed as so permeated by the effects of a fallen creation that it is almost impossible to imagine who they might be in the healing that is resurrection. In other words, disbelief in the wonder and "strange vocations" consigns some lives to be lived entirely in the shadow of the problem of natural evil.[64] When modern Christians believe this, whether unwittingly or explicitly, they have decisively broken with the patristic rule of human solidarity.

The theological tradition surveyed in part 1 highlights this fracture within Christendom by raising an alternative question with expansive heuristic import. To experience something that might well be explained in wholly naturalistic terms as a wonder or wonderful is to transcend the frame of natural causality. When Christians admit the question, "What is the Creator saying here?" they are ultimately enacting a hope for the advent of that signal wonder, the incarnate Word, the resurrecting and liberating Jesus. That liberating word is announced in every human birth. Augustine and then Luther's proposals emphasized that point with their enjoinder to listen for this merciful and promising word in many forms of creaturely mediation—even in those lives that seem marked by lack or incapacity. Reclaiming the revelatory capacity of people labeled disabled today is crucial if the *political* potency of the term is to be preserved. Like so many Christians down through the centuries, those people who today carry the label "disabled" may understand better than most why a God who *interrupts* the certainties of the age is a God who inspires *hope*. Thus, far from being "prompts" for the wonderment of the able bodied, people who carry the label "disabled" today can be appreciated as reviving wonder at the Creator's intentions for *every* human life.[65]

Only because the Christians of the patristic era viscerally experienced themselves as having been forgiven and redeemed, to an extent they could never repay, were they able to roundly reject the Greco-Roman matrix for assessing the worth of human lives—even if it cost them their own lives. In a world where this experience of radical forgiveness is no longer widely shared (even among church members), forgiving debts becomes increasingly difficult to comprehend. Debt relations inevitably codify into rules about socially acceptable minimum levels of performance or ability, demanding that some lives justify themselves. Christians have little reason to expect Christian accounts of care, compassion, or mercy to survive conversion into secular terms like "services" or "rights."[66] Where this linguistic translation has occurred and crystallized in institutional practices, genuine Christian (and so human) compassion will appear transgressive.[67]

Moderns have internalized ways of seeing themselves, and themselves with others, that minimize the importance of attending to bodies. If Christians have not seriously attended to the diversity of human bodies, it is in no small part because they have not taken their own bodies seriously enough. *Moderns have been trained into an insensitivity to bodily life, having come to understand even their own bodies as clusters of organ systems and risk factors. In such a world, to rediscover the implications of the confession that Jesus Christ became incarnate in a body offers precious analytical insight into contemporary Western culture.*[68] Human beings are beings of flesh. God knows human bodies, has known humans in the body, and teaches a faithfulness to bodies that opens communication by attending to bodies. Fleshly lives can be saved by the actions in the flesh of another, and can save the flesh of others, if not their souls. Divine mercy orients human bodily compassion for those bodies. Thus, the evident bodily suffering of the other points a way out of the predicament of the age, its deafness, and addiction to ways of listening that devalue the voices and body experiences of others.

In a theological account, the vulnerability of human bodies is no longer a "problem" or a "need" but a bodily sign from God, a *divine call*. A new "ought" has been established not generated by a rule, but by a body, a body through which God directs human action. The call of the body opens an alternative understanding of justice and faithfulness as well as revealing a new form of sin: the sin of ignoring the body's claim, of coldness, of looking away. Medics, parents, and caregivers are challenged to preserve the priority of the unique voice of each person in expressing their own bodily experience. Supreme efforts will be needed from medical professionals to set aside the idea that the body of the other can be known well without knowing the story of their corporeal sensations, and to overcome them will expose the paternalistic (if unconscious) impulses of caregivers to preempt the halting and often nonverbal voices of disabled people.

To reappropriate these traditions of mercy and gratuity today will require relinquishing some deeply ingrained modern intellectual habits, most obviously the modern progressivist assumption that the Christian tradition is antiprogressive. Engaging in an intergenerational conversation within a shared tradition is a distinctively Christian mode of self-criticism, one that begins by dispensing with the modern conceit that truth and a just society are best achieved by constantly throwing overboard the legacy of a murky past less true and insightful than our own.[69]

When Christians study the writings of dead Christians, they engage in an act of intergenerational listening within an extended community gathered by a single Lord. Such listening offers Christians a footing in the trans-temporal and transspatial community that Augustine called the City of God and offers a view of the contemporary world through *their* eyes. Engaging the Christian tradition in this way carries on the Christian community's expectancy that ancient texts can be the conduit of an animating Spirit. Through this attentive reading, voices of believers can be heard, who worshiped a God they did not believe to be silent. Their voices can breathe life back into our dead, disenchanted secular world, a past once seeming archaic springing to life as it sheds new light on contemporary perplexities.[70] Such listening is a preparation for listening to people today who seem incapable of speaking in the hope that through them, too, the Trinitarian God still speaks.[71]

The deepest reason to listen to the tradition is that it is the site of Christ's crucified body in this world. The most fundamental location of the Christian is within the body of Christ, as often as this is forgotten. But the Western Christian is also emplaced in a highly developed secular polity. The patristic awareness of gesture and gaze presses contemporary theologians never to forget the positionality of all thinking, living, and theologizing. Modern theology has inherited a blindness to the relevance of place and discursive practices, as well as to the social protocols that continually shape and position our instinctive awareness of licit and illicit action.[72] The theological task is to parse what this ecology of gazes and gestures reveals about the human hearts out of which it is born, and which hold it in place. The experience of disability today cannot be understood without constantly attending to the field of gazes and gestures characteristic of the public world of secular liberalism. We turn now to that cultural world and the gazes and gestures that make it sometimes hospitable, but often threatening, to those carrying the label "disabled."

PART II

WELCOME AND SCREENING

Doxology and Anti-Doxology

3

Practicing Welcome in the New World of Genetic Testing

BEING HUMAN IS A PRACTICE

Societies organized around the supremacy of personal choice ought to greet the choice to bear and love a child with disabilities with a shrug. That's not quite how things have worked out.

Modification of the human genetic inheritance is generally assumed to be as unstoppable as the spread of the internal combustion engine or the internet, despite some residual foreboding. What is clear is that these techniques are already directly impacting people with minority genetic conditions, and not always for the good. Many see these techniques as marvelous new tools for the progressive elimination of human suffering. A few others see them as the lethal machinery for ridding the world of disabled people.[1] It is no accident that the perfection of techniques to find and eliminate in utero human beings with unwanted genes happened at the very moment activist movements began to form to demand civil rights and social inclusion for people with disabilities. The incommensurability of these clashing narratives hints at what is actually under dispute: rival proposals for enacting the human.

Being human is a practice carried out each and every day, in small and large gestures.[2] Only rarely do people pause critically to analyze the shape of this ongoing practice. The practice of medicine is a difficult subject because it so deeply shapes modern Westerners' understanding of what constitutes a good society, a good life, and even a good body. It has become a taken-for-granted environment vital for security and wellbeing. Medicine is about identity in the West. Thus, when a dispute about a discrete suite of medical technologies comes out into the open, it affords a rare opportunity critically to examine the ethos of the Western medical project. Disputes about medical procedures make it possible to peel back layers of linguistic cloaking to study the sort of humanity modern Westerners are currently performing. What is revealed is a refusal of wonder so deep that the question does not even arise about what God might be up to in the life of an anomalous new one. Without this wonder, in a technological society, there is no real question that this natural tragedy will need to be fixed.

This chapter focuses on a specific technology, prenatal genetic testing, which presents its own special problems of analysis. Machines do not work themselves, and modern technologies demand exacting institutional and infrastructural support. To study technological change thus demands studying the forms and characteristic common sense of the societies in which they are imbedded. "Technology" too turns out to be a type of self-description of the humanity being performed in a given place, but one that highlights the apparatuses that sustain that way of life. To get at our technological present demands close participatory examination of the contours of real lived experiences.[3]

Before diving deep into one story of that impact, it is important to note that the overarching ethos of the landscape in which the action is set is that of the neoliberal market state. Modern democratic governments promise to keep their citizens secure. Security takes wealth. Technologically advanced societies are therefore econometrically engineered to maximize the happiness and wealth of the greatest number of its citizens. Western governments are adjudged to have succeeded or failed by this measure. "Liberalism" names the political and legal commitment to maximizing citizens' domain of free choice, while "neoliberalism" or the "market state" names the politico-economic policies that harness the engine of consumer choice to the maximization of the wealth of the citizenry.[4]

Modern democracies can be called "biopolitical" to the extent that their routines of governance do not *repress* but aim to *foster* and *augment* the forces of human life.[5] With this shift has come a far-reaching alteration in the role played by norms in political life. High modern accounts of moral and legal norms understood them as forbidding or prohibiting certain actions through prescriptive injunctions such as "one should not lie" or "stealing is illegal." Today norms work differently, neoliberal societies priding themselves in the freedom they allow their citizens. Simply forbidding actions and suppressing infractions by force draws too much attention to the limits of freedom. Lighter-touch norms preserve the illusion of citizens' freedom being essentially untrammeled.[6]

Ultimately, however, the mandate for states to provide security demands imposing some limits on personal autonomy. Citizens' freedom of choice needs to be steered toward some actions and away from others. At the same time, some norms are needed to keep such highly fluid societies from disintegrating into disorienting atomization. The rise of statistical modes of capturing what is going on in modern societies provides those who govern with tools for shaping individual behavior without appearing to limit the freedom of citizens. Internalized norms are far more subtle and powerful tools for keeping order in liberal societies. Older "normative norms" that bluntly decree limits to behavior enforced by the threat of state violence can be laid aside in favor of econometric approaches. Econometrically organized governance understands norms as more flexible, graded domains of more and less acceptable behavior. These norms are more accurately called "normalistic" in no longer being externally set rules or laws, but time-bound and fluid *comparative processes*. Point norms (best visualized by the traffic light which establishes behaviors as either legal or not) have been transformed into range norms best visualized using statistical curves. *"Normality" has now become the behaviors most citizens assume to be normal and which are capable of statistical documentation.* A biopolitical governance regime moves people by inducing conformity with majority behavior. Normalistic norms can only be generated within highly data-oriented societies—the societies in which, in fact, most Westerners now live.[7]

The utility of normalistic norms is the ease with which they allow cultural practices to be interweaved with legal protocols. A normalistic social norm, "most people expect me to behave this way," thus paves the way for an ethical norm: "Everybody (many) does (do) that; that's normal." Political governance no longer needs to shape citizens' behavior by outlawing unwanted behaviors. The masses can now be directed by far less confrontational social messaging.

> Completely voluntarily, in line with ideals of autonomy and self-determination, we orient ourselves to the middle of society, to average norms. We want to live the way that other people do; most importantly, we want to be "normal." If we feel enjoyment in deviation, it is only because we want to "march to the beat of a different drummer"—but, only for a little while. By no means do we want to be permanently localized at the negative pole of the spectrum of a certain behavior or characteristic.[8]

The behavior of the majority constitutes the power of normalistic moral and legal norms.

The eradication of some congenital disabilities has only been accomplished with the rise of normalistic governance. As technologies of prenatal diagnosis become ever more sensitive and reliable, flexible norms become the natural mechanism for relocating the eugenic choice from policy makers to parents, a decision springing from the stated objective of governance to augment economic security of the state. The older eugenic norm that attempted to legally decree that the twisted branches of the human genetic tree be cut off has given way to a eugenics that achieves the same end by asking families to make free (and rational) choices.[9]

A normalistically governed society allows some to "march to the beat of a different drummer," knowing that the deck has been stacked against them. This chapter offers one real-time snapshot of the forces genetic technologies bring to bear on the disabled and their families. It is the beginning of our story with Adam. His mother, Stephanie, and I are both privileged, white, and highly educated. I am an academic theologian and medical ethicist, and Stephanie a neonatal nurse. Ours is a story of negotiating all the typical joys and frustrations of first-time parenthood. But it is also a tale of the impact of genetic testing that reaches deep into the lives of many who are far less privileged.

GENETICS CHANGES EVERYTHING

Adam was conceived in England, three months before a planned move to Germany. Since the move coincided with the time when prenatal consultations usually begin, Stephanie waited to begin this process until we reached Germany. It seemed easier to enter the bureaucracy of antenatal care in the country where Adam would be born. Stephanie was left free to experience our growing child in the traditional way, by marveling at the changes in her body. Neither of us felt the lack of antenatal care, confident that we would have timely access to the right professionals should any problem arise. We were happy, and all seemed well.[10]

Stephanie was nearly four months along by the time life settled down a bit in Germany. Not knowing where to begin formally to enroll in the health-care system, she visited the prenatal department in a hospital (Frauenklinik) and was allocated a first examination. That examination included a direct and insistent urging to have a sonogram as quickly as practicable. Stephanie was puzzled about the insistent tone and asked whether the doctor's worries concerned baby or mother. When pressed, the examining doctor admitted skepticism about Stephanie's stated conception date, and the legal cutoff date for an abortion appeared perilously close.[11] She discovered that the doctor's anxiety rested on a set of assumptions she did not accept about the purpose of prenatal examination, but which were not presented up front. Having entered the clinic to arrange antenatal care and to discuss birthing arrangements, Stephanie was instead offered medical treatment that she neither sought nor desired. She received it anyway as part of the institutional, legal, and social location of women's medicine within the "norming norm."

The episode crystallized our theological belief that only one criterion for diagnostic action made sense. From here on out, all proposed healthcare investigations and treatments of mother or child should be correlated to the medical interests of both. This turned out to be an increasingly difficult line to maintain in its implicit denial of termination as a "treatment." We might have discussed termination were the case an issue of Stephanie's safety, but there was no hint of such a scenario. This first conflict with the medical profession thus raised the question of what and who medical testing is *for*. The strong emotional engagement in establishing an accurate date of conception by the medical professionals involved pushed the question of the reasons for the intervention into the foreground.

Dissatisfied and shaken by her experience at the Frauenklinik, Stephanie contacted a midwife to discuss a home birth. Simple examinations ensued: measuring growth, asking how Stephanie was feeling, looking at her color, asking about specifics like aches and pains in the teeth and bones.[12] The twenty-week ultrasound scan in the hospital raised no questions at all. Stephanie was still relatively young (twenty-nine years old) and visibly healthy, both before and during her pregnancy. A home birth was agreed upon without question. To the day of birth, no countersigns indicated that anything but the most normal of babies was soon to arrive.

Adam emerged into the world just before dawn one stormy August morning, three weeks ahead of schedule but apparently healthy. Mother, father, and midwife greeted the dawn with relief at the short night of labor and the arrival of a son sporting a complete complement of fingers, toes, eyes, and ears. As might be expected of an early arriver, he was not large, but immediately and easily took to the breast. Brimming with fatherly pride and completely untainted by worries or doubts about the future, I vividly recall walking to the nearby bakery for breakfast rolls, announcing the good news of Adam's arrival in the early morning sun to the ladies behind the bakery counter. The next three days were spent at home, adjusting to the unpredictable biological cycles of our new family member, interrupted only by the daily checkups of the midwife.[13]

On the fourth day we ventured out for Adam's first scheduled medical checkup. We were glad for the chance to see a doctor, since Adam seemed to be developing a minor infection around his navel and a light skin a rash. The doctor checked him over and reassured us that new babies often have skin rashes that are completely normal and most often quickly disappear. The cursory nature of this doctor's investigation reassured us that Adam's premature birth had no special significance; Adam was a wholly normal baby. He was going to have all the unexceptional ups and downs of all the other infants with which we had been acquainted—Stephanie having been acquainted with many, as a neonatal nurse.

Lying on the examination table at midday in the brightly sunlit examination room, Adam was still a normal child with a normal rash. Soon Adam would become "disabled," his every symptom rendered ominous. Soon the troubled future that had not yet even been mentioned would balloon to dominate every medical examination and discussion of treatment.

Seven hours later I was in the middle of a phone call filling in my family back in the United States about their new relative. As Adam lay on my lap, he went from being a bit listless and blotchy to grey, limp, and lifeless. Though reviving and recovering his color within a minute, we were rattled. We called our midwife, who suggested we wait a bit and watch him closely, but Stephanie was convinced that we needed to take him directly to the local children's hospital emergency room for examination. We both still assumed that Adam was a normal child who had an infection and had perhaps choked on some milk, but something was certainly not quite right. Thus, it was *Stephanie's* insistence on medical *testing* that in the end broke through the tacitly and explicitly stated opinions of medical personnel and even her husband that day: the doctor at noon, the midwife at seven in the evening, and soon the doctors at the emergency room. All shared a single message: "If it will make *you* (i.e., the mother) feel better, we will check him over." It took some persuading for the doctors in the emergency room to investigate a baby with a rash. Eventually his blood saturation levels were assessed, at which point it became apparent that this was no first-time-parent panic. Despite his relatively unremarkable visible appearance, Adam was in critical condition.

By midnight he was in intensive care with what turned out to be a serious blood infection (sepsis). The doctors were unwilling to predict the outcome. Adam's odds of survival were simply unknown. Forty-eight hours later, and to our unimaginable relief, he had turned the critical corner. It was during the period of his ascent back from his drugged and betubed existence in his tiny incubator that Stephanie first noticed the words "verdacht Trisomy 21" in his chart—"suspected Down syndrome." After asking the doctors if this meant what we thought it did (and trying unsuccessfully to discern when they planned to tell us of their suspicion), we were left to absorb our dark discovery: Adam is not normal.

LIFE IN GENETIC LIMBO

The emotional turmoil provoked by this discovery cannot be understated, and not simply because we hadn't expected it. Rival futures immediately crowded our minds. One was having to face grieving the loss of a beautiful, healthy, firstborn son. The other was living with a disabled child. We swung wildly from practical questions about how to go about burying a child in a foreign country to amorphous fears of never being able to do the things we loved with our son. It was disorienting. We shouldn't have been surprised, either at that time or in hindsight, to have contemplated the horrible and yet predictably human question: "Would it be better if he died?"[14]

On the tenth day of Adam's hospitalization, we had our first discussion with the head physician about Adam's suspected Down's. He admitted that they had taken blood and had it genetically tested on admission to establish whether Adam had Down's or not. The test, however, had failed, and they planned to repeat it immediately. We were legally literate enough to be shocked by the missing request for our consent. We asked whether it was legal in Germany for genetic testing to be undertaken without permission, and he admitted without explanation or apology that yes, parental permission is legally required.

We immediately clarified our position. We were unhappy that they had taken blood and done a genetic test without our permission and were now simply informing us the test would be repeated. On those grounds alone, it seemed to us that it was not in Adam's or our best interests to conform to an apparent status quo which included ignoring legal consent. We clearly stated that we did not want the retesting to proceed.

We got into the habit of repeating our simple question whenever a diagnostic procedure was proposed: will it aid Adam's treatment? The doctors urging Adam to be genetically tested in the hospital suggested it would be good so that we could plan for his future. Once his diagnosis was confirmed, other problems often suffered by children with Down's could be investigated, such as problems with sight and hearing, intestinal troubles, and thyroid disturbance. Again, we had the sense that the energy being expended to persuade us to test was incommensurate with the benefits being offered. If these problems are known comorbidities of Down syndrome, we asked, won't he be examined for each of these problems without the genetic test? This was the question that flushed out the real reason for pushing the testing.

General appeals to our and Adam's best interest easily gave way to the real reason for their interest in having Adam genetically tested: you wouldn't want to have any more of "these children." Only if we knew what *kind* of

Down's he had would we be able to calculate our chances of having more healthy children. We could not help but wonder if this genetic information was also being sought for the purposes of gathering genetic data for genetic population studies. All these considerations suggested that we would do well to refuse consent to the repeat genetic test, which we did. Adam's suspected Down's remained just that—suspected. We were later very pleased to have taken this route since it reasserted our central priority: that Adam be understood as first a patient, and perhaps only then an experimental subject or case for clinical teaching.

Subsequent experience has highlighted how widespread the assumption is that no one would choose to have a child with Down's if it could possibly be avoided. It is a claim we have heard repeated with some insistence and in good faith even by well-meaning medical professionals in our own families. During Stephanie's second pregnancy in Scotland, one of Adam's primary medical caregivers was outspokenly certain that we were making a mistake not to test comprehensively during Stephanie's second pregnancy as it would "put your minds at ease." This from a specialist in Down's and whose care for Adam has been exemplary. When Stephanie gently attempted to evade discussing this prenatal testing (without explicitly stating her reasons), the doctor then reassured Stephanie that, "your risk is only one in a hundred now, and they'll do very detailed scans on you anyway."[15] The scans she had in mind might not have been invasive or dangerous to our second child. But the suggestion that we wouldn't want another child like Adam and the "treatment" we were being invited to contemplate for the newest member of our family shook us deeply.

We grew increasingly secure in our belief that Adam was best served by insisting that all testing to which he was subjected be justified by the possibility of it leading to treatment of a presenting problem. Two main considerations appeared to animate medical resistance to this position. Since testing is routine and yields interesting and potentially useful information, it should be pursued as part of the wider project of advancing medical science. While Adam might not directly benefit, his "donation" of genetic material might help cure others in the future, perhaps even of Down's. Furthermore, the security imperative demands it. Parents must prepare for the future, and the birth of another child with Down's or some other genetic anomaly is a devastating harm to avoid. It is probably not coincidental that both suggestions lead to the augmentation of medical power through increasing knowledge. While that increase in medical power might not always come at the expense of a given patient, we wanted to know whether it would be to Adam's benefit.

With Adam's growth came an irrepressible and increasingly psychologically draining obsession with parsing his physical features. The ambiguity of his being "suspected" was clearly affecting us. Until the genetic age borderline cases like Adam's could only have been resolved by the unfolding of time. We were learning the hard way about the phenomenally wide range of symptoms that may accompany Down syndrome. Many of these are widespread among the general populace: extra creases in the palms, premature birth, extra muscular flexibility, small size. We alternated between scrutinizing his symptoms and trying to push them from our consciousness. Two competing responsibilities lay behind that relentless mental oscillation. "Do I betray my normal child by suspecting him of defect?" fought tooth and nail against another: "Do I betray my disabled child by withholding some treatment which he might need at this early stage?" These two questions cut across almost every detail of caring for an infant. This all-too-present future unsettled us, a fear learned from Adam's doctors. The genetic test promised resolution.

Modern tests bring the future to bear on parents and doctors alike in a new and forceful way. Before the advent of genetic testing, parents could fear little more than an early death from unknown causes. What is remarkable about the current landscape of parenthood is the expansion of the domain of what can be feared and how parents today can feel as if they are dangling on the edge of a dangerous precipice even while feeding and caring for a happy, growing, and developing infant.

Many parents experience these anxieties after being told their new one has Down's. The difference between our case and the typical case is that we had crossed *the* moral boundary in the age of legalized abortion: our child was outside the womb. The birth canal had been his gateway to citizenship, rights, and personhood in the fullest sense. We find it hard to imagine facing these questions with his face not yet visible and surrounded by the voices of reasonable authorities, families, and friends telling us, "Don't risk it. Start over with a clean slate."[16] In a cultural and institutional context that systematically maximizes the precarity of some lives to minimize their grievability when the decision is made to kill them, the burden of proof is firmly on those who wish to accept all life. It is easy to imagine how moral scruples about aborting a genetically anomalous fetus could fade into insignificance.

That Adam was only "suspected" had forced us into a hermeneutic exercise. To parent Adam well demanded our discerning the aims, skills, and interests of the doctors examining him. This meant discerning whether their fears and hopes coincided with ours as parents. We brandished his body like a divining rod as we hunted for a doctor who could care for his particular needs. His body unnerved doctors increasingly unfamiliar with nonstandard infants. And they instinctively reached for genetic testing as a diagnostic panacea.[17]

When combined in a medical context, his ambiguous body and our probing questions could sometimes become explosive. Adam was five months old when Stephanie took him to the doctor for treatment of a runny nose, having learned enough to know that children with Down syndrome are prone to respiratory tract infections. In the examination room the doctor opened her file, then glanced at Adam. Then a question laced with moral outrage: "Why haven't you had the genetic test done?" A heated exchange of views yielded a deadlock over what should come next, so the doctor tried to get Stephanie to admit that it would have been prudent to have had Adam genetically tested. "You know, don't you, that Adam will never go to normal school." This pronouncement turned out to be the entirety of the advice offered by a medical expert on this occasion; no further examination was undertaken, and no treatment suggested. The ideology of genetic testing had again managed to crowd out attention to the symptoms of infection even in unexpected quarters. Stephanie had intentionally sought out this female homeopathic physician precisely in hopes of receiving more holistic and caring attention. Adam was denied medical attention for his presenting illness, and Stephanie was left to weather Adam's cold and discomfort, alone and shaken.[18]

Yet again our parental priority was unchanged. Adam deserved treatment for his specific needs, on this occasion his cold. Our interest in meeting that specific need ran up against a belief, or a fear, that treatment was not advisable without a proper, scientific (read genetic) confirmation of diagnosis. By pressing for the specific need rather than the global need to be treated, we positioned ourselves within the dominant framing of medicine as parents resistant to admitting blatant facts about their child and irrationally avoiding a routine diagnostic procedure. There could be no genuinely rational reason to resist a test that would both dispel parents' illusions of health and concretely document that the child belonged in the social and medical role assigned to children with this genetic condition. All parties ended up poorly served by this heavy-handed exercise of medical authority: the doctor did not have the satisfaction of turning a truculent parent into a conforming one, Stephanie was offended by the implicit disparagement of her parenting, and Adam was not treated for his cold. The existence of the technology of genetic testing, combined with the vast numbers of people who utilize it without protest, established a norming norm that was the *condition* for this conflict.

After several months of searching and through a recommendation by a friend from church, we finally met a neonatologist who was also the father of a child with Down's. He examined Adam during an informal meeting at his house and told us that, for several reasons he patiently explained to us, he felt there to be something like an 85 percent chance that Adam had Down's. For the first time we felt like someone with medical training had actually *looked at Adam*. We had finally met one of a dwindling number of medical practitioners with firsthand experience of this increasingly rare condition.[19] He was able to assess Adam with the eyes of experience as he listened to our account of his progress and ailments, and to patiently and kindly articulate the reasons for his diagnosis. It was a delightful bonus that he and his wife could give us the kind of parental advice we so desperately craved about how to deal with Adam's particular health difficulties. Our inner conflicts were beginning to resolve. It was looking more likely that he did have Down's than that he did not. More importantly, we were beginning to feel that we would be able to handle whatever was to come. We passed the news on to our families across the Atlantic who, never having met Adam, would now also have to embark on their own journeys of acceptance.

To our eyes Adam seemed to be developing well, if slowly. Whether he had Down syndrome or not, he was showing only mild versions of the classic symptoms. During his first hospital stay we had been warned that he had a characteristic hole in his heart, again common amongst many genetically typical infants. We hoped it would close, and whatever the worries the medical professionals might have harbored, they did not express them to us. We were therefore unpleasantly surprised by the results from his six-month cardiac ultrasound. The holes between Adam's atria and ventricles had not closed, leading to dangerously high blood pressures. He would have to undergo open-heart surgery as soon as possible if irreparable damage to his lungs was not to occur from the massive imbalances developing in his intersystemic blood pressures.

By this time, we had privately decided that if Adam would already be having routine blood work as part of his surgery, we would no longer fight the genetic test. No new conviction that Adam would receive better treatment as a result was to blame. The doctors, with our express permission, were simply treating him as having Down's, and had quit asking us to do the genetic test. When Adam went in to have his heart operation, we reversed our position, not under the pressure of the medical professionals but as a concession to two of the softer social "normalistic" pressures.

The desire to be part of the playgroup circles where trade secrets about child rearing are handed on is endemic to the maternal tribe. Not knowing the exact state of Adam's condition meant that from the beginning Stephanie struggled to answer basic questions that are put daily to new mothers: "How old is he?" or "What is he doing now?" As Adam's growth and development were progressing less quickly than that of other children, Stephanie felt she was constantly having to answer such questions without really knowing what to answer. The crucial point, however, came shortly before Adam's operation when another mother, after looking at Adam, said to Stephanie, "my son has Down syndrome too." Stephanie needed out of this limbo. She needed to know to which community Adam belonged, and so herself as his mother. Marching to a different drummer had finally worn her down.

Once we "knew," we could begin to seek out other parents of children with Down's and throw ourselves into learning about the condition without reserve. A biological test could solve a crisis of belonging. We would be released from conflict with a medical establishment unwilling to say outright that Adam had Down's without a genetic test, and the puzzled silence he continually evoked from most people on the street, both inside and outside the church. We soon learned that Adam would come to be admired for an equally uncomfortable reason—as a particularly photogenic exemplar of a race experienced by many as less than easy on the eye.

If it was social norms that ground us down, it was ultimately legal norms that dealt the crowning blow. As in most Western countries, so too in Germany: only people medically certified as disabled receive social benefits. A genetic test would be required to certify Adam's diagnosis and so secure benefits.[20] Only later, in Scotland, were we properly inducted into the more detailed negotiations of medical labels necessary to secure different types of social benefits measured on sliding scales related to extent of incapacity.[21]

Thus, in the end, it was not the pressures exerted by medical professionals, but by other parents and the legal frameworks around social care, that led us to agree to a test which we felt had no direct benefits to Adam's health. Our decision rested on the much messier and less defensible sense that the test would provide social benefits primarily to Adam's harried parents. Within the context of another hospitalization Adam would be caused no new suffering, but it would resolve social conflicts for *us*.

The test was duly administered during the course of his hospitalization. We were surprised at the relief we felt upon receiving the diagnosis. Six months of either/or, of the crossroads of two looming alternate futures, had weighed on us more than we could have articulated at the time. The social pressures for a "definitive" diagnosis had been stronger and more varied than we could ever have imagined. Our acceptance of Adam, just as he is, was made easier for us because the truth of his bodily constitution was finally unveiled only in life or death moments. While still in the shadow of a life and death crisis, to hear that a living child has Down's can only seem a reprieve. Whatever the challenges that were to come in Adam's life, they paled into insignificance beside the altogether more threatening possibility of his not existing at all. Against the backdrop of death, the wonder of his life was remarkably luminescent.[22]

"UNLESS THE LORD BUILDS THE HOUSE"

Though the econometric government of modern societies implicates everyone in the drama of prenatal testing, our family has been involved in a more direct and visible way than most. Adam pushed us up against the ragged boundaries of the new genetic world. The practical realities of receiving Adam as a divine gift to our family have yielded a wealth of new perceptions of how society (and marriage) work.

Coming close to the almost unbelievable powers of modern medicine, we discovered firsthand the importance of mustering critical resistance to some of its dynamics. At times we felt we were wrestling with powers larger than ourselves, what the New Testament calls "elemental forces of this world,"[23] as we sought to remain true to Adam, the Creator who entrusted him to us to parent, and those who also felt responsible to care for him.

One of the hints that something bigger was afoot was the pervasive and palpable fearfulness present across our different skirmishes with medical professionals. The remarkable recurrence of this fear felt to us something close to the "soul" of the genetic age. The mismatch between the great anxiety medical professionals felt about testing Adam was particularly obvious when set alongside the meagerness of the medical problems that it could be expected to resolve. Noting this disproportion allowed us to see the way our refusal to test could be experienced as a challenge to medical authority. The challenge was not our desire to question their authority: it sprang from our refusal to agree that we should share the anxiety of medical practitioners—and thus automatically comply with their recommended course of action. Diverging fears and hopes are apparently as threatening in the twenty-first century as they were in the first.

These were fears with long tentacles. Fears about lack of diagnostic information bred paternalistic fears that we could not be trusted to do the "best" for our child. Doctors found us oddly devoid of the anxiety they thought it was appropriate for us to feel for denying them information they felt they needed to do their job. Nor did we share the fear that we were undermining medical expertise by asking professionals to present their medical recommendations in terms we felt we could embrace. The tragedy they feared was simply not a tragedy to us. In short, our very different fears and hopes appeared in the horizon of modern medicine as challenges to the techniques which reassure medical personnel of their social position by bolstering their sense of mastery or control.[24]

No demonization is intended of the various medical professionals who played bit parts in our story. On the contrary, all but one were kind and conscientious. The chilling truth is that it is the very best and most conscientious performances of medical professionals that sustain the norming norms of the genetic age. They were living into a vision of humane medicine and responsible parenthood with fundamentally different contours to ours. Believing in the neutrality of genetic information, they were unaware of the normativity implicit in their assumption that no *good* parent would resist genetic testing.

Some have protested that our story betrays an unwarranted suspicion of medicine. The objection overlooks the fact that Stephanie is herself a medical professional and that we kept *returning* to medical professionals for advice about Adam. We took this to be an important aspect of parental responsibility. We are grateful and consider medicine a form of God's grace in having saved Adam's life not once (during the first week), but a second time by repairing his heart, and a third time much later. The most intensive and invasive techniques yet developed by modern medicine were deployed in these episodes. Yet the pervasive dogma that citizens of liberal societies are free to make their own choices is belied by our experience that *any* questioning or refusal of proposed courses of treatment were cause to place *us* under suspicion as recalcitrant, unreasonable, deniers of facts, etc.[25]

The ascription of irrationality seems most readily applied when the only medical reason for a test is its being routine. HIV testing during pregnancy provides a telling example. The transmission factors for the disease are well known. If faced with a pregnant medical professional (Stephanie being an example), one might expect their word to suffice that an HIV test is unnecessary. Yet the test is routine because medicine systematically distrusts people's statements about their health status. Good reasons can no doubt be offered for this distrust. But similarly, substantial considerations suggest that this suspicion corrodes the patient's belief that their words are being taken seriously in morally serious ways. Faced with a medical professional who refuses to trust the words of a patient, individuals feel themselves swallowed by larger forces. Only the irrational could raise questions and only the suspicious would think to.

In the face of this atmosphere of pervasive anxiety we have found Luther's meditations on Psalm 127 provocative and comforting.

> Unless the LORD builds the house,
>   those who build it labor in vain.
> Unless the LORD guards the city,
>   the guard keeps watch in vain.
> It is in vain that you rise up early and go late to rest,
>   eating the bread of anxious toil;
>   for he gives sleep to his beloved.
> Sons are indeed a heritage from the LORD,
>   the fruit of the womb a reward.

Luther sees in these verses a contrast: between human activity flowing out of trust, faith, and appreciation of the variability and fecundity of God's love through creation and human activity driven by anxiety about creating goodness. "Because God gives him nothing unless he works, it may seem as if it is his labor which sustains him; just as the little birds neither sow nor reap, but they would certainly die of hunger if they did not fly about to seek their food."[26] The same, Luther says, is true of human procreation.

The dynamics of modern genetic testing can be read as a symptom of modernity's near-complete loss of the sense that human action is only *discovering* God's ways of sustaining and continuing the human species, nation, or family. Luther positions medicine as an embodied discipline flowing from gratitude for the concreteness of the particular bodies that God has personally created. Human beings who think that they are creators, or that they are absolutely indispensable for sustaining the human fertility or preserving the lives that already exist, become anxious with the anxiousness that marks those without faith. Medical devotion to ameliorating all peoples' physical problems is heightened by gaining a clearer view of how either faithful gratitude or fear, and the desire to manage outcomes, shape human practices.[27] In at least the surprisingly large cultural space associated with genetic testing, our experience suggests that contemporary medicine finds itself more determinatively oriented by a framework of fear than gratitude. When medicine is annexed to serve the political imperative to secure biopolitical security, it will be difficult if not impossible to separate medicine as a project responsible for creating "normal" children from medicine as a human technique for caring for each person's physical problems.[28]

Children are the wellspring of all society.[29] It is inevitable that the bearing of children will be a region of human activity that constantly provokes anxieties, fear, and the promethean lust for power. Everything here turns on how the new one will be named.[30] Procreation is either humanity's most important resource to be technologically "managed" at all cost, a site of ultimate power struggle and angst, or it is a particularly rich seam of God's gift to humanity, the "jewels in the mines": "Like arrows in the hand of a warrior; so are the children of youth" (Job 28:1-6; Ps 127:4).

A significant strand of the patristic view of human life emphasized how human variation is God's way of keeping humanity from falling into the wonderless idolatry of homogeneity. For them the spiritual fault line runs between those who see diversity as a good gift and those for whom it evokes anxiety.[31] The doctors assumed Stephanie and I had no choice about genetic testing because they assumed a metaphysics of biologically grounded tragedy that we felt to be undermined in the work of Jesus Christ. Anxiety about a child being a burden does not produce a richer way of being human but descends into the violence that goes with quests to perfect races or produce perfect families. A Christian vision of the human places a high value on all those consigned to outsider status by merely human visions of perfection and human community.[32] In other words, to draw attention to this spiritual fault line is directly to engage questions of social justice from an unfamiliar angle.[33] What is unfamiliar about this approach to questions of justice is its starting point in the confession that justice is not first a human invention, but flows primordially from *God's* justice. To frame justice as first God's allows the affirmation that the value of a life like Adam's "is God's secret. Those around and society as a whole may not find anything in it, but this does not mean that they as a society have a right to reject and liquidate it."[34]

A genetically anomalous child can be experienced not as "negative pregnancy outcome" synonymous with personal misfortune, but as joyous and enlightening liberation.[35] Given the negative stereotypes that circulate about the lives handicapped children will lead, to experience an anomalous child in this way will require the merciful disruption of a wide range of cultural narratives which position the lives of children labeled disabled as a tragedy.[36] The only real alternative is to make plans and build systems to ensure that parental desires for perfect children will not be let down. And that, it seems, is the world we have built.

4

Prenatal Testing as Anti-Doxology

INFRASTRUCTURES OF EXCLUSION

It feels perversely risky these days not to test pregnant women for conditions that are potentially catastrophic for the health of the child, such as toxoplasmosis, AIDS, or hepatitis. The development of noninvasive, cheap, and safe prenatal genetic tests will soon render it equally nonsensical not to test future generations for genetic defects.[1] The public debate about these techniques was apparently over before it started.[2] Any moral qualms that might remain are being quietly ignored by the managers of modern states who are attracted to the promise of fetal genetic testing to trim mounting healthcare costs, and think that public debate is unnecessary since they consider it an extension of routine prenatal testing.[3] These additional tests are attractive to modern parents for remarkably similar reasons.

It is easy to forget how new this state of affairs is, as the history of Down syndrome reveals. The genetic basis of Down's was first isolated in 1959 and the first prenatal diagnosis achieved in 1968. Clinical amniocentesis procedures were perfected in the late 1960s, the very period when abortion laws were being liberalized across the developed West. Amniocentesis began to be widely diffused in the mid 1970s, and the first legal action by parents against a hospital for not providing the test was lodged at the end of the decade. Only in the mid-1990s did the less invasive chorionic villus sampling test come into common use, though only today becoming the standard screening procedure. Widespread Down's screening began in the UK in the late 1980s, with complete penetration of NHS prenatal services achieved in 1998.[4]

A starring role was played by Down syndrome in the rise and public acceptance of these techniques. The visibility of the condition was pivotal: most people recognize it on sight and assume that these lives will be of lower quality and a burden for families. The condition was therefore uniquely culturally motile.[5] Once relatively noninvasive techniques had been developed to detect the condition in utero, researchers knew it was the ideal condition around which a cultural and material screening infrastructure could be established.[6] The medical consensus that the condition is compatible with life was the only wrinkle in sight.[7] Down syndrome became the black box at the heart of prenatal screening culture: everyone assumes that everyone else knows all they need to in order to act responsibly. Such "public secrets" are a powerful social glue. Careful sociological work, however, can bring those secrets into view in the service of genuine moral scrutiny.[8]

Such scrutiny seems more than warranted given that soon being born in a Western democracy will mean having passed a life or death test. In such circumstances it is tempting to paint prenatal screening in black or white terms, as the dawn of a new, less burdensome age, or as a nightmarish evil.[9] Disability studies has highlighted the recurrence in popular narratives of "kill or cure" tropes in which disability is presented as a condition that cannot be meaningfully lived and so must be cured or the sufferer killed off.[10] Emotionally loaded accusations that all prenatal screening is by definition eugenic likewise stifle discussion, leaving the moral issues at stake uninvestigated. The aim of the old eugenics—to improve national gene pools—may be out of favor, but the previous chapter suggested that moral black boxes may still be at work to achieve not dissimilar ends by less offensive methods. Many reasons lie behind decisions to abort a genetically anomalous child, and there are all sorts of reasons why parents are drawn to engage the screening process. The fact remains that Western democracies have made substantial economic, legal, and emotional investments in the infrastructure of prenatal testing. Any society that constructs disability as removable and marginal, associating full citizenship rights only with the nondisabled, must eventually face the moral implication of such policies.

The task of this chapter is to face the full conceptual and ethical implications of the Western world transitioning out of the stance of welcoming acceptance of all nascent human life that was, at least formally, affirmed in Christendom. An accounting needs to be made of the society that has emerged as its successor, which has embraced the practice of extending a conditional acceptance based on agreements about human lives worth living.

Any such accounting demands moving beyond simple antithetical binaries like pro-choice versus pro-life, or eugenics versus choice. Since bodies have an invariably public dimension,[11] the real issue is how this public dimension is constructed and when human beings are considered to have emerged as public figures.[12]

The distinction between full political rights and conditional rights is usefully explored by thinking about the ways walls order political communities. Walls highlight the decidedly binary character of political recognition. Someone either is or isn't granted the right to pass through a wall or border to join the community. Reflecting on the boundary-keeping behaviors of political communities also raises the question of what a given society defines as a legitimate deployment of lethal violence. To ask about prenatal screening as a social practice is to highlight characteristic attitudes and institutions across modern liberal societies. In these societies, the moral baseline of abortion discussions has been the presumption that the right under discussion is that of an individual woman to defend herself against an unwanted intruder.[13]

Border walls are hybrid material and social entities. The Berlin wall exemplifies this mixed social and material reality. It was both physical—constructed of concrete, topped by barbed wire, and surrounded by exclusion zones—and all too human. Gates had to be guarded and a vast intelligence system erected to ensure only the select few were certificated to cross. To maintain the wall required the continual efforts of vast numbers of soldiers, police (secret and explicit), judges, and legislators. Thus, the wall became a way of life, seeping into every nook and cranny of the society that it purportedly protected.

The power of the Berlin wall to determine the perspective of the people within it led the East German theologian Wolf Krötke to characterize its brutalizing presence as a paradoxical living nothingness. The wall finally demanded that the whole social order be organized to maintain its lethal impermeability. Embodied human lives were being lived to the end of keeping people separate and punctuated by lethal violence. At the same time this became an unremarkable aspect of mundane daily existence.

> When I looked through the window I could see the Berlin Wall scarcely five hundred meters away. . . . What was playing itself out before my eyes was absurd. A boundary which threatened the natural communication of its citizens, families and friends was drawn right through the middle of a vibrant city. It was spectral, but exactly as such also real in brutal ways. In itself it was *nothing*, but exactly as such it was dreadfully significant. And yet, it was passed off as something truly good by a great

> mass of shameless lies. The same structure clearly repeats itself wherever people do that which we call "evil."[14]

Human beings need walls to carve out habitable spaces in which life can flourish. At the same time, they need to be able to spot walls that choke off the lifeblood of human communion. The trick is to discover which is which. In any given case, the question of whether a wall is life protecting or life destroying will take looking more closely at the ways that the boundaries of moral concern are being practically enacted.

It was a praying community that played the decisive role in the fall of the Berlin wall.[15] Only a praying and worshiping community can legitimately hope for the reversal of the powerful cultural and institutional forces that are currently arrayed against genetically anomalous lives. But Western Christians have no option but to think about disability within an ethos already saturated by culturally elaborated hopes and fears. The emotional upheavals unleashed by the announcement—"your child is not normal"—reveals with great emotional force how deeply those dreams and fears have been internalized. The burning question is how any nonstandard lives can break into a cultural space that seems so emotionally and practically invested in resisting their arrival.

The Christian tradition proposes considering these emotional reactions as emerging from the songs of praise that are constitutive of human lives.[16] The field of faith is comprehensive, since every human action honors or dishonors God's name.[17] Since living entails being in movement, it is impossible for faith to be idle.[18] The term "doxology" helpfully draws attention to this *global*, *embodied*, and so *articulate* nature of lived Christian faith. The term also highlights the role of affect and hope in animating human action. The language of doxology unites theologies of witness with the politics of praise. Christian life is rendered a making public of the miracle of divine self-revelation.[19] If doxology is the expression of emotionally engaged and bodily expressed praise of the true God, those bodily practices and emotional investments that are its antithesis must be understood as anti-doxologies. Sin is more than guilt and transgression. Sin is something people *do*. And it can become a *life*. Refusals to praise generate living, articulate, and institutionalized embodiments of fears and misdirected hopes that drive out the praise of a good Creator for the good gift of new life. Against these filled-out and personified anti-doxologies, the saints find themselves drawn together in magnifying the Lord alone: "The right hand of the Lord has done mighty things" (Ps 118:15-16). It is a song that must be concretely sung and constantly relearned, given the global nature of faith and the need to live it out amidst a world order to praise very different powers.[20]

Believers are drawn to the community of praise precisely because they do not know how to praise. Not being able to see how to embellish God's works with their lives is a sure sign that some of the glories of the creaturely realm are being exalted as themselves powerful and self-creating.[21] In short, "we cannot deal with God in more than two ways, namely, by giving thanks and by voicing our petitions. By thanking him we honor him on account of the blessings and gifts of grace we have already received; by praying we honor him account of the blessings and gifts of grace we would henceforth like to have."[22] This is the Christians sacrifice of praise and prayer, and "you cannot do more for God, nor render him greater honor."[23]

To be caught up in God's work is to be learning to live into an embodied recognition of God's grace and care and unlearning idolatrous anti-doxologies that exalt other powers as salvific. As genetically anomalous bodies enter the domain of prenatal testing, they present an invitation to expand our welcome. The new one announces a gift not only to the families most directly involved, but to all humanity. This chapter will begin to explain the reasons why Christians might hope that the worshiping community's patient but insistent prayer for the unseating of the powers that resist such lives might in fact be a work serving the assault of Jesus Christ on human sin. Praise analysis offers a mode of social criticism through which people's reasons for resisting praising the Lord for some human lives can be made audible.

POLICING THE BOUNDARY

The evil of the Berlin wall was invented neither by the guards who stood at the border with guns, nor by the officials who issued passports, nor by the legislature that decreed the norms for entry and exit. But all upheld it. Medical researchers develop prenatal diagnostic tests. Legislators, acting on the advice of managers, accountants, lawyers, and physicians, legislate permissible and desirable modes of policing the boundary of human life. Sonographers test and personify the new one in the womb. Genetic counselors explain and validate the notion of protective borders to parents who often have ambivalent feelings about bearing a disabled child. And at the end stand the techniques of violence wielded by the medical practitioners who perform abortions.

Prenatal testing is controversial because there is no consensus about when decision legitimately enters the scene.[24] Western democracies have agreed that being born makes one unambiguously a citizen and rightsholder but being conceived does not. Between the two lies prenatal testing's black box. The lack of consensus about when and under what conditions it is licit to think about ending a human life emerges from sweeping and largely unexamined assumptions about what sorts of lives are thinkable and which are not. In the absence of years to reflect on the matter, the value placed on a given body in the context of a prenatal clinic will tend to reflect common assumptions about a community's sense of the good, how people gain legitimacy within it and achieve social recognition and worth.[25]

Seen from this angle, the standard answers to what makes a human life appear valuable are far too superficial because they rest on several intellectual and emotional evasions. Human beings are embodied creatures from conception, but they kill some bodies without grieving them, most obviously those of animals, human fetuses, and enemy combatants. To observe this reality is to raise the question of what it means to *recognize* a life, a body, as *worthy* of grief. It is a question that can be evaded, but only at our peril as bodily beings. All of us have emerged from absolutely dependent vulnerability to, and reliance on, other bodies—and *remain* ineradicably vulnerable to and dependent on one another. Moderns may wish to imagine themselves as self-contained and self-determining from the time of their earliest memories, but the longings and anxieties that attend even their adult lives betray them. At one moment human beings are being drawn out of themselves by others and at another they are finding themselves involuntarily subjugated to others. *This externalized aspect of human selfhood is constitutive for human beings to emerge as individuals*. Given the complexity of this process, individuation must be understood as a hard-won accomplishment, not a given. Achieving it is certainly not guaranteed.[26]

Given these interpersonal aspects of human personhood, attempts to resolve the question of the boundaries of legitimately recognizable persons by invoking testable cognitive criteria are merely a stopgap.[27] Most Western law takes the morally relevant passage of bodies to be the crossing of the cognitive threshold.[28] If only bodies that have crossed a threshold of cognitive capacity are legitimately grievable, then the passage of those bodies into and out of existence is morally irrelevant and should leave those involved unmoved and unchanged. In reality, however, human cultures have many ways of supporting, feeding, and clothing the most vulnerable human lives, whatever their capacities. Other rituals are often developed which render some lives not worth protecting (including highly cognate lives) and therefore *not* legitimately grievable.[29]

Every society sets conditions for public grieving. These conditions can be breached by grieving lives that have been decreed ungrievable. The rules and limits of Western public discourse are revealed by the impossibility, for instance, of finding a newspaper that would publish an obituary for an aborted new one diagnosed with Down syndrome.[30] Genetically anomalous lives draw attention to the limits of liberal public toleration and with it the liberal political theory on which it rests. Faced with these limits, and unwilling to define human lives by appeal to capacities, many liberal theorists find themselves forced back upon irreducibly religious accounts when attempting to defend human lives as valuable while still in the womb.[31]

Christians in secular societies have access to theologically defensible reasons (such as a Christian view of freedom of conscience) to support legalized abortion as a public policy in cases where the only alternative is a politically unpalatable criminalization of abortion.[32] To admit this is to cast an even more unforgiving light on the social values and structural inequalities that position aborting a genetically anomalous child as a rational act.[33] Here the implications of that rationality become painfully obvious when the marked imbalance between investments in genetic research and technologies is compared with the resources devoted to supporting the living disability community.[34]

Some will protest that a defense of prenatal testing and the routine abortion of genetically anomalous new ones has no bearing on citizens currently living with those conditions.[35] No one so far, however, has mounted a public defense of the benefits of screening that foregoes *all* appeal to perceived negative impacts on society of living disabled people, or at least the health of the human genome.[36] In practice, virtually every mother or couple faced with a diagnosis of genetic anomaly draws on anecdotal experiences and accounts of the lives of the disabled and their caregivers as they decide whether or not to abort.[37] That these mother's or parents' decisions often entail judgments about some lives being unlivable and so ungrievable is suggested by the way murders of learning-impaired children by their parents are culturally figured. One of the dominant tropes for such stories presents them as tragic works of compassion by devoted parents (typically mothers) ground down by the burden of caring for the very children whose own stories disappear within the "tragedy" that their lives are presumed to embody.[38] This rendering of some lives as ungrievable in the cultural domain breeds violence against living people, law often falling into alignment with popular sensibilities about lives worth grieving.[39]

If violence undermines the political nature of human life, there can, by definition, be no genuinely *human* freedom to destroy humans whose genes appear to differ from an assumed norm. *Selective abortion destroys human community at its foundations by setting up a criterion against which every human life must be justified before being granted the right to enter human society*. When seen in this light, prenatal screening and abortion of the disabled looks very much like a classic case of nothingness, in that if one is labeled "disabled," one is forcibly denied entry into the community of the living. Screening is, by definition, a screening *out* of those considered defective, a burden, and so a threat. And it is never solely a parent's choice to bar the gates to an individual life: such denials can only be carried out by a whole social order.

These two strategies—setting up criteria to judge the unborn and then attempting to disengage these criteria from living disabled citizens—are embodied anti-doxologies. But they are not the only ones sung in the prenatal testing clinic. To hear what else is being praised will entail attending to the ways people in modern society understand themselves to gain control over their lives. Here anthropological studies offer more supple purchase on the lived reality of boundary policing.[40] In the next section I draw primarily on Rayna Rapp's seminal study of the drama of amniocentesis in New York in the late 1980s and 1990s and Gareth Thomas' qualitative study of two screening clinics in a major city in the UK from 2011–2013. Despite there being significant differences in prenatal testing practices and ethical construals of these practices within the Western cultural clearing, substantial *moral* continuities emerge when these different practices are studied anthropologically.[41] A composite picture with definable contours of the cultural ethos of prenatal testing within the medicalized Western world emerges clearly. Behind the technical and cultural variations in prenatal testing clinics, a relatively homogenous epistemological and moral regime can be glimpsed.

The core of that moral regime is a collective agreement that there are boundaries between "us" and "them" that need to be protected. It is this "wall in the mind" that precedes and sustains prenatal testing practice. If selective abortion of genetically anomalous new ones is indeed a sinful collective illusion, it is theologically interesting to ask what sustains it.[42] To look into a black box and to unveil an illusion will be to ask how boundaries form in the collective consciousness, what makes them solid, and what drives the final decision to enact the denial of entry of the supposedly substandard human to the body politic.

Tracing the paths of three sets of actors in this drama will allow the doxologies that animate this ongoing barrier maintenance to emerge. We begin with the *sonographers* who bring the body of the new one into view, and with them the *geneticists and laboratory technicians* whose technical expertise supports the claim that there is a clear boundary here at *this* point. Next, we turn to the *genetic counselors* who explain this boundary and how pregnant women should understand it. We end with the *pregnant woman* herself, who now must decide how she will view the life she is being asked to decide whether to end. Other supporting actors will remain offstage—the medical personnel who schedule and carry through the decision to abort, the researchers and technologists who push testing techniques forward, and the legislators who frame laws on abortion, prenatal testing, and the social provision which would support parents raising a disabled child—even though each of these other actors play vital roles in sustaining the environment in which these three main groups of actors meet to police the border between "us" and the disabled.

PRACTICES OF NEOLIBERAL EUGENICS

Many pregnant women in highly medicalized Western societies feel strong, sometimes coercive, resistance to their decisions not to abort a genetically anomalous new one. Leisa Whitaker has a form of dwarfism and elegantly describes how the common sense of the prenatal testing clinic can clash with the lived experience of disability.

> I remember sitting in the [genetic specialist's] rooms listening as he explained that there was a 25 percent chance that our child could still inherit the dominant achondroplasia gene and the dominant pseudo-achondroplasia gene—a combination that they had never seen before anywhere in the world. They had no idea of what effect this would have on the baby . . . Having told us this the specialist offered us an abortion. He asked us to think about whether we wanted to bring another dwarf baby into the world. It was something I hadn't even thought of. This was our child! Why would we not want her? Why would the world not accept our child?[43]

For some pregnant women the scene of this conflict begins in a darkened room with a sonographer.[44] When a pregnant woman enters the exam she knows her body in one way, and certain aspects of the new one's body who is nevertheless visually unavailable within her.[45] The sonographer overlays the bodily self-knowledge derived from the woman's own sensation with a new layer of visual imagery. The effect is to grant the new one a more independent standing. This is a cyborg experience since all parties will now focus not on the new one's body itself, but on its image on a screen that will in important respects overshadow the earlier forms of relating to the new one. The visualization of the new one takes place in Western societies in which visual images, especially live video, have become the dominant medium for proving that something "really happened."[46] In such a society the rituals of parents viewing moving, real time images of the new one are viscerally powerful, and "taking home baby's picture" initiates a public quickening, transforming the social reality of parents. Publicly intelligible proof has been provided that a publicly nongrievable fetus has now transitioned into being a viable baby who can be welcomed without qualms.

Being cross-slice images, these visually cryptic sonographic images require explanation for nonexperts, and this is one of the most important social roles played by the sonographer. The mother herself can often see the screen and may be accompanied by a partner and even children or a grandparent. As they produce the ultrasound scan the sonographer is thus traversing highly complex social, emotional, and evaluative territories. Because the imagery is live, and both the mother and the sonographer must be in bodily proximity, the sonographer is bound to conversation during a scan. The woman with the probe pressed to her belly needs to be calmly reassured as the sonographer looks for anomalies, and in this context long periods of silence can easily be interpreted as ominous.[47] A pastoral task intersects here with an evaluative task. The whole time the sonographer is deploying his or her medical training to spot defects, he or she must continually reassure the pregnant woman and promote bonding with a "normal" child in the womb by utilizing descriptions that emphasize its vigor and personality. The new one's representation on the screen is often described in terms of parental, gendered, and childlike personality traits ("look, she's excitable like dad") that invariably suggest culturally coded images of competence as productive members of society. Should an anomaly be uncovered, however, the task immediately shifts to the much more fraught work of directing attention away from a "fetus" about whom a "termination" will now have to be discussed while attempting quickly to discern whether this is what the mother wants.[48]

One of the most decisive operations of the wall has already happened in the first minutes of the ultrasound scan. The test's power to reconfigure the parent–new one relationship has been called the "one-two punch of birth in the technocracy."[49] Having separated the mother from her initial sense of knowledge and bond with her own body and that of the new one, the sonographer's performance comes to be positioned as an indispensable part of the bonding process between mother and new one, and increasingly, the father, other children, and even grandparents and friends.

For the last few decades the sonographic discovery of a suspected genetic anomaly has been followed by amniocentesis. Amniotic fluid must be extracted, cells cultured from it, chromosomes separated, and then a judgment made about the health (or otherwise) of the new one's genes. The testing laboratories where this processing is done have been called "laboratories for fact construction."[50] The aim of these labs is to produce a clear genetic diagnosis, but to achieve a clear result requires not only good lab technique but substantive knowledge of human genetics. It has typically been less educated women who do most of the bench work in this process while the geneticists who oversee the work and make the final diagnoses are most often highly trained men specializing in cell biology, embryology, and pediatrics (disciplines in which the rhetorical positioning of genetic anomalies is overwhelmingly negative and whose scientific literature is noticeably free of any consideration of the life experiences of people with specific genetic conditions). Though both lab workers and expert doctors are very aware that each stage of the process involves craftwork, and that false moves may be made which may invalidate the final diagnosis, there are strong reasons not to admit the interpretative nature of this work.[51]

The problem of the negative positioning of genetically anomalous new ones is compounded by the reality that medical science still has very incomplete knowledge of how any given genetic anomaly will be expressed as a child matures. Autopsies are routinely carried out on selectively aborted fetuses to study genetic anomaly expressions. Since genetic testing is typically presented as a binary, factual, and purely technical matter, it is only at this point that some parents discover its evaluative nature. The shock of this discovery is palpable in one woman's eruption of grief upon hearing that her aborted new one's body was being sent to pathology. "When the doctor took a tissue sampling I asked him why, and he said, 'To send to pathology to confirm the diagnosis.' And I started howling, I was just screaming my head off: 'If there's anything that even possibly needs confirming, what am I doing here?'"[52]

In earlier phases of genetic testing practice, geneticists dealt directly with parents, but much of this work has been handed over to genetic counselors. Their stated aim is to assist women's reproductive choice by providing information about hereditary risk.[53] In practical terms they prepare parents to take the test and to explain the meaning of laboratory results. Counseling sessions therefore have four main goals: to establish the primacy of scientific discourse, to establish the authority of this discourse, to communicate risk, and to construct a family history narrated in medicalized terms.[54] Anthropological research suggests that genetic counselors play a prominent role in disseminating the ethos of Western medicine that positions bearing a disabled child as an irrational choice. Given the highly complex relation of genes to phenotypical expressions later in life, the stories that are told by educators about the implications of a given condition will always be grounded in choices about which representations to present—and thus no story they tell can be neutral or value free.[55] What is assumed in related peri- and neonatal fields must be explicitly articulated by the genetic counselor.

Genetic counseling is a subfield that grew from research genetics in the 1970s. It took over the task of transmitting knowledge from the scientific laboratory to parents, with the stated purpose of assisting women's reproductive choice.[56] As a discipline, genetic counseling espouses a nondirective ethos and aims to provide value-neutral information. Its basic aim was conceived of as uncontentious: the genetic counselor provides information about hereditary risk to prospective parents. Parents need to be prepared for the test and then have laboratory results explained. The social role of the "scientific expert" helps accomplish that task. Establishing the primacy of scientific discourse involves explaining what chromosomes are, how they work, and how "defects" produce disabilities. In this sense genetic counselors are science educators who simultaneously establish and maintain the authority of the scientific expert. As the accuracy of the geneticist's diagnosis is the premise of the counselor's work, a strongly proexpertise bias is built into genetic counseling.

Until prenatal genetic testing is universally administered, genetic counselors first need to make sure that high-risk pregnancies are scanned. The main goal of the early part of the counseling session is to teach and guide parents in renarrating their family history in medicalized, "diagnostic" terms by which they discover whether they are in a high-risk category and in need of a scan. To orient the laboratory's investigation of specific anomalies, parents are asked many questions that could be considered surprising or unsettling in normal life, such as "Have you recently come into contact with cats?" or "Have you taken drugs or had unprotected sex?" and even "Could the child's father be your relative?" The counselor is teaching the pregnant woman to reconsider her own biography within the terms of the medical self-understanding.

Explaining the functioning of chromosomes is a prelude to introducing the crucial concept of risk. Though thoroughly statistical territory, the aim of introducing the discourse of risk is practical: to construct an "appropriate" or "numerically rational" sense of anxiety in the mother that is linked to those features of the body of the new one that are capable of being genetically tested. The genetic counselor needs to bind an individual woman to a universal account of the normal, based on a statistical average, while not giving any specific advice about how she should respond to it. Former generations of geneticists boldly pronounced on which lives were and were not viable, but in a context when speaking directly of aborting genetically anomalous fetuses is becoming more politically incorrect, it may be sufficient for genetic counselors to do no more than "help clients to identify their own positions in the broad terrain of normality and deviation."[57]

Genetic counseling is thoroughly wedded to this medicalized and statistical understanding of pregnancy. Even though the technology of prenatal diagnosis was explicitly developed for the location and abortion of new ones whose atypical chromosomal configuration hinted at future disability, the language of genetic counseling tackles the issue obliquely.

> The language of genetic counseling is intended to enhance awareness of the age-related risk of chromosomal problems, but counselors rarely speak directly about disability or abortion decisions unless a problem is detected. Counselors describe their goals quite differently: to give reassurance. . . . This language of "added risk," "background risk," and "reassurance" is consistently deployed by all the genetic counselors I have observed at work. It thus foregrounds a statistical, medical, age-related, universal and wholly individual model of risk.[58]

Risk can be communicated in more or less sophisticated ways, depending on the mother being addressed.

> To someone perceived as scientifically sophisticated, at Middle or Elite Hospitals: "At 35, a woman's risk of bearing a live born child with Down syndrome is one in 385; at 40 it increases to one in 106; at 45, it is one in thirty." . . . Another counselor said of advanced maternal age: "It's like crossing a street with each pregnancy, and when you are older, it's a little easier to be hit by a car. But suppose there is a traffic light. Then, you want to cross on the green. This test puts you back to the green light. Oh, you might still get hit by a crazy hit-and-run driver, but it's not too likely. At the red light [without the test], your age makes you a more likely target for an accident."[59]

Though the heavy use of statistical language lends an air of objectivity and value neutrality, the comparison of some births with an "accident" that ought to be avoided highlights the value-laden and historically peculiar nature of the exercise.[60] The moral valances of risk language are revealed by the alternative language of "chance" favored by some midwives. To say that "a fetus is at risk" concentrates attention on supposed negative outcomes, while the language of "chance" highlights the givenness of an already existing baby. The language of risk thus lands responsibility to achieve a good future on a mother in a way that chance does not, which admits the existence of the child as well as the possibility of that child having one or another life challenge to come.[61]

The biomedical and public health establishments that employ genetic counselors assume that some conceptions are expendable or even burdensome.

Yet the genetic counselor thinks of herself as value neutral even while playing a gatekeeping role. Genetic counselors, in short, are "trained to offer a value-charged technology in a value-neutral manner."[62] This lack of self-reflexivity is highlighted when genetic counselors are surprised or offended by parents who recoil from their proposal of abortion, or dispute their account of the implications of specific disabling conditions.[63] This unknowing of the genetic counselor functions at an institutional level to mask and ameliorate the very purpose of the whole institutional setup: to eliminate new ones bearing anomalous chromosomes before they become costly burdens to themselves and others.

Most of the unknowing of the genetic counselor is hidden away in the language of risk and normality.[64] Normality is based on quantitative data and calculations of averages, but risk adds an additional layer of analysis: the measurement of probabilities. Statistical averages say something about the present (distinguishing bodies that are as they should be from those that are not) while the language of risk says something about the future. It is the category of risk that transforms events in human life into "accidents" capable of statistical tabulation, and whose odds of recurrence can be calculated. Nothing is a risk in itself but anything can be labeled a risk: everything turns on how events are understood. Just like workplace accidents and highway fatalities, "birth accidents" can be labeled risks and managed according to an insurance rationality. Attaching this label also levies moral claim—someone is now "responsible for it" or is made "responsible to reduce its incidence." To label something a risk is to engender political responsibility. Thus "seemingly natural and uncontrollable events, such as disease and congenital impairment, assume the character of social facts and, as a result, legitimize social solidarity (and intervention)."[65]

The statistical rationality that is the root metaphor of the discourse of genetic counseling can in some cases limit its effectiveness in teaching people to think of their lives in biomedical terms; "ironically, the very populations most at risk—less privileged 'older' women having more pregnancies with more partners; experiencing more reproductive, perinatal, and infant mortality; and higher death rates throughout their life cycles—may least be likely to live by the numbers precisely because they understand their risks to be spread over a greater territory than chromosome analysis in pregnancy describes."[66] Such mothers expose the evaluative horizon of biomedical construal of risk by implicitly, and sometimes explicitly, doubting the self-presented expert's claim to be able to predict risk, the real risks that matter for their lives, which lie far beyond a new one's genetic palette.

The genetic counselor thus constantly faces tricky code-straddling tasks. The fiction of "just describing a scientific finding" must be maintained while still effectively conveying that there is a risky pregnancy afoot that a parent might do well to consider aborting. Conveying risk while not appearing to offer advice cannot be accomplished without first reducing the new one in the womb to an entity that is nothing more than a package of genetic characteristics.[67] At the same time, the scope of risk must be expanded to encompass not only the new one's life, but the life of parents and families as well as society as a whole.[68] The anomalous new one will need to be positioned as a genetic package injecting a stain of risk into the wider web of the social order if ending its life is to appear as a rational act. Western society as a whole has learned to "live by the numbers," and the genetic counselor's prime task is to ensure that pregnancy is also understood in these terms. If the cutting edge of the medical apparatus is the sonographer's probe, the critical decision on the mother's part is whether or not to internalize the notion of risk. Much of theological interest appeared in these cases where some parents could or would not evaluate their pregnancies in terms of this metanarrative.

It appears then that prenatal diagnosis as just described expresses a biomedical account in which *prenatal screening precedes and is more fundamental than prenatal care*. Theologically we need only note that the paeans of praise to concepts like value neutrality, individual choice, risk avoidance, and the authority of expertise are problematic in themselves, and they become a deadly cocktail when unreflexively teamed with decisions about whether to eliminate humans perceived to be a burden. While each concept might conceivably find a place in a song of praise to the creating and redeeming God, in the contemporary usage just described they clearly preface any sense of wonder and thankfulness for the gift of conception with a prior anti-doxology lifting up the promises of perfect control, benevolent expertise, and a life free of "accidents." Not only is this to praise gods of fertility and quality assurance who are bound to disappoint when children do not conform to expectations, but also to undermine with a benevolent smile the hurdles facing the socially marginalized, for whom "genetic risk" is a very small part of their daily life challenges.

In systematically directing attention away from the concrete responsibilities facing mothers (that is, the work of caring) and suggesting that their hopes and fears are most appropriately attached to a realm of possible choices (the task of testing), genetic counseling illustrates a classic instance of how evil is both a nonreality and embodied in concrete words and actions. The substitution of the imagined for the concrete is a familiar political ploy, in this case played out by perhaps unwitting genetic counselors speaking for a state (or for-profit medical system) whose offer of help to those mothers who most need social support has been reduced to the offer of an abortion. Even as they serve the widespread use of the technologies of elimination, the genetic counselor's self-perception as apolitical is preserved by their self-understanding as nondirective. In theological and pastoral terms, the net effect of this antidoxology is the loss of attentive empathy and concern for the whole of life in service of the state's interest in minimizing economic cost.[69]

Prenatal testing presents mothers with a bewildering set of social pressures. The earlier definitive test, amniocentesis, yields a diagnosis late in pregnancy. Mothers were put in the position of having to distance themselves from new ones they may have wanted and were certainly beginning to experience as independent living beings.[70] Many women who had borne live disabled children told of having been the object of anger and disappointment from medical staff, and expressed their own amazement and disgust at the rapidity with which adoption or institutionalization of their children was offered.[71] In the United States, poorer women are often not tested simply because the prenatal care available to them is so poor and time consuming to procure that they give up in frustration.[72] A similar dynamic recurs in the United Kingdom, when women who are not comfortable speaking English are given sonographic scans without English translators being present.[73] New noninvasive prenatal genetic tests will resolve the fetal health risks of undergoing amniocentesis as well as its relatively late verdict on a pregnancy. But it will not make interpreting test results any less difficult for mothers for whom comprehending the language of science and risk is daunting. The sexual politics of the decision to test or abort will also remain highly complex: women will deploy the personification of the new one accomplished by the ultrasound scan to draw ambivalent partners to commit to relationship, and men will invoke patriarchal privilege in turn to deny testing—the permutations in this contested domestic territory are myriad and unsettling.[74] For all these reasons and more, mothers deserve compassion and social support.

The reality remains that they, too, are drawn into the role of gatekeepers, whether by choice or simply in acceding to a culture that demands the final judgment on a pregnancy be pronounced by the mother or both parents. The theological task is to discern the doxologies that orient parents, especially mothers, as they digest a diagnosis of a fetus with an anomalous genetic inheritance.

Mothers whose new one has been designated genetically anomalous are pushed toward a transformation of their self-image simply in being forced to articulate their reasons for continuing a pregnancy. Women are expected to collate the information on which a "rational" choice to continue a pregnancy can be made, or to explain why, against the grain of the medical establishment, they ought not be asked to make such a decision at all.[75] As one mother put it, "I felt like a voice in a Greek chorus, chanting, 'Your choice, your choice, your choice is upon your shoulders.' I felt like a minor character in a major tragedy."[76] The potency of this moral dilemma suggests why clinic professionals tend to position testing as wholly routine, and genetic diagnoses as unambiguous and definitive.[77] As one doctor put it to a pair of parents wrestling with an unwelcome test result, "That isn't a baby. . . . It's a collection of cells that made a mistake."[78] When routinization and the desire to spare mothers a painful choice (that is nevertheless being pressed on them) in ways that obscures the life and death questions at stake (and in a context where genetic conditions like Down syndrome are treated as abnormal and negative outcomes) women may not even realize that the moment has arrived when they must shoulder the burdens of being a "moral pioneer."[79]

While it may be true that prenatal testing aims at parental bonding with some unborn children, it also quietly encourages distancing from others. A world can be imagined of sonography booths ringing out with joyful wonder at the genetically anomalous child, followed by serious discussions of what care needs will need to be in place to ensure such children's flourishing. Much more often, however, the onus is on mothers to make the "responsible" decision and to save everyone money and grief by asking for an abortion. Liberal society calls this a situation of private choice. In truth a tacit collective agreement has been reached to thrust women into the role of lone gatekeepers.[80] The vast majority of mothers are left confronting an unwanted testing verdict, isolated from any tradition of explicit thought about how to respond to it. Living within an enforced but at times empowering privacy, these "moral philosophers of the private" must think through their decision surrounded by the cacophonous opinions of medical professionals, newspaper pundits, friends, family, and other children.[81] Being offered the right to make a "personal choice" intentionally leaves the questions open about how that choice *should* be discharged.[82]

Two priorities recur in the answers mothers give today to why they would consider aborting a new one diagnosed as anomalous: their capacity to mother a disabled child, and the impact of a disabled child on the mother's most intimate relationships. Four broad types of justification typically underlay these two reasons to consider erecting a lethal border against a genetically anomalous fetus. Aborting might be repositioned as an act of love, in praise of "protecting the children."

> Some people say that abortion is hate. I say my abortion was an act of love. I've got three kids. I was 43 when we accidentally got pregnant again. We decided there was enough love in our family to handle it, even though finances would be tight. But we also decided to have the test. A kid with a serious problem was more than we could handle. And when we got the bad news, I knew immediately what I had to do. At 43, you think about your own death. It would have been tough now, but think what would have happened to my other kids, especially my daughter. Oh, the boys, Stephan and Alex, would have done ok. But Livia would have been the one who got stuck. It's always the girls. It would have been me, and then, after I'm gone, it would have been the big sister who took care of that child. Saving Livia from that burden was an act of love.[83]

In such reflections we see women being forced to imagine the outer limits of their maternal embrace.[84] Given their understanding of their responsibilities as mothers and women, and imagining life with a disabled child, mothers are forced to articulate a set of values ostensibly located in the private realm but formed by, and forming in turn, the life of society as a whole.

While sociological studies of the practice of prenatal testing suggests that women are in a privileged position in our societies to push back on contemporary assumptions and practices of prenatal testing, it has also highlighted the ways in which the medical and legal guilds discourage any such critical resistance. Medical cultures foster the expectation that testing, especially for older mothers, is not optional.[85] And important defenders of women's rights are so intent on defending women's right to choose that they have little space to question the abortion of genetically anomalous new ones.[86]

ANTI-DOXOLOGY AS REPUDIATED ANNUNCIATION

The anti-doxologies that have emerged in the domain of prenatal testing practices are "common sense" and pervasive. The ubiquitous praise of "protective limits," "insuring the future," "knowledge as power," "acting to improve life," "protecting the children," and "free private choice" are salvific promises lived into by people far beyond the prenatal clinic. Lost to the singers of this anti-doxology is any notion that new life is a gift that is inherently enriching. To become a philosopher of the limit in practice almost always excludes serious consideration of *positive* effects that might accrue to siblings of a disabled child or to themselves as parents.[87] The two songs are incompatible.

These particular anti-doxologies also subvert the collective will to support women, parents, and families, since they position the decision to embrace a disabled child as tantamount to economic and personal suicide.

The anti-doxologies of women who abort out of love thus mesh with the anti-doxologies that demonize the desire to share medical costs or the cost and labor of childrearing. They likewise hide the voices of parents who have raised children with disabilities and understand their experiences in terms of a journey toward acceptance, appreciation, and enrichment.[88]

Theologically described, prenatal testing culture rests on the assertion that decisions must be made about who will be accepted into the human community in order not to overstretch finite resources. Iron curtains, it turns out, are just as much a problem for liberal secular societies as they were for communist states. In the same way that the sonographer's processes establish the new one as an "individual" while inviting the parents to form a new "bond," modern neoliberal political philosophy separates people from human community with its initial premise that all people are essentially individuals who might *choose* to join communities. A single ideology grounds both: the individual is understood as fundamentally preceding the community. "Thus we begin with individuation, separation, and distancing and move towards unity and relationship, a unity and relationship that is *optional, tentative*, and *dependent* on the child fulfilling certain criteria."[89] The rapturous praise of free markets characteristic of neoliberal societies can offer no resistance to the anti-doxology of prenatal testing. Feminist critics have added that it also rests on a highly masculine account of the controllable body that finds the abject dependence at the origin of every human life a problem, even as offensive.[90]

In such a landscape, prenatal testing is just one of many mechanisms serving the worship of freedom defined as "choice." It harmonizes perfectly with the praise of techniques that can save individuals and families from "accidents" that will destroy the lives they have imagined for themselves. When preventing these "accidents" means the elimination of some sorts of human beings, philosophies of limit are, by definition, anti-doxologies articulating an internalized belief in the human *right* to screen out those who don't belong. But if human beings are never "accidents," then instructing people that they have a choice and how to make it is an induction into an anti-doxology that refuses to praise the Trinitarian Creator for fertility and new life. They cannot be glosses on the song "The right hand of the Lord does valiantly"; rather they sing, "We must act to save ourselves from 'them' or be drowned."

When these anti-doxologies are dominant, the appearance of the genetically anomalous new one can only appear as an aporia, a dark option to choose meaningless suffering. Perceiving such a new one as a wonder becomes politically subversive in such a context. The new one we label disabled is not silent but presents a positive word of grace and liberation to those entangled in the glory of their own fetters. From this angle of view new ones appear as angelic messengers inviting secular humanity to attend anew to the strange ways of God's working. It was the annunciative character of a genetically anomalous new one that transformed the privileged academic Rayna Rapp from an abortion activist into a genuine inquirer. She ends her sociological study with this elegiac dedication to her aborted offspring, a lament that strains the limits of allowable public grieving.

> Mike named the fetus XYLO, or X-or-Y for its unknown sex, LO for the love we were pouring into it. Together, we watched XYLO grow; together we chose to end his life after a prenatal diagnosis of Down's. My personal pain and confusion as a failed mother led me to investigate the social construction and cultural meaning of amniocentesis. . . . XYLO's short life pointed me toward these vital concerns; his ending marked the beginning of my search for contextualized knowledge. If the work accomplished in this book helps others to think about these evolving issues, his short life will have been a great gift.[91]

In the light of God's self-annunciation from the manger in Bethlehem, the Christian is enabled to say in faith—without the intervening and instrumentalizing "if"—that XYLO was indeed a great gift. With the cultural landscape Rapp has described now fully in view, it becomes clear that his appearance should be narrated theologically as an *apokalypsis* or *krisis* drawing the curtain back on a wide swath of the shameless lies covering a society's collective decision to refuse him entry into life with his parents. In XYLO the angel's message to Mary and the shepherds is reiterated: "Fear not." Such an annunciation threatens to sever the cords of enslavement to the control that wishes the disabled not to exist. Some Christians have experienced new ones like XYLO in precisely this way.

> Annunciation—a sign. Even when that to which it points is unwelcome, it can be a grace. Whether it becomes a grace depends, in part, upon whether we possess the humility and grace to receive the message well. Witness Mary, a young girl, probably not older than fifteen . . . Perhaps she did not understand what submission to this scheme would cost her. She would have to bear his death. Could she have grasped the great sorrow of watching Him die? . . . All of heaven and earth waits to hear her response. And Mary speaks, "Let it be to me according to your word." She would bear God, she would give him her flesh. . . . We did not receive our annunciation from a messenger of God. And the message signaled nothing good. . . . Trisomy 18. Lethal. Inevitable. Death. Would

> we terminate? Annunciations can be intrusions. They leave us expecting the already inevitable but not yet.[92]

That group of human beings gathered today under the label "disabled," whether born or unborn, announce an end to the need to draw boundaries between them and us. Their living, moving, and growing are gestures insistently repeating that human community is not maintained by violence, but by openness to being surprised by the birth of the unexpected.[93] These babes speak Jesus Christ's own message: "For he is our peace; in his flesh he has made both groups into one and has broken down the dividing wall, that is, the hostility between us" (Eph 2:14).

The term "disabled" stands as an invitation to human beings to give up defining themselves by means of any violent separation from those believed to be "unlike us." *We are constituted in recognizing and being recognized. There is no human "I" outside of the constant granting of recognition and being recognized in all our need and vulnerability*. The self is not a static entity but is formed through the configuration of recognition and refusal of recognition. The woman who aborts is a different woman from the one who chooses not to, and neither is the same after the "one-two punch of pregnancy in the technological society" that accelerates the individuation of the new one. The new one is an invitation to recognition, and therefore to all around to become someone different by recognizing their presence. The only alternative is to cut themselves off from her or him. Human beings stake their own being in this struggle for recognition, a struggle that in every case demands transformation of the one who recognizes an other.[94] *What is today called "disability" is a crucible for Christian theology because it is the domain in which human beings enact their fundamental beliefs about what it means to be, and to recognize, another human*. Though highly problematic in common usage, the language of "disability" thus points to the heart of currently enacted images of worthy life and the image of God.

Christians should welcome the fact that technologies developed to aid screening can now be used in the service of care.[95] Marked differences will be visible when those technologies are deployed out of desire to care for children in the joyous receipt of a divine gift, and their deployment as expressions of the ideologies of control, management, expertise, and risk avoidance, by which they are subjected to grading according to laws of satisfactory performance. Even here, though, under the judgmental light of the sonographer's probe,[96] the annunciative call can emerge from grainy imagery and the stony silence of a disappointed sonographer.[97] Given the internalized fears of the other that Christians share with other developed Westerners, as well as the ever growing imperative to control chance and deviance, *the church's witness to the annunciation to "fear not" will remain a task first of all of receiving our redeemed selves*. The self that is announced to everyone in the sonographer's booth calls for that confession on which the church is continually founded: *in receiving them, we receive Him, and so ourselves*. Self-protective habits are exposed as a denuding refusal of life with God. Enclosed behind walls of our own making, we are trapped in a living death—isolated, homogeneous, and wonderless. A stone has been rolled over a tomb.

***

CODA: PART 2

In contemporary society, the terms "prenatal care" and "prenatal screening" are taken to be synonyms. In practice they become antonyms when the refusal to test is portrayed as unnecessarily risky and aborting a disabled child a relief. To become aware of this inversion is to be invited to explore what it might mean faithfully to continue the early church's "rule of human solidarity" in the modern developed West. God's merciful and saving presence through the Spirit presses back on the habits of the secular West in the body of the new one, disabled or not, whose very existence is an appeal for recognition. Jesus located such appeals as the call of the vulnerable neighbor. Vulnerable bodies proffer so many invitations to a form of life together characterized by gratitude for concrete human otherness in all its bewildering and sometimes frustrating diversity.

Embracing the full diversity of human life is beyond the natural capacities of fallen human beings. The fears of parents that they will not have the resources to raise a disabled child are by no means groundless. No one who lives with the mentally ill or intellectually disabled would dispute that the task is often overwhelming in modern societies that often isolate caregivers.[98] At the same time, the stereotype that a disabled child is an unsupportable burden to a family is certainly overblown, as substantiated by the testimonies of many parents of children with disabilities—notwithstanding the wide currency of these stereotypes among practitioners of medicine, public health, bioethics, and the inventors of testing technologies.[99] Those who embrace children (any children) as having been *given to them* come face to face with their own self-protective urges. To recognize a human being as a gift is a work of hospitable embrace of a relationship with the Giver in the very act of receiving. Our own bodies stand as invitations into relationship with their Giver, and to recognize one's own body as a gift is incompatible with seeing embodiment as a burden, since it is the condition of human existence.[100]

Recognizing the limits of human powers of recognition is to be thrown on the support that only the Holy Spirit can provide. The most surprising and essential *work of the Spirit is to transform people's ideas about who they are and what they can do*. Human beings need to discover ever anew that the abilities they need to flourish are ones that must be *given*, and therefore must be *asked* for. The Spirit's help is not coerced in this asking nor by acting in faith that it will be given. Theology needs to abandon its false modesty about the resources promised in the Spirit. When it does not, it cannot avoid the trap of wishing for perfection from humanity. Either the Father brings peace and flourishing through the Son and aids people to receive it through the Spirit, or all human beings can do is hope for the least complicated experience possible of parenthood, marriage, work—of life. *The problem of not being able to receive every human being with open arms turns out not to be an insufficiently inclusive anthropology, but an atrophied pneumatology*.

A church that takes this message to heart will have to *learn to pay new forms of attention*. A new attentiveness to social gestures is necessary to respond to the crisis of recognition in liberal societies that is especially acute in relation to the most vulnerable. A whole Western ethos lying behind and going far beyond specific ethical debates is being questioned at this point and will be no more easily accomplished as an armchair exercise than it was for patristic Christians. Very active self-critical disciplining and engagement, and intellectual and practical labor, will be required to unlearn deeply ingrained patterns of exclusion and denial.[101] To do so is to discover what it means to inhabit Christian praise.

Christians must confess their *sinful attraction to the promise of an easier life* to become this church. The desire to make life easy is the door left wide open to the judgments of medical experts and insuring calculators of risk. If it is never right to view children as a risk, threat, or natural tragedy, then children must be free not to conform to parental and societal expectations. To the extent that the neoliberal ideology of (economically) rational choice defined by the statistical norm has penetrated the church, it too will find itself torn between the logic by which it "manages" and "stewards" its resources in most areas and the logic of prenatal testing. Christians are liberated to name the forces that enslave humanity in confessing the self-annunciation of Jesus Christ to be the lifeblood of the church. In witnessing that this child, too, reveals the mercy of Jesus Christ, the church serves society by bringing the anti-doxological fundament of this slavery to light.

Together these two alternative paths generate an *alternative suite of ethical questions*. Christians will find themselves resonating with surprising fellow travelers also raising serious questions of the status quo.

> Rather than simply conflating disability and suffering, we can ask, How have these particular forms of attention to suffering precluded the analysis of and response to *other* causes of suffering? To what extent does emphasizing prevention, elimination, and cure of intellectual disabilities divert attention and resources away from the many ways in which persons with intellectual disabilities and their families suffer at the hands of a society that devalues them, economically disadvantages them, and subjects them to social stigma and discrimination? How will suffering be increased in promoting practices that are purportedly aimed at eliminating it? And to what extent does the tragic portrait of the inevitable life of suffering obscure other dimensions of disabled existence?[102]

The theological themes only introduced in this coda will move to center stage in parts 4 and 5. In part 3, attention turns from investigation of how developed societies greet the arrival of anomalous new lives to how they treat them, in sickness and health, once they have arrived.

PART III

SYSTEMS, NORMS, AND MODERN MEDICINE

Attending to Creatures

5

Two Critiques of Orthodox Medical Ethics

DISABILITY AND MEDICAL ETHICS

Medical ethics was born as a subspecialization of Christian ethics. Its seminal texts highlighted the extraordinary nature of setting people aside to dedicate their lives to caring for the ill, and the roots of that moral commitment in the work of Jesus Christ. It is a distinctively *moral* achievement for any culture to institutionally imbed a refusal to abandon the ill, dying, or disabled. One signal that Christians in medical ethics have broken faith with the vibrant concern with the outsider so characteristic of the patristic era is the discipline's apparent lack of interest in disability. The almost total absence of interest in intellectual disability is even more striking.[1]

The bioethics community and the disability rights movements may appear to share a single goal of promoting health and flourishing for all people. They have in fact been locked in a protracted dispute for some decades.[2] The nub of the criticisms of disability activists is that bioethicists are so wedded to medical models of disability and embedded in medical institutions that they are no longer capable of critically challenging the institutions the discipline was originally developed to hold to account.[3] A narrative is needed that shows doctors why, and how, attending to lives labeled disabled can help loosen the noose they so often feel around their necks. Academic medical ethicists have all too rarely taken this to be their goal.

Empirical studies suggest that modern medical training often turns the most caring, educated, and mentally resilient students into professionals who are depressed, burn out at high rates, and are in one of the highest brackets of suicide risk.[4] Chapter 4 has outlined a range of acute moral paradoxes in one domain of modern medicine, the prenatal clinic. The burden of this chapter is to broaden that account to show how the dominant account of medical ethics intentionally closes the door on substantive theological thinking about disability. In doing so it undermines any moral grounds for medical professionals to question problematic aspects of the healthcare systems in which they work.

The body of this chapter is devoted to a close engagement with *Principles of Biomedical Ethics*, by Tom L. Beauchamp and James F. Childress.[5] For several decades, the approach they present in successive versions of this book has defined the moral parameters of medical ethics in the English-speaking world. The depth of the influence of this text on the academic discourse of medical ethics is unsettling, given its implications for those called disabled. Close attention to the social, political, and legal context of contemporary medical decision-making reveals that the principleist style of medical ethics promulgated in this text not only fails to provide satisfactory resolutions to the hardest cases, but also systematically disempowers physicians as political actors. Though originating in a discipline once directly drawing on Christian truth claims, the position developed by Beauchamp and Childress has played a crucial role in breaking down the rule of universal human solidarity that was the central characteristic of the Christian view of human life from the earliest Christian eras.[6]

The ethos characteristic of the approach of Beauchamp and Childress is best grasped by beginning where their book ends, with their description of the ideal medical professional. An ideally moral medical professional knows that "what counts most in the moral life is not consistent adherence to principles and rules, but reliable character, moral good sense, and emotional responsiveness."[7] Compassionate, discerning, trustworthy, and possessing moral integrity—it is inconceivable to think of someone having such virtues in their professional duties and yet be callous, undiscerning and untrustworthy when off the job. By focusing on virtues a medical professional must possess, Beauchamp and Childress are clearly suggesting that these character traits cannot, indeed must not, be confined to professional life alone. To be a moral healthcare professional is to be a certain kind of person. Medical professionals who live out these caring virtues in a consistent manner will be seen as "persons of high moral character [who] acquire a reservoir of good will in assessments of the praiseworthiness or blameworthiness of their actions."[8] By offering this thick account of the moral aspirations of medical professionals, Beauchamp and Childress attempt to erect a buffer against overly rigid or heartless applications of the system of rules and principles that the bulk of their treatment is devoted to explicating. The question is whether the moral agents who formed in these virtues will be able to recognize the virtues of their patient's decisions.

The core offering of *Principles of Biomedical Ethics* is a set of four principles that are presented as universally applicable and so at least in principle capable of resolving any potential ethical dilemma. This ethical framework admits, however, that a given doctor might find himself or herself facing a situation in which an act seems to be morally incumbent and yet goes beyond the sorts of action that could be defended on the basis of the four principles. Beauchamp and Childress label such acts "superogatory." Their decision to do so offers a window into what sort of theory they are offering, and what sort of medical practice it assumes.

A supererogatory act is considered to have four features. A supererogatory act is optional, neither required nor forbidden by common morality standards. Such acts exceed what is expected or demanded by the common morality. They are praiseworthy in intentionally seeking the welfare of others. And they are objectively morally good and praiseworthy, not declared good simply because they are undertaken out of good intentions.[9] Supererogatory acts go beyond the ordinary standards of behavior expected of everyone in society. They are heroic and so morally unique acts that in their very heroism could never be described as a universal duty.

When combined with the practices of prenatal testing surveyed in part 3, the common assumption in the secular West is that, all things being equal, it should be considered obligatory for the average pregnant woman to continue an "unaffected" pregnancy. Continuing an "affected" pregnancy, however appears quite differently. If it can be considered good at all, it cannot be considered a universal duty. This makes it a paradigmatic supererogatory or even a heroic act, in being "intentionally taken for the welfare of others." But given that many mothers today experience carrying a genetically anomalous new one as burdensome or a meaningless act, it is more usually the case for their choice to carry such a child to term to be understood as serving no one's welfare, not even that of the unborn child. In this light, the criterion that for an act to be supererogatory it must be *actually* good and praiseworthy, and not just good in *intention*, begins to look distinctly problematic. In a medical context in which all the dominant discourses position the bearing of a disabled child as an avoidable accident, it becomes almost impossible to imagine that someone could ever qualify as "heroic" by doing something the majority understands as patently irresponsible. Their definition of supererogation could therefore not morally valorize such an act, but could only designate it as a morally allowable individual choice to take on parental burdens that go far beyond what the system of prenatal screening assumes parents can reasonably be asked to bear.

Furthermore, Beauchamp and Childress explicitly define the threshold between morally obligatory and supererogatory acts by asking how much *risk* is taken on.[10] An act which is *risky* is, by definition, one that is not universally morally prescribed, and the role of the concept is to allow medical professionals to allow themselves and patients to forgo any procedure or act that is deemed risky. A judgment of an act to be risky is precisely the sort of moral judgment that is difficult strictly to confine to the professional sphere. When faced with a pregnant woman who has entered the domain of medical care, maintaining this separation of professional and private moral aspirations is difficult. Maintaining that continuing a pregnancy is risky as a purely professional judgment is doubly difficult if the woman resists the suggestion that perceived risk is the determining feature of the moral situation. Given the systematic accentuation of a narrow accounting of the riskiness of pregnancy characteristic of contemporary practices of prenatal testing, it becomes clear that the dominant account of medical ethics must present some forms of human vulnerability as presenting risks any reasonable person would avoid. *The concept of supererogation is a moral get-out clause that combines in powerful ways with conceptions of genetic risk to render the carrying of a disabled new one to term at best, heroic, and at worst, callous and socially irresponsible.*

THEOLOGICAL CRITIQUE OF SUPEREROGATION

Protestant moral theology raised a set of sharp worries about the concept of supererogation. In the medieval tradition, the concept of supererogation had been part of a wider presumption that it was legitimate for some in the church to be understood as following a higher path of holiness beyond what was expected from the great mass of believers. What the Kantian neo-Protestant uses of this term take forward is the presupposition that, though there is a "regular" duty to the neighbor, moral elites have the option to embrace more stringent "special" duties not incumbent on everyone.[11]

During the medieval period the distinction between following both Christ's commands (charity, understood through the cardinal virtues) and his more strenuous counsels (poverty, chastity, and obedience) had been increasingly solidified. As it did so it inevitably aligned with the monastic-laity distinction, with the label "vocation" coming to be reserved for the higher way alone.[12] It would not be an overstatement to read the whole Reformation as an elaborate protest against this distinction.[13] Luther insisted that in truth Christians could obey *neither* Christ's counsels nor his commands, and so are constantly thrown back on grace and into love of the neighbor without hesitation or moral hairsplitting—completely without reserve.[14] Such moral exception clauses appeared to confine a vital transformative faith to clerics and monks and to leave a culturally conservative and conformist Christianity to everyone else.[15] One of the characteristic features of the theologies of the Reformation is their subsequent reformulation of the concept of vocation, which was applied to activities as apparently different as the work of the priesthood, trade, parenthood, and government.[16]

The English term supererogation is a direct descendent from theological uses in being derived from the Latin *erogare*, meaning "to pay" or "expend." The term appears at a pivotal moment in the Latin (Vulgate) version of the parable of the Good Samaritan. Having rescued the injured neighbor, the Samaritan takes him to an inn and asks the proprietor to care for him. He also promises to reimburse his expenses, "and whatever you spend besides" (*quodcumque supererogaveris*) (Luke 10:35). The passage came to be a paradigm of supererogation in the medieval tradition, along with Zacchaeus' superabundant restitution (Luke 19:8-9) and Paul's using his own funds to support his ministry (Acts 20:34; 1 Thess 3:8-9).

Luther's doctrine of spontaneous good works presumes that it was no accident that Jesus answered the question of what it means to love one's neighbor with the story of the Good Samaritan. Jesus is overturning the Pharisee's question "Who then is my neighbor?" to resist its underlying assumption that morality begins with trying to define the other "out there" to whom empathy and solicitude is due. His question is wholly different: Who *turned out* to *have been* a neighbor? Faithfulness here appears as a transformed consciousness in which one's own self-interest is wholly tied to the well-being of the other. Jesus is suggesting that this specific form of attentiveness to others is morally irreducible and is trying to inflame this sort of attentiveness in his hearers. It was his emphasis on this single-tier morality of attentiveness to the neighbor that bequeathed evangelical ethics a sensitivity to all moral logics that justify two-tier moralities.

The spontaneous responsiveness of the Good Samaritan turns out not to be "irrational" or "unpredictable," but a distinctive and very practical rationality. Jesus is inviting human beings to become people whose relation to human vulnerability begins not with a distancing from others as "subjects," but the response of a glad heart to the vulnerability of the neighbor. To discover such spontaneity is a gift of the Spirit that cannot be ensured or legislated by any law but begins in the prayer which requests it. Such love, as Jesus' parable suggests, requires conversion, not simply information or education.

The parable of the Good Samaritan suggests that a steady emphasis on the occasional, gratuitous, and personal nature of Christian responsiveness need not be opposed to more hardheaded institutional thinking (*pace* Reinhold Niebuhr), but in fact demands it.[17] The Samaritan's response to the neighbor was a personal act that developed into a search for an appropriate caring institution, in this case an inn. The very same attention that led the Samaritan to the need of the other was the criterion of judging whether the inn was the right place to leave him for care. Public institutions are not somehow competitors to personal spontaneity. Personal care should be the criterion of the good care institution. Institutional configurations may serve or resist moral agents being turned out of themselves and toward others. When the hermeneutic of the body Jesus is offering is lost, institutions change, reorganizing themselves around other purposes. In Christian terms, rightly directed hearts are essential if institutions are to remain humane. An inn as a meeting of economic, political, and interpersonal cultures may be a better or worse place for the Good Samaritan to leave his ward. And institutions can be organized to maximize this personal attentiveness.

L'Arche is a witness to the rooting of institutional structures in a personal spirituality of attentiveness.[18] Christians living in communities like L'Arche are primarily offering a witness to the engaged presence that sustains real relationships, a witness that is far more important than providing "industry-standard health care." Beginning from a need for caring institutions, L'Arche institutionalizes the response of people to serve their opening up toward one another, not the "provision of care services." L'Arche seeks to be a community where people can discover the fecundity of divine love through personal attentiveness to others. Such an institution simultaneously challenges the assumptions behind the ordering of healthcare institutions today in their intertwining with the characteristic forms of individual attention that they demand. Its witness is to a *politics* that Christians have a duty to offer to a secular political society, but which it cannot conceive on its own terms.[19]

Christian ethics so positioned is at every point a public social ethic in which individuals must constantly exercise the personal attentiveness of the Good Samaritan. A properly Christian political ethic strives to witness to a political ethic with definable contours and growing from its own characteristic tradition. The Christian understanding of neighbor love combines with Christian commitments to the good of noncoercion in political affairs to yield a refusal of any suggestion that such Spirit-enabled spontaneity can be imposed on all of society. At the same time, it will advocate for public social structures that can protect and promote the space for spontaneous attentiveness to occur, in full awareness that the Christian focus on Christlike attentiveness to the neighbor cannot be reduced to, or translated into, the language of secular rationality. The appearance of the most vulnerable human lives, and the claim they make on those who wish to bear and live with them, constantly cries for the witness of this rival way of life.

HOW MEDICAL ETHICS DISEMPOWERS

What Christians call "witness" Beauchamp and Childress have called "risking an accident." Their judgment springs from their having positioned medical ethics not as growing from the Christian tradition, but as orienting itself within the domain of universal rationality. Some medical professionals may be aware that there are problems with fostering a gaze that looks on vulnerable lives as risky, but medical ethics orthodoxy forces them to compartmentalize any such worries. Even if in their private lives they have a heart for the most vulnerable, in their professional lives they are adjudged duty bound to make efforts to prevent the "accidents" that are the lives of the most vulnerable. An exemplary case study displays how the four principles of Beauchamp and Childress morally disempower the physician in borderline situations.[20]

Consider this relatively common example of a request for a late-term abortion of a genetically anomalous new one. Mrs. X is a thirty-seven-year-old married woman with two children aged five and seven. She has fallen pregnant though she and her husband had not intended to have any more children. For a variety of reasons prenatal testing has been delayed. Routine antenatal screening and a blood test indicate an increased risk of a fetus with Down syndrome. Amniocentesis is performed, and Down syndrome is confirmed at thirty weeks gestation. The fetus appears to be developing normally otherwise, and there is no evidence of associated major congenital malformations. Mrs. X is counseled by her obstetrician about the problems faced by children with Down syndrome. The question is whether she should she be offered the option of a feticide.

According to current British legislation, a termination may be performed at any stage beyond twenty-four weeks of gestation if two doctors agree in good faith that one of the following conditions is met:

1. If the child were born, there is a substantial risk it would suffer from physical or mental abnormalities that would leave it seriously handicapped.
2. It is necessary to save the life of a pregnant woman.
3. It is necessary to prevent grave permanent injury to the physical or mental health of the woman.

Enter the four principles of orthodox medical ethics.

Beneficence. Mrs. X has a duty of beneficence to the fetus, to her other children, and to herself. The duty to the fetus is ambivalent given that it is possible that the quality of life with Down syndrome can dip into negative net benefit. Death might in some cases be preferable to a continuing existence. The duty of beneficence to her children encourages her to protect them from the adverse effects of having a sibling with Down syndrome. The emotional energy spent by parents on a child with special needs is a loss to the siblings, as may be their having to live with the possible social stigma of disability. Mrs. X also has a duty of beneficence to herself and may legitimately feel that there will be negative effects of the child on her own psychological welfare and the strength of her marriage.

Nonmaleficence. Again, the duty to the fetus is ambivalent. To terminate the fetus may be viewed as an act of maleficence, but only if the net quality of life is seen as positive. If the future net quality of life is negative, then killing can be understood as an act of beneficence. The possibility of fetal sentience at this late gestational age can be considered a legitimate harm, as is the associated psychological distress to staff, mother, and other children associated with a late feticide. Since the survival of the fetus may have negative consequences on the siblings and on Mrs. X herself, its survival could be perceived as an act of maleficence.

Autonomy. Since the fetus is generally regarded as having no self-awareness, it has no power to act autonomously, but termination will foreclose its future exercise. The loss implied in this foreclosure is less than in unaffected pregnancies since people with Down syndrome have lower potentials for autonomy (in comparison to healthy individuals) given their learning and cognitive disability. The autonomy of Mrs. X is the most significant of all the individuals concerned, and she should be free to exercise her own choice free of overt or covert persuasion from professionals and other interested parties. The fact that the pregnancy is unintended, and the diagnosis has unintentionally come late, are crucial factors on the side of Mrs. X's right to exercise her own autonomy about the continuation of her pregnancy. She should be provided with information about options and likely outcomes in a neutral and value-free manner, and no preferences should be expressed by health professionals as to likely choices and outcomes.

Justice. The principle of justice particularly addresses the allocation of scarce healthcare resources in society. A surviving child with Down syndrome will probably consume greater healthcare resources than the norm and thus survival may contribute to injustice. It is similarly unjust for a surviving child with Down syndrome to deprive the other siblings of parental attention and resources. On the other hand, people with Down syndrome are entitled to receive as many resources as others in society, and the destruction of the fetus on the basis of this diagnosis may be perceived as an act of injustice or discrimination against individuals with Down syndrome, reinforcing negative attitudes toward existing people with the syndrome.

At this point a doctor will have to make a decision about whether or not to offer the option of a feticide, and it is clear that the woman's choice will be the determining factor, since substantial considerations have been tendered on both sides of the equation. Most obstetricians feel personally ambivalent at best about providing the option and yet feel pressured by the law to make the offer due to the very real risk of a wrongful life suit if the obstetrician fails to inform the mother that feticide is a medical option.

The most obvious reason for reluctance to offer a feticide is the prospect of horrified parents hearing the offer as a proposal. The consequences are disastrous for the trust of patients. As one sufferer of an inherited brittle-bone condition commented after one such conversation, "that unsettling meeting with a doctor on a mission to destroy my offspring ruptured the sacred bond of trust between physicians and patients that underpins a humane healthcare system." He continues,

> My respect for hospitals also took a bullet. I suppose it is hard for able-bodied people to grasp their significance to OI-affected families: I can recall gatherings from my youth where we discussed hospital staff in the same way other families chat about revered schoolteachers, soccer coaches or piano instructors. Dad often praised his favourite orthopaedic surgeon, while his siblings would wax lyrical concerning the ENT surgeon who miraculously restored their hearing. I might pipe up to extol the wonderful "Plaster Room" Nursing Sister who had a knack of cracking jokes, immobilising broken limbs and administering pain-killers in a way that sent a downcast lad safely on his way thinking he could face the world again. Because we knew they cared for our welfare, we grew to love these hospital staff. It never crossed our minds that they would intentionally harm or trick us into attending unwanted consultations. Why would it? Our reverence for hospitals had accumulated over generations of a shared family experience of living with OI. By contrast, the slick, manipulative workers in the genetics clinic seemed to hail from another planet. A "healthcare revolution" of far-reaching significance had clearly occurred in the years since I last needed orthopaedic assistance.[21]

From the perspective of someone with a genetic condition, the revolution in genetic testing has brought a seismic shift in the moral presumptions of medical professionals. Yet Beauchamp and Childress have obscured this transformation by having drastically limited the reasons and aims permitted for doctors to bring into discussion contentious cases like late-term abortions. Some physicians believe that because their professional life has been devoted to reducing suffering in the world, lives full of pain should be prevented. Thus, potentially disabled lives should be terminated whenever possible. Others never want to offer abortion and are deeply torn by feeling forced to do so. Finally, doctors are often frustrated that after a full course of fetal screening, some mothers refuse to follow through on what they see as a consent to abort implied by their ongoing participation in an extensive procedure. They consider it obvious that screening is designed to find untreatable conditions which will be treated in the only way that they can be treated—by abortion.

The elision of these aspects of the decision to offer feticide constitute a significant deficit in the common mode of moral reasoning which Beauchamp and Childress espouse, and the practical, political, psychological, and finally, moral ambiguities which their account systematically leaves to the practitioner. A whole range of other morally relevant practical questions are also systematically screened out by Beauchamp and Childress's moral procedure. In fact, many of the forms of judgment physicians commonly apply in making decisions are positioned as unnecessary or even detrimental to what is taken as a satisfactory resolution of an admittedly problematic case. For instance, such late-term requests for abortion are unusual because fetal abnormalities are normally detected much earlier. Why has this not happened? If this is a systemic failure, is the doctor duty bound to offer a termination they find personally abhorrent?

Nowhere do Beauchamp and Childress define how a moral dilemma is recognized *as* a dilemma. No reasoning is offered to distinguish between a practical complication and an ethical dilemma that should be resolved through explicit moral deliberation. Their goal is to provide the tools for the resolution of ethical problems, and all problems are assumed to be *prima facie* present, ethical (as opposed to political, religious, economic, etc.) and in need of a solution. In the final analysis, because their moral thought is pragmatic and seeks social harmony rather than an explicit view of justice, embraces a high level of ambiguity, and minimizes the place of the physician's conscience, it is bound to leave doctors feeling that the substantive moral questions surrounding such a tough case have been evaded.

The persistence of these ethical loose ends and the inconclusive nature of the analysis deserve further scrutiny. The looseness of the moral analysis is in fact intentional. Beauchamp and Childress aim to create an ethic fluid enough to accommodate changing social mores in liberal, pluralist society. They therefore derive their four moral principles from a metaethical construct they refer to as the "common morality."[22] "Universal common morality" is taken to rest on "a plurality of customary moralities" which include all the moral positions held by different religious and secular groups. Ethical theory amounts to a description of the grammar of this universal common morality, distilled from the points of overlap of many customary moralities. The four principles are presented as an attractive ethical method in being able to affirm the strong consensus about the universality of human rights shared by all common moralities while avoiding making strong moral claims on issues where the various customary moralities are at loggerheads (offering as an example of a topic where no moral consensus exists the question of animals as research subjects).[23] Because the substrate of their ethical principles is the pluriformity of ethical positions, they take "disunity, conflict, and moral ambiguity as pervasive aspects of the moral life."[24]

Locating moral deliberation in the overlapping territories of pluriform customary moralities only works if any absolute moral claims that might emerge from customary moralities are not admitted.[25] The four principles are norming norms designed to set up fields of obligation that exert limited and nondeterminative moral pressure on action. The assumption is that *all* moral questions will be resolved based on a shared commitment to casuist problem resolution, even the most divisive,[26] and that if practitioners then violate these rules it will mark their character, leaving "'moral traces' which should be reflected in the agent's attitudes and actions."[27]

THE DISEMPOWERED PHYSICIAN

The feeling that standard accounts of medical ethics are evading the real moral questions is not the only dilemma principleist medical ethics lays on the doctor's conscience. Much as the pregnant woman in the prenatal clinic is placed under great, if indirect, pressure to "choose" whether to abort a genetically anomalous new one, the doctor-patient relationship has become a catch basin for a range of moral, political, and practical questions that the courts, legislatures, and the public have chosen to defer. Aware of these competing and manifold pressures, doctors feel the weight of being asked to resolve them by making wise "professional choices." Orthodox medical ethics reinforces this cultural settlement by framing medical ethics as a tool set for medical professionals to resolve complex individual medical choices. The wider scope issues layered onto the doctor-patient relationship are systematically screening out as legitimate ethical considerations. This society-wide moral evasion becomes positively perverse when some suggest revoking the physician's right to conscientious objection.[28] Physicians, it seems, can have opinions about morality and immoral medical practices as long as they keep them in the private domain. Acting on them would disrupt medical systems. No wonder so many medical professionals feel trapped.

The last two hundred years have seen an exponential growth in the complexity of the physician's role in Western society. While the professionalization and specialization of medicine has exponentially increased its political power and capacity to direct the shaping of society (by commanding funding, shaping policymaking, etc.), this has also attracted actors who aim to guide and commandeer aspects of this social power for their own purposes. It may be that the apogee of the social power of medicine has already been reached. Physicians now retain a modicum of social power but are increasingly shorn of the freedom to wield it for what they see as the good of patients and their own conscience.

The disempowered physician may well be the perfect social glue in neoliberal societies. Pharmaceutical and medical technology companies, hospitals, and governments would be delighted to transform physicians into employees who uncomplainingly follow centrally dictated policy. If they can be persuaded that the only ethical questions that pertain to them are narrowly defined problems of patient care, they will be discouraged from protesting management restructuring for maximum efficiency. The recent growth of pharmaceutical advertising provides a case in point, a problem especially pronounced in the United States. No longer legally allowed to influence doctors through lavish personal gifts or entertainment, pharmaceutical companies have turned to influencing the public.[29] "Do you suffer from indigestion? Ask your doctor to prescribe Zantac for quick relief." Governments and HMOs simultaneously demand doctors achieve ever greater efficiency with drugs, treatments, their time, and personnel.[30] Unique problems also pile up in particular medical domains. Growth in the belief in "consumer choice" lands obstetricians with skyrocketing rises in elective cesarean births. Neonatologists face a deluge of complicated pregnancies as a result of exponential grown in fertility treatments.[31] Since highly desired IVF babies often experience much higher rates of medical complications, a double standard arises for the care of "natural" and "assisted" pregnancies.[32] Having so heavily emphasized the importance of patient autonomy, medical ethics leaves doctors powerless to raise moral questions about such trends, including about the commercialization of reproduction.[33]

The positioning by Beauchamp and Childress of the late-term abortion case typifies all these problems. They have simply assumed that a request for a late-term abortion represents an "ethical dilemma," eliding the role of the physician's conscience in assigning this designation. Medics who think the fetus is a "mistake" will see no ethical dilemma. Other medical professionals will find their consciences disturbed by a much wider range of societal implications of late-term abortion, understanding the ethical dilemma as far more than a question of choice for the mother, or pastoral tact for the practitioner who is squeamish about offering termination. By hiding the role of the medical professional's conscience in designating a moral dilemma,

Beauchamp and Childress present ethical problems as self-evident. They also do not seriously engage the question of conscientious abstention. The result is an account of the virtuous conscience as internalized ethical and professional standards. Virtue is equated to living up to the roles that have been assigned doctors by the healthcare institutions in which they serve.[34]

While Beauchamp and Childress do admit cases of conscientious objections and abstentions from practice, these are presented as relatively rare and extreme cases, such as a hospital's refusal to be conscripted in preparation for nuclear war. Beauchamp and Childress consistently assume that moral objections to certain practices are conflicts to be resolved, not politically weighty attempts by medical professionals to participate in the formation of a humane society.[35] The end result is the intellectual straitjacketing of physicians in a pure social conservatism. Doctors are allowed, as professionals, to "resolve" cases using the deliberative tools provided, but this is the limit of their justified political engagement. All problems are resolvable through mutual discussion, the resolution of particularly vexing questions by physicians providing the casuistic case log enabling society at large to hone its social consensus.[36]

The conscientious refusal of a particular medical professional is positioned in this account as an irrational and unjustifiable behavior growing from an irascible character or the unwanted influence of a "customary morality" which has not reconciled itself to the hegemony of the common morality. The grounding of the method in "customary morality" can now be seen as a strategy of marginalization of the actual moral narratives which have grounded the ethical lives of social groups for all human history. African, Asian, Hindu, Buddhist, atheist, and agnostic alongside Christian stories about the nature of the universe and where humans fit in it are labeled "customary" from the "universal standpoint" which Beauchamp and Childress presume themselves to occupy. From that vantage point customary moralities inevitably appear less tolerant and therefore less morally serious than their common morality.

An unintended consequence of this moral theory is that in practice it seems to refuse physicians any moral right to deviate from the common morality. That the theory seems unable to contemplate physicians questioning common morality suggests an assumption that compliant physicians are necessary to hold together a range of delicately balanced competing political and moral forces. Disempowered physicians are socially useful in being intelligent agents to whom morally tricky questions can be systematically delegated.

The various attempts of U.S. and U.K. legislators to provide sufficiently clear and robust legislative guidelines which value and protect the physician's right to conscientious objection illustrate the difficulty of sustaining this situation. Late abortion is morally interesting because British law has slowly limited the scope of a physician's professional judgment. At least in Britain, public ambivalence to late-term abortion has not been matched by offering any legal protection of conscientious objections by physicians.[37] Legislators avoided directly addressing this moral divide in society by refusing to let doctors make the same choice not to decide. Since late abortion is defensibly legal in almost any conceivable case of fetal malformation or disease, the physician has no legitimate or publicly defensible reason to refuse the request for a legal abortion, and indeed has a professional duty to raise the possibility with the pregnant woman. Moral and legal responsibility is concentrated on the physician. Countless doctors are therefore legally obliged to make and remake the same morally draining decision legislators refused. Hospital management, government managers—each goes on providing what is necessary to keep doctors working, while at the same time applying subtle or not so subtle pressures to keep physicians from substantive protest. Questions of the moral responsibility of the legislators who constructed the legal structure for late-term abortion has been swept from the table. All that is left is for medical ethics to hold the doctor in place and force him or her to forgo the call of conscience, having been informed by experts which moral factors are legitimate to consider, and which are beyond the scope of "legitimate" ethical deliberation.[38]

That is not quite true. Doctors can fill out feedback questionnaires. Feedback forms are one of the defining features of governance in an econometrically ordered society. What is less often noticed is the political utility of letting people air their grievances. Workers can be kept in unsatisfying factory jobs by being given the opportunity to express their grievances without much change on the shop floor.[39] While the physician's work certainly entails intrinsic rewards not available to the factory worker, it is not too fanciful to suggest that Beauchamp and Childress have understood discussion of the "ethical dilemma" less as a genuine moral deliberation and more as a safety valve for preserving the status quo. On closer examination their main interest appears to have been in guiding doctors to internalize the audit culture, defining this conformity as virtue. While encouraging the sharing of pangs of conscience within this formal structure, they carefully stipulate, among other things, that this discussion ought not lead to the overriding of the wishes of the patient except in extraordinary cases. Doing well is being positioned as a fulfillment of the law of the audit above the law that arises from the body of the patient. They thus provide an all but complete undermining of the grounds upon which a physician might register the practical absurdity of neonatal wards, where increasingly sophisticated neonatal care proceeds literally across the hall from the provision of late abortion procedures. The moral unease generated by such practices of the human deserve to be recognized, but "managing" them may alleviate the problem by forcing people to submit to them more completely.[40]

The systemic refusal of the doctor's capacity to respond to the systemic pressures on people with disability has significant liabilities not only for individual doctor-patient relationships, but for the coherence of medicine as a moral enterprise.[41] Rather than empowering the dilemma-resolving capacity of practitioners, Beauchamp and Childress' four principles approach systematically separates practitioners from the resources they might call upon to resolve ethical dilemmas. In so doing it unravels the moral fiber of the practice as a whole. Physicians' powers of judgment and their conscience must be sacrificed to a medical consensus that denies the importance of their very particularity. *Principles* purports to be solving ethical questions but is in fact systematically insisting that medics legitimate the presuppositions of the dominant social paradigm. And in doing so all rival ethical viewpoints are delegitimized.

LIBERAL *PRINCIPLES* AND CHRISTIAN MARTYRDOM

The claim of Beauchamp and Childress that they can maintain their pluralist equipoise because they propound no substantive anthropology has become common in liberal political philosophies.[42] The foregoing analysis suggests that rather than yielding the "neutral" ethical tool they intend, Beauchamp and Childress have in fact built their theory on an implicit anthropological grounding that is far from morally neutral. Faced with the inconvenience of a morally conflicted and thus inefficient physician, Beauchamp and Childress offer a mechanism to resolve perceived moral dilemmas and keep doctors working. The legitimacy of their ethical hybrid method rests on an appeal to the thicker cosmologies or anthropologies of particular moral frameworks that they studiously avoid more closely investigating. They seem wholly unaware that it might falsify some moral systems to situate them as pragmatic and provisional hypotheses about the nature of the universe. Only because their own anthropology is so substantive can Beauchamp and Childress ignore the substantive claims of other thought systems. For them humanity is comprised of autonomous problem solvers who are tolerant of others' beliefs, and who simply need a technique for reaching what they consider the only worthy goal of moral deliberation: practical agreement.[43]

In their metanarrative, personal beliefs, or the beliefs of communities, are assumed to be parochial, "customary" in the sense of unreflectively held religious beliefs and personal aspirations. These beliefs and aspirations are among "a host of other considerations that must be accommodated" in ethical deliberation.[44] Beauchamp and Childress admit that individuals can choose to "accept and submit to the authoritative demands of an institution, tradition, or community that they view as a legitimate source of direction,"[45] and that these commitments might warrant an individual's refusal to participate in certain procedures (such as abortion). But they have firmly positioned such beliefs as inherently the views of marginal communities rather than universal and rationally binding. With this deflationary move the central claim of customary moralities is rejected: that they represent *rivals to*, not simply *sources of* the universal reality descriptions grounding the metanarrative of *Principles*. Theories like that of Beauchamp and Childress are "simulacra of morality" because any gravitas their position possesses is derived from the very thick moral traditions that their own position marginalizes in practice.[46]

Christianity is one such customary morality, and its story begins with a martyrdom.[47] Something unique about reality and humanity was revealed in the figure of Jesus Christ on the cross. Two thousand years of Christian thinking on this subject have not yet summarized its implications, but one is certain: Christian ethics is not primarily a discussion designed to secure practical agreement in a pluralist society. In the Christian story, God is remaking humans so that they can discern their place in the cosmic struggle that culminated in the cross. In the cross God also reveals that the ways of peace and violence are at loggerheads, which is why Christians have long recognized that following Christ may get one killed. Because it so often did in the first Christian centuries, martyrdom played a formative role in the process of self-definition of the earliest generations of Christians. From the moment the disciples gather at the foot of the cross (including Jesus' mother), *community is created in that suffering death*. Jesus' promise of blessedness for those who hunger and thirst after righteousness and who "are persecuted for the sake of righteousness" founded a trust among these Christians that with their suffering with Christ would come life, joy, and the presence of the kingdom of God. These themes echo through the rest of the New Testament and were woven deeply into the life and theology of the early church.[48]

No encouragement to seek martyrdom was implied in this account, and Christian theologians never allowed biblical passages such as Samson's suicide attack on the Philistines to justify seeking it out. Christian martyrdom is a passive display of the power of Jesus Christ to overcome the fear of death. Holding fast to the promise that "I am the resurrection and the life" renders the Christian's undergoing of martyrdom the final conclusive mark of life lived in the peace of God. Christian martyrdom displays what it looks like to live without fear of death, trusting in God's merciful action. In so doing it reveals the *purpose* of life, death, and all human action.[49]

Ultimately Christians are not responsible to publicly acceptable canons of morality, but to God. Thus, the Christian should expect to be called upon at times to see truths, and pursue ways of living, which are unpopular and even diametrically opposed to the political rulers of their time and place. In publicly praising Jesus in Christian worship as *Kyrios*—the "Lord" with authority over all political rulers—they are taught that the claims of social consensus and political power are not as ultimate as they claim to be. What Rome called an absurd irrationality the martyrs understood as revealing the derivative nature of the Roman rulers' own claims to authority. Martyrdom was politically potent in exposing that the lethal force of Rome could kill Christians but not victimize them. Christians died in confidence that the story of martyrdom as defeat that Rome was trying to weave around them was not the true story of their death.[50]

The allegiance of the church to God alone freed it to foment the coming kingdom within the kingdoms of this world. Such conflicts can always arise as the church militant struggles toward the justice of Christ's kingdom that has not yet been fully achieved. Where Christ's kingdom has provoked open resistance, Christians have suffered it in their yearning for that kingdom that is coming. Martyrdom is thus a work of a civilization that lifts its hand against God, and a church that is too at home in the world will be unprepared for this and so unprepared for mission.[51] Conversely, where the church finds rulers sympathetic to its practice of humanity, it is glad to join them in mutual service. *The church that no longer believes martyrdom possible has wrongly equated its own society with God's justice. To think that conflict can no longer arise between Christians and political authorities is the real defeat of Christ's kingdom.*[52]

The strong moral assumption of Beauchamp and Childress that humans are best understood as problem-solving beings capsizes on the rock of Christianity's strong moral claim: that being human consists in conformity to the likeness of the divine human, Christ, who is establishing a kingdom of peace amidst the political kingdoms and powers of this world. On the basis of common morality-based ethical theory, one might die for that which one believed in, a death which might even be called supererogatory—though Beauchamp and Childress seem skeptical that one is *ever* justified in giving up one's decision-making ability in this way.[53] Within the Christian description of reality, however, in addition to dying for the good of someone else one might also suffer, and even die, rather than be forced to act in ways that repudiate the service of others embodied in Jesus Christ. This is the strong moral claim that gave Christian ethics the necessary moral force to so deeply reshape the ethics of the Western world. It was a witness that pointed to a paradoxical truth, to an alternative reality.[54] *Out of martyrdom's crucible the universal rule of human solidarity arose to stand against every utilitarian view of human life*. The rule of universal human solidarity was one concretization of the totalizing claim of Christian knowledge.[55]

CHRIST AND THE VOCATION OF WITNESS

Christians in medicine who resist commonly accepted moral beliefs, like the unfettered right to abortion, court loss of status or even their profession. When faced with such prospects, the Christian understanding of martyrdom offers some purchase on the spiritual work involved in resisting powerful social norms. The term "martyrdom" is not restricted to dying for the faith but names the location of a Christian in any conflict between God and a resistant society. The term therefore also draws attention to the self-renunciation and perseverance characteristic of the martyrs of the patristic era.[56] Never an end in itself or a way to accrue merit for Christians, martyrdom was always understood as a communicative act of witness. In dissenting from the orthodoxies of a given age, it points to the futility of opposing God and directly testifies before human political power of its nonultimacy.[57]

Christians can always be martyred by a world in rebellion against God. But because martyrdom is an act of witness to Jesus, it cannot be performed as a defiant gesture. It performs a general invitation to join the martyr's worship of the one Lord of heaven and earth.[58] The martyr acts in faith that the God of love will prevail over the forces of evil and dissolution, refusing to do evil to insure a more comfortable future. The moment to resist in a world filled with moral compromise may not be easily perceptible. What is sure is that calling out an injustice will provoke resistance in implicating the behavior of others. It would be paralyzing and pedantic to call out and resist every evil or injustice, but if Christians wish to maintain a working conscience they cannot afford to invest their lives in systems they come to see are antichrist.[59]

This chapter has highlighted the particular injustice of selectively aborting the genetically anomalous new one. Christians can and must speak out for social policies that uphold what they understand to be the moral truth of human life. Silent acceptance of majority behaviors is the fundament of the econometrically governed society. In such societies the silence of Christians is abandonment of the hard-won lessons that yielded the rule of human solidarity. But devising norms for public life is a subsidiary concern of Christian ethics. Winning legislative battles is not the primary witness of Christians. Their lives are that more basic witness. Martyrdom is always a personal calling or vocation that becomes visible when the individual Christian is pressed to do evil. In such moments responding is not supererogatory. It is being a Christian.

Every Christian discovers their vocation as they are drawn more deeply into God's story with creation. Vocation is the place of discipleship and can become, at times, unexpectedly arduous. Self-denials will be demanded that could never be converted into a social norm, not even among Christians. In embracing this invitation believers give up genuine created goods due to them, in the process glimpsing the truth of Christ's living rule more clearly and sharply than before.[60] The language of vocation takes the believer out of the place of moral reasoning occupied by Beauchamp and Childress, of the expert applying principles to cases. Moral agents are instead situated as human beings attempting faithfully to discern a course of action amidst the swirl of life as a whole. The language of vocation allows Christians to talk intelligibly about the utterly unique place in which each individual is responsible to discern the good works that have been given to them alone to do for the good of the world.

In some cases, Christian faithfulness might well mean shoring up the institutional structures that are in place while in others demand mounting opposition to cultural protocols, institutional guidelines, and legal orders. Here Dietrich Bonhoeffer's reflections on the conflict of Christian doctors during the Third Reich are especially instructive. Even in cases where the scope of professional responsibility is being progressively restricted, the medical professional remains responsible to other human beings, to their coworkers, and to their family. This responsibility is never abrogated when laws and regulations become unjust. In precisely such moments, these relationships of interpersonal responsibility beyond all human law become all the more important.[61] Bonhoeffer offers an alternative to the view of conscience proposed by Beauchamp and Childress. *The Christian's conscience is clear in Christ alone, and not in any fulfillment of the duties decreed by a professional guild. To attend responsively to the call of the neighbor is to welcome Christ.*[62]

The Christian medic's freedom of conscience liberates them for the witness of genuine political protest by clarifying their moral perception. It was the witness of Christian medics that helped Bonhoeffer name the Nazi extermination program for what it was from the very start.[63] The program began by "liquidating" those in institutions for the insane and mentally ill.[64] Bonhoeffer visited one of the institutions under threat by this policy, The Bethel Institute for the Physically and Mentally Handicapped, a Christian institution run by a doctor he deeply respected.[65] The church he saw there was the real church that he had been looking for, its congregants being mentally impaired, sufferers of mental illness, as well as the poor from the community alongside the doctors, nurses, and their families. Here he could see the diversity of human life and the redeemed community of mutual support that is church. The concreteness of this community revealed the euthanasia program and the whole Nazi ethos of strength and uniformity as madness.[66] "Christianity has been blamed ever since its early days for its message to the weak," Bonhoeffer preached a few years later. "Christianity stands or falls with its revolutionary protest against violence, arbitrariness, and pride of power and with its apologia for the weak. Christianity has adjusted itself much too easily to the worship of power . . . [and] should give much more offence, more shock to the world, than it is doing."[67] Bonhoeffer would not have encouraged Christians to think that twentieth-century Germany staged the last conflict of Buchenwald against Bethel, nor that those who worship power and security ought to no longer find the view of Christians offensive.

Unlike contemporary political theory with its tendency to reduce political action to voting, Bonhoeffer never loses sight of the medical professional as an actor who is constantly engaging in and shaping the political life of the state through his or her vocation, with the aim of contributing the lessons of his or her encounter with Jesus Christ.[68] The Christian medic enters the political stage with a message and a clear idea of the shape of reconciled humanity, resolved to act for others and on their behalf.[69] In so doing they remind every Christian that their own vocational responsibilities are the locus of their participation in the political life of society, the concrete place where they express God's resistance to dehumanizing forces.[70] The inner wellspring of Christian vocational faithfulness is the positive experience of God's appearance to which Christians respond within the concrete particularities of the vocations of citizen, worker, parent, spouse, and church member.[71]

The annunciative call of the genetically anomalous new one radically challenges Beauchamp and Childress' framing of the "problem" of late-term abortion. Christian witness at this point exposes the contradictions the secular liberal West wishes to hide, forcing them back into the public consciousness. This witness may echo patristic practices by adopting and fostering children, and by thinking creatively about how to receive unwanted children with disabilities.[72] It may also take the form of the Christian medic's refusal to abort the genetically anomalous new one, as costly as this might turn out to be. The smooth functioning of medical institutions and societies that believe themselves dependent on the provision of abortion on demand is threatened by insisting that Christians be allowed to speak of this life, too, as valued in Christ. Such acts shine the light of Christ's love for the least of these on the humanity being performed by the secular technological West.

6

Quality of Life in an Industrialized Age

THE LAWS OF AVERAGES AND SYSTEMS

The vast cultural edifice called modern medicine is designed to relieve human suffering. The suffering that it inflicts, especially the suffering of those labeled disabled, is its festering wound.[1]

Modern medicine is a bureaucratic domain. The pragmatic problem-solver anthropology surveyed in chapter 5 demands an existential stance in the world that lives within and perpetuates a distinctive politics.[2] Medics today approach patients within terms set by bureaucratically organized spaces. Time with patients must be minimized, and the number of patients seen maximized. Some forms of listening to patients are accentuated and others ruled out. In all this, medicine is by no means unique, the prosperity and security of North Atlantic societies having long ago been hitched to the industrialization of labor processes and the computational management of information.

As those who confess that they are schooled in worship by an external word of God that is life-giving, Christians possess an important clue about how to live humanely in the world of modern medicine. A church that regularly practices listening to God's Word may well foster a practice of medicine that listens more closely to the stories and bodies of patients than the current configuration of medical knowledge seems to admit.

What has been gained and lost as a result of this heavy cultural investment in specialization is most easily displayed with a quick detour through modern agriculture, which has also been reconfigured according to the laws of industrial manufacture. The aim of this reconfiguration is the maximization cost per "product" unit. The transformation of "harvest" into "product" is accompanied by the transformation of "farmer" into the "agricultural production expert."[3]

The main casualty of this process is the loss of the ability of the farmer to respond to variability and individuality. Reconceiving poultry farming as a process of "meat production" demands standardizing chicken growing time, emphasizing temperamental placidity in the breed being used, maximizing disease resistance for animals kept as closely together as possible, and so on. The limits of what can be done to improve animal welfare will be defined by this quest to maximize efficiencies in feeding and breeding. Breeding and genetic manipulation shape chicken bodies for survival in a battery-cage system. Chickens who cannot thrive in such an environment die or are killed. The reconfiguration of poultry farming by experts whose goal is continual cost reductions for ever increasing "final product" display why, in bureaucratized systems, it is inevitably the nonstandard body that suffers most.

The changing landscapes of the industrialized West also display the reality of the law of efficiency. Farmable land demands the use of large equipment, and hilly, rocky, or small plots that might easily be made productive by a farmer are left fallow while the hedgerows and fences that once divided the land are torn down. Land that is machine farmable is then treated as a mechanical system of input and outputs that can be reliably controlled. The presumption of such control justifies the planting of vast fields of single plant species which are as uniform as possible to be machine harvestable and easily machine processed. Because monoculture farming is more susceptible than mixed plots to catastrophic illnesses and predator depredation, insecticides must be sprayed to kill unwanted insects and herbicides to kill unwanted plants. By the same logic the uniformity and predictability of chemical fertilizers displaces natural fertilizers such as manure for staving off unproductive fallow years or crop rotation.[4]

The ideal of expertise drives inexorably toward normalization: the achievement of high production depends on every part of the system approximating a predictable statistical average. Crops need to be of uniform size, shape, and color, the land of a predictable and uniform chemical composition, and all threats to the now-uniform crops exterminated.

The expert's narrow focus on efficient production elides questions of sustainability and the value of the particularities of place. Agribusiness measures its success in terms of ability to produce a marketable surplus, whereas husbandry is concerned with sustainability, the health and fertility of the soil, and the communities that farm and live off it. A different skill set is demanded from the type of intimate knowledge of a particular place and soil characteristic of earlier forms of farming. Sophisticated premodern farmers learned that the productivity of the land increases when crops are intermixed with one another and different varieties cultivated in different regions and ecological niches so that, should there be a bad year or an extremity of weather or infestation or disease, the farmer can find another plant which has survived and use it to begin cultivation anew. But these earlier forms of farming also depended on a larger and more varied stock of tools, more manpower, as well as intimate knowledge of the plants and animals that might be able to flourish and enrich the fertility of particular places over the long term.[5] Rival portraits of agricultural technology are in fact rival answers to the more basic question of what human beings are doing as they alter the earth and its organisms.

Caring for particularity is inseparable from valuing diversity, and modern conceptions of expertise devalue both. The knowledge of the expert is general and generalizable and centers in the skills of gauging statistical probabilities, spotting laws of averages, and minimizing outliers and uniformities. But this knowledge not only drives out other more particular forms of knowledge, but also the cultural virtues that attended its attainment and maintenance. Similar forms of rationalization and technical expertise have been deployed to increase production in almost every sphere of work in the developed world.

MEDICINE UNDER THE LAW

In the early 1960s Michel Foucault had already begun to discern the same tendencies in modern medicine. The ideal of expertise called forth new forms of medical rationality and new ways of perceiving the patient. The ancient account of medicine as the study and restoration of health to an individual particular person was displaced by a new interest in normal functioning and deviation from it.[6] The development of generic accounts of normal function went hand in hand with the development of new modes of information gathering. The new forms of information gathering no longer centered on the taking of a patient history but on the constructions of charts capable of mapping changes over time. Deviations in temperature, fluid intake and output, weight, heart rate, and so on, could be studied for the first time with these new techniques. Medical knowledge shifted onto a new ground for perceiving the body; what was important about the individual patient was a statistically structured data set. Average values were established as the central conceptual framework directing the medical gaze.[7]

These observations begin to suggest why the modern hospital and the "healthcare industry" with which it is inevitably intertwined rely so heavily on the law of averages to establish "normal" types of human life. "Normal" disease etiologies must be established by research which indicates what is most statistically likely to occur in a given case. Drugs and treatments are aimed to shape the bodies and minds being treated to conform as closely as possible to this "normal," which also serves as an allocation mechanism to divert medical resources to the majority rather than more complex minority sets.[8]

The globalized scope of instrumentalization is a problem for everyone in modern societies. Parents and caregivers for nonstandard children learn this lesson very quickly. Their children are the outliers not studied in medical research and place demands on modern medicine which it cannot meet. Modern agriculture can afford to leave uncultivated those parts of the land it finds difficult to fit into its mode of care, but medicine cannot. Disability exposes the tensions between medicine understood as technical expertise and medicine understood as care for the flourishing of individuals in all their diversity.

THE SUFFERING OF THE STATISTICAL OUTLIER

Whatever their demerits, modern information systems can also reveal the cracks in those very systems. In response to a scandalous case of mistreatment in the Winterbourne View home for mentally disabled people uncovered by the BBC in 2011,[9] the British prime minister, David Cameron, convened a wide-ranging special inquiry into the state of care given to learning impaired or mentally disabled people in the U.K. Its findings were released in March 2013 as the *Confidential Inquiry into Premature Deaths of People with Learning Disabilities*, the CIPOLD report.[10] A research team from the University of Bristol comprehensively studied two years' worth of mortality statistics for a population of over 1.6 million people in the southwest of England.[11] Their aim was to build a picture of the incidence of premature or preventable deaths among mentally disabled people. Building on a string of similar reports going back well over a decade,[12] the commission sought concrete data on whether mentally disabled or learning-impaired individuals were being systematically discriminated against by the National Health Service (NHS).

The report found that mentally disabled people still die much earlier and more unexpectedly than the majority population.[13] Researchers also found that, statistically speaking, the more severe the mental disability, the higher the likelihood of an early death from a preventable cause. Broader analysis revealed, in addition, that people with learning disabilities were statistically underweight (a contributor to early death), suffered from more preventable conditions than the general population (such as pressure sores or acid reflux), and were unlikely to have had regular health checks or health plans. For the minority of individuals who had been given integrated health plans, the commission found that the use made of these "personalized health plans" was more often to hold patients to account for self-care than for the purpose for which they were originally designed—to coordinate disjointed health-care provision. Most importantly, "reasonable adjustments" to the normal ways of providing health care for those with special needs were rarely and certainly not routinely made, meaning that a whole range of practical barriers often derailed effective diagnosis and treatment.[14]

After examining 247 deaths of people with learning disabilities during the study's two-year window, the commission found that the majority of what they called premature or preventable deaths were not caused by caregivers overlooking or ignoring the distress of an ill person.[15] The fatal problems arose when medical professionals failed to offer a timely and accurate diagnosis and/or a workable treatment plan.[16] Two cases illustrate recurrent difficulties. The first concerns a *problem of information flow*. When taken to the hospital with respiratory problems, Robert had no one who knew his story present during the diagnosis process.

> Robert was found to be unwell by his care home staff and they called the out-of-hours doctor. He was taken to hospital unaccompanied, so the information that he had possibly been aspirating food and fluids was not passed on. Robert had an ECG but no chest X-ray or blood tests and was then returned home. His assessment at that time was deficient, given the lack of a clear history and his significant co-morbidities. Robert continued to have respiratory problems and was seen twice over the weekend by the out-of-hours doctors and prescribed antibiotics. On the Monday morning his own GP was asked to visit. She recognized his deterioration and admitted him to the hospital, but his pneumonia was described as "severe" by this stage with a complete "white out" of 1 lung. Robert's condition deteriorated and it is possible that an earlier diagnosis of his pneumonia might have prevented his premature death.[17]

A second case reveals a related aspect of the problem. Even when medical personnel do have some version of the story of a patient's sickness, the limits of people with learning difficulties can lead to *hasty or incorrect diagnoses* of their presenting symptoms.

> Henry was taken into A&E at about 8am. His sister reported to the CIPOLD nurse that the hospital staff had been convinced that Henry had had a seizure and did not listen to his family when they said that it

> was something different. His sister recalled suggesting to the hospital staff that Henry had either had a stroke or a brain haemorrhage. His sister said: "I am no medical expert but I said he's bleeding from his nose and from his mouth and they said that he had probably bitten his tongue while he was fitting. Mum kept saying that she didn't see a fit and it wasn't a seizure bearing in mind that she has been doing this for however many years . . . I said to the nurse something is not right . . . he is in pain . . . and they said no he's not . . . They took him up for the MRI scan. It all changed then didn't it? They were very nice to us then, let's go into the side room and all that business . . . Of course, it was a haemorrhage wasn't it? All she could say to us was that she was very sorry. It seems like yesterday because I felt that I had let him down. I hadn't fought his corner hard enough to say it's not what you think it is. You are just looking on the papers, in the textbook . . . he has collapsed so he has got epilepsy. You are not listening to my Mum and she was his main carer but all they could say was that they were sorry. They were sorry because they had missed it and that it had taken so long and that he had been in pain from 7am until 5pm."[18]

The authors of the report indicate that this was not an isolated story and concluded, "For some people, it appeared that once a provisional diagnosis had been made, it prevented doctors from having an open mind and challenging the provisional diagnosis as symptoms developed."[19]

For similar reasons people with intellectual disabilities have very low rates of participation in routine medical screening regimens. Without "reasonable adjustments" to routine protocols being made, procedures like the preventative screening that is offered to all patients when they reach a certain age can easily become too unwieldy for staff or caregivers, or too distressing for patients. Similar problems emerge when doctors prescribe complex treatment regimens or assume that everyone is capable of keeping up with difficult hospital checkup appointment schedules.[20] In many cases mentally disabled people's "social care providers appeared to be neither equipped nor resourced to chase up appointments or monitor [the person's] progress through so many different systems, and there was no one else to do this on [his or her] behalf."[21] In addition to these hurdles, many people with learning difficulties and their caregivers were often unaware of the services that might be available to ameliorate some of these difficulties.[22]

It is now evident in a more rounded way how, at least in southern England, the culture of hospitals is configured in a manner that assumes that the "average" patient can be counted on to present their own symptoms and deal with the waiting, discomfort, and logistics it takes to secure their own care. The system as a whole is geared toward the statistically normal patient, and if an individual's specific mental disability makes the system threatening or inaccessible, the evidence suggests that the statistical outliers will simply be ignored, solidifying their invisibility as appropriate recipients of the routine health care statutorily due to every citizen of the modern nation state.

One of the report's most pointed conclusions was that a core deficiency in healthcare provision for mentally disabled people is a desperate lack of advocates. Advocacy at least entails presenting the story of the patient's suffering, but, the report suggests, would also include being willing and capable of pressing medical professionals to revisit and revise diagnoses and care plans. Yet the evidence stands that those who did play the role of an advocate in this way regularly reported that they felt they were not listened to.[23] To make matters even worse, the commission found that over a quarter of intellectually disabled people have no one who even knows their story over a long enough period to act as their healthcare advocate.[24] The report suggested several structural changes, but one core aspect of the commission's recommendations was that more formal ways had to be found to remedy this knowledge deficit, a solution that would need to be combined with a willingness on the part of medical professionals to listen first to the patients themselves, then to advocates, and to adjust their usual practices in order to circumvent some of the more obvious problems that normal routines cause for individual people with mental disabilities.[25]

FROM LISTENING TO SYSTEMS

Becoming a doctor today means being socialized into "care systems" that demand thinking within an algorithmic diagnostic logic. The rise to dominance of the expertise model of medical knowledge has made the research physician king, displacing older apprenticeship models of medical training. The prestige of the master clinician has deflated as their pedagogical role has been squeezed out of medical training. It is difficult to be a high performer at both laboratory bench and bedside. As a result, the role of trust and clinical listening is rarely modeled for medical students and is not treated as an essential aspect of good diagnostic procedure.[26]

The shifting of pedagogical practice toward testing is grounded in the evolution of medical knowledge. Examination has shifted from listening to the patient's account of their body's changes to the skilled deployment of tools to listen to body parts or systems. A dangerous illusion now easily arises among recent generations of doctors: that medical tests can mechanically determine correct treatments. This is to misplace diagnostic certainty. Comprehensiveness in medical testing cannot itself yield diagnostic certainty, as if the sum of all known tests would yield an unambiguous diagnosis. Modern medical tests are calibrated to detect normal ranges of human functioning, though the *fact* that large numbers of people's bodies work one way establishes no *normative* claim about how any one body should be.[27] It is thus impossible to prove how general normal ranges relate to the normal range of an individual body, nor do anomalous value ranges automatically indicate any linkage to a presenting complaint.[28] The often observed tendency for tests to proliferate marks the impossibility of generating diagnostic certainty by tests alone.

> Remember that tests are defined according to 95 percent of people who fall into the "normal" range, meaning that 5 present of people who actually have no problems will end up being "abnormal" based on their test. . . . [in addition] rules [for routine administration of tests] are established on populations, not on individuals: they may work for "most" people between ages twenty and fifty, but not all—and you may be the exception. Also, rules typically have arbitrary cut offs. Many rules, for example, use a specific age as a criterion, or heart rate. But does it make sense that someone who just turned 65 has to have an X-ray, but if their injury occurred last week, they were OK without one? Or that a patient with a heart rate of 99 beats per minute is fine, but if the heart rate goes up to 100, they suddenly need a blood test?[29]

In short, medical tests may well reveal "abnormal" values, but this may be unrelated to or not the source of the presenting complaint. Close attention to the specific contours of the presenting complaint may suggest tests that routine protocols may miss.

In the final analysis, modern diagnostic testing can never achieve certainty without recovering older practices of close listening to patient histories. The "open listening" demanded by taking histories does not come easily to medical students who have been systematically trained to ask yes-no questions as they proceed through diagnostic decision-making trees. But this retraining remakes the partnership between doctor and patient, because the modern algorithmic account of diagnosis evacuates patients' self-descriptions of medical meaning. Because the symptom has become a *proxy* for patient narratives, only engaging patient histories can offer a firm basis for building working theories about the illness at stake. Working hypotheses are in fact the ground of any diagnostic certainty because they should *guide* the ordering of medical tests. Supple history may even reveal that the "chief complaint" does not even have a physical cause. There is a moral imperative for doctors to keep asking questions until they have a working diagnosis *before* they order tests, and patients should gently tempt their doctor to look more deeply into a patient's history to aid better diagnosis.[30]

Some doctors may find this description of the problems that attend medicine-by-test, and the proposal that doctor-patient relationships require much higher levels of communication and openness, a seductive fantasy, since "most acutely ill people just want an experienced person to take over, to do what has to be done and do it fast."[31] It is certainly more psychologically complex for a doctor to approach a patient holding the mantle of expert lightly. For medical professionals to admit up front that their diagnoses are hypotheses shakes the carefully constructed edifice of medical expertise. But when the medical professional dons the mantle of doctor-as-expert, he or she also quashes the free speaking of patients (and caregivers).[32] In the final analysis, there are substantial moral reasons to avoid donning the role of the scientific expert. When medical professionals assert the "inviolability of expertise" they set up barriers to the honest communication that is crucial to good health care and which is a significant contributor to litigation against doctors when things end up going wrong.[33]

The CIPOLD report also highlighted the lack of advocates for mentally disabled people, the difficulties surrounding their communication of pain, and their apparent inability to advocate for their own interests in healthcare contexts. It is unlikely that a patient who is incapable of narrating their own complaint would be capable of the even more taxing work of pushing doctors to get a correct diagnosis or to follow a complex treatment regimen. Such problems multiply when caregivers find themselves in the position of feeling morally responsible to undertake this work. Such caregivers may not even be legal guardians in emergency situations. The CIPOLD report concludes that the inability of a patient to speak is no excuse for a medic to forgo trying to discover a patient's story. More knowledgeable advocates are needed, and adjustments simply must be made if a more serious, extended, and open-ended listening is to be achieved among doctors.

Yet such close listening to particular patients not only goes against the grain of the practical processes in modern medical systems, but even against the internalized self-understanding of most doctors and patients. A historical account can clarify how this has become the default setting in modern medicine and therefore where a response to it might fruitfully begin.

What is often called Hippocratic medicine (medicine before the eighteenth century in the West), understood the task of medical diagnosis to be a matter of listening to nature. The modern concept of health did not exist, and it was assumed that bodies healed themselves. The patient's narration of their experience of their own bodies thus offered the necessary clues to find the blockage keeping a natural body from healing itself. The physician was listening for a clue about how to help a patient open that blockage and using the power of the healing word (counsel and sympathy) to encourage and reinforce nature performing its own work of healing. Only occasionally were pills or powders (which today appear highly poisonous) or other basic treatments prescribed.

In the late eighteenth century, medicine was reconceived as a practice of using tools to listen more closely to aspects of the body (such as the heartbeat, though counting heartbeats arose only in the nineteenth century) and of using tools to intervene in the functioning of some organ understood to be malfunctioning (such as surgery or forceps). Thus, the picture of the body and of the doctor-patient relationship radically changes. A doctor is defined as someone who deploys tools to fix organ systems that the expert knows how to diagnose but the patient does not.[34] The doctor is both the expert in developing and deploying diagnostic tools (and here we must understand the development of these tools into the whole sophisticated battery of mechanical and chemical means of testing the body) and the expert in intervention via tools into the functioning of bodily parts or systems (whether chemically, through drugs, or surgically).

The tool-using model of medicine is now in the midst of a third turn, the turn to the body-as-system. Here the body is conceived as an extraordinarily complex arrangement of feedback loops. The fundamental feature of the body so conceived is that it is understood as driven to survive by maintaining an informational balance.[35] Machines that can visualize changes in biological functions over time become necessary to make the feedback loops and information flows of the body visible to both the patient and doctor. Now a healthy body is *only* knowable best through the tools of testing and the conceptuality of probability and is, *by definition*, not susceptible to meaningful narration by the patient. The probabilistic account of health yielded the contemporary assumption that the patient's account of their own experience only points to testable patterns lying beyond the patient's perception of their own body arises. To be healthy is reduced to patterns of the firing of the muscles of the heart, for instance, or of the body reaching optimal states of chemical balance or temperature.

The doctor as systems analyst has arrived at the opposite pole to the Hippocratic doctor, who had engaged the body much like a good theater audience at a tragedy. The Hippocratic doctor listened to the complaint of the patient to perceive the singularity of this distinct patient, with his or her uniquely configured palette of physical sensations and mental narratives about the sequences of those sensations. Such engaged attempts to narrate the body of the patient have been displaced by the tragicomedy of modern medical practice in which patients and doctors alike are both far too comfortable using yes-no question-and-answer modes of relating "symptoms." Patient and doctor alike have internalized views of the body as seen through medical tests and visualization techniques. Listening to the experience of one's own body has been so devalued that neither patients nor doctors know any longer how this experience is relevant for medical caring. Both have been decisively configured by the contemporary framework of knowledge.[36]

If the experience of one's own body was in fact irrelevant for diagnosis and treatment, we would expect those who are unable to articulate their experience of their own bodies be the perfect patients of modern medicine. That they are not exposes the reality that the modern diagnostic emphasis on the function of bodily systems and organs is, in fact, always precariously suspended above, and reliant on, the safety net of the earlier modes of diagnostic listening. Though modern physician training has in effect deskilled practitioners in the practical arts of listening to patient stories and whole bodies, the attempt to live by testing alone is so fraught with complications that these older and more time-consuming forms of listening remain indispensable in health care of real quality. The CIPOLD report is not only revealing of a range of injustices in modern systems of care for people with mental disabilities, but in fact exposes a problem at the heart of modern medicine: *devaluing listening makes it impossible to respond to nonstandard cases*. To begin to unravel the unnoticed brutalities of modern "humane" medical institutions will demand reexamining the configuration of medical knowledge and its role in constructing the bodies and patients that are assumed to be normal and functioning in our modern developed societies. Doctors gentled by engaging patients with disability might be the promise of a gentler medicine.[37]

RECOVERING QUALITY LIFE

These problems are not new. Solutions have been offered from within the systems-logic characteristic of modern healthcare institutions as well as the doctor-patient relationships that unfold within them. In a medical context, the phrase "quality of life" is an umbrella term for a wide range of efforts continually to improve modern health care.[38] The so-called Quality Adjusted Life Year (or QUALY) is a mode of economic assessment that aims to scientifically rationalize economic allocation decisions within larger medical institutions. The basic assumption of the QUALY is that it is possible for healthcare institution managers to calculate how many good years can be purchased for the most people by making judicious funding allocation decisions.[39]

The phrase "quality of life" has many nuances of meaning in the English language, a rich universe of connotations overlaying its deceptively simple basic reference to "a good life." More so in American than in British English, the phrase refers to "the degree of emotional, intellectual, or cultural satisfaction in a person's everyday life as distinct from the degree of material comfort."[40] In popular usage the definition expresses a quest to discern how money can be spent in a way that produces an overall effect that is aesthetically pleasing—discussions that the financially comfortable middle classes enter when dreaming of vacations or buying second homes. But even the narrower usage of the phrase in British English highlights the term's linguistic capacity to designate lives of "quality" as distinct from less desirable lives. The drive to compare life with life likewise underlies the more technical meaning that the phrase has acquired within healthcare sectors.[41]

Disability and especially mental disability are a dark background for this language, the worst-case quality of life scenario that allows a "good" life to stand out as a bright and attractive foreground.[42] The clashing of the semantic fields of "quality of life" and "disability" is a clear marker of a rift in the contemporary social order. One of the paradoxes of modern QUALY language is that it has arisen to serve allocation decisions in the medical domain, the very domain in which those it assesses to have the lowest quality of life have the worst experiences of their lives, however stoically they may bear it.[43]

To remain present with the mentally disabled is to discover a radically different order of values than those assumed in the continuums that drive both the bourgeois and the QUALY moral calculus. Yet both the QUALY and the sense of a good life available to the intellectually disabled remain concerned in their own ways with *livable* lives. An investigation that remains present with people labeled disabled will call for a less pragmatic and more comprehensive account of quality of life.

Most intellectual disabilities make themselves visible in gesture, gait, and speech, and to live with these conditions is to live a life of being the object of the stare of passersby in most public spaces. To be different is to stand out, to attract attention. To be a member of a tiny group is to be a statistical outlier and therefore to attract a certain curious gaze that may be a normal human reflex, innocent and involuntary. One's very body consigns one to the fate of living life as one who is looked at.

At the same time, in a medical context this same statistical outlier status renders people with disabilities *invisible*. Social and political systems, and most medical systems, are organized to meet efficiently the medical needs of the masses. Standardized health care demands standardized patients. Modern medicine is so powerful and rife with normalizing trajectories because it is industrially organized. But it will never well serve people who cannot answer letters or get to doctors' appointments or vote on their own. Disabled people are rendered invisible, and this invisibility will become routine. It is this routine invisibility that is the most determinative feature of the quality of lives available to people with disabilities in modern societies which has for some decades now been the target of disability rights movements.

These considerations render it prudent to resist quality-of-life language. Its deployment as a technical term in medical contexts must be strictly contained by a highly nuanced set of caveats. If these are not in good order, the language will drive toward severe truncations of healthcare allocation decisions. Furthermore, the phrase is only useful if it remains firmly connected to an older tradition in medicine, in which the core task of medical care is understood as serving the well-functioning of corporeal beings holistically understood.[44] The quest of utilitarian moral theorists to find an algorithm that can ensure the health of that institution subtly ceases to ask about the "quality of life" of patients in favor of a question of the quality of *the healthcare system* typical of industrialized systems theory.[45] System logic strips the somatic experience of living in a body out of quality-of-life definitions since such experiences can only be articulated by patients in day-to-day language. It is a shift into system thinking that inevitably generates comparisons between people that are prejudicial to people with disabilities.

The QUALY allocation mechanism thus imbeds the devaluation of listening and attention that characterizes system-think at the level of the doctor-patient relationship. "Quality" is broken up into portions to allow lives and even parts of lives to be weighed against one another and then aggregated with the aim of making healthcare systems function more efficiently and economically.[46] Even medical care is broken up, no longer residing in a doctor-patient relationship but in the provision of discrete caring acts that can be performed by anyone. The interpersonal and political are thus removed from the definition of medicine.[47] With its reliance on algorithms, the QUALY allocation mechanism promises to render obsolete the close listening to *political* discussions that alone can decide what a given society will account as acceptable health care. Rational healthcare allocation is not any more susceptible to automatic processing than are medical tests. There are configurations of healthcare systems that we might defend as *rational*, but which are nevertheless *unjust*.[48]

Which sorts of healthcare expenditures should be prioritized in healthcare systems is a question that will never be reducible to sheer medical criteria, as the QUALY model assumes.[49] The fact that people do continue to recognize and give care to those who will only minimally benefit from that care, most obviously the elderly and disabled, makes the claim of justice on the shape modern health care has taken all the more visible.[50] To offer the care and attention that will help a stroke patient relearn to button their own shirt may never make sense within reasoning that aims for maximal economic rationalization, but a wide range of people nevertheless do still think this is care worth rendering. The covert understanding of justice that underlies this constant stream of gratuitous human care bears explicit articulation: precisely because some people are vulnerable and outliers, they are owed a special solicitude. Even, *especially*, when very little can be done, this moral burden lies most heavily.[51]

The felt obligation of many people to care for the most vulnerable is not intelligible within the logic of modern medical systems, in which it inevitably appears as an inefficient or unproductive use of healthcare resources. It is more theologically appropriate to understand such efforts as instead lying at the heart of a humane medicine. The sympathy, compassion, and care that keeps faith with those who are approaching death or are mentally disabled represents a refusal to define the human as being fit, strong, and productive. Once again, a link emerges between justice and human fidelity that rests on God's merciful fidelity to humanity. To care in fidelity to those who seem hopelessly unable to repay that care is a response of gratitude for God having already shown Godself to be faithful to us.[52]

***

CODA: PART 3

Over forty years ago Jacques Ellul proposed that it was essential for Christian political witness that Christians provoke common people to push back "upwards" against the systems that impose denuding orders on human life. Addressing common people without great education or ambition, but who remain open, spontaneous, and compassionate, is politically promising. If given a little teaching, "he or she is relatively better prepared than intellectuals, technical experts, and executives to take the values of life seriously."[53]

Parents, caregivers, and allies of people with disabilities almost certainly find themselves in a disproportionately important role today. From the Christmas party to the funeral, any gathering of families, caregivers, or friends of the severely disabled will find conversation eventually turning to tip swapping about how to negotiate the intricacies of healthcare systems. In the United States this discussion often orbits around the severe problem of securing adequate funding for complex care, and in the United Kingdom, to the labyrinth of Self-Directed Support or Direct Payment infrastructures. Knowledge about hospitals, schools, and government officials who listen well, or do not listen at all, is laboriously collated. When caregivers and companions themselves do not feel heard, they will find it safe to assume that those officials will not be attending closely enough to the vulnerable and inarticulate lives to whom they are bound. A motley but politically promising group finds itself drawn together across all kinds of other ideological differences in this politics of hope.[54]

Parents, caregivers, and allies by necessity must become experts in resisting the *tyranny of the expert*, since their lives are deeply shaped by the quest to find a professional who can take the particularities of a unique person seriously.[55] To the extent that medicine has been configured on an expertise model, the burden of proof is shifted onto parents who might suggest (whether erroneously or not) that any given child has in the past not conformed to the expected laws of averages. Medical professionals will very often assume that laypeople's perceptions of etiologies and drug effects may not be informed enough to serve as a basis for medical judgment. Behind this will often lie the deeper, sometimes legitimate suspicion that the views of parents and caregivers have been clouded by their investment in the person needing treatment. Constantly up against such challenges, parents and caregivers sooner or later give up hope for miracles, in exchange for the far more mundane quest to find caring professionals who will treat them or their loved ones like a person.[56] Parents, caregivers, and allies of people with disabilities are at bottom seeking something that lies at the heart of any interpersonal act of care: a proper collaborative discussion in which both parties recognize the value of the other's knowledge.

The conversations of the gathered community of parents and caregivers confirm Ellul's insight into the political power of the nonexpert's more rounded view of health. Such conversations are the deepest stratum of *politics*, because it is out of such forums, in which goods held in common are discovered and shared, that all truly political engagement must come. The political impact of such conversation is immediately discernable. Parents and caregivers are learning how to advocate for their loved ones' best interests more probingly and intelligently. They are learning to articulate in concrete healthcare settings the inadequacies of generic healthcare regimens and systems.

The *politics of hope* embodied in this investigation by caregivers and companions rests on an acute awareness of the need to find actors within the institutions of modern health care who genuinely care—and that this is essentially not only for the flourishing of their loved ones but even, in some cases, for their very survival. A politics of hope so configured cannot but challenge the smooth and efficient functioning of medical-care systems and even the medical model itself. Medical personnel are challenged to invest themselves in getting to the root of the bodily suffering of mentally disabled people, and to be prepared to bend or subvert the medical system if necessary. The politics of hope is also an implacable enemy of the complacency that makes no special efforts to fight systemic features that keep disabled people boxed out and invisible or offer "more testing" or pacifying treatments instead of taking the time to hear stories and build a patient history.[57]

The politics of hope is also political in a more subtle and far-reaching way. Such a community gives succor and encouragement to those in modern (industrialized) healthcare systems who sense that somehow all is not quite as it should be. Where medical systems might roll over the nonverbal or inarticulate patient relatively easily, the advocate who speaks on behalf of the patient can help to provoke healthcare professionals to slow down, to look and listen again. In this way advocates offer a service to the whole political community. In resisting the smooth and infinite expansion of standardizing and efficiency-seeking behavior in modern industrialized expertise-driven systems, this resistance ultimately benefits everyone.

Part 3 has highlighted how the interface between the *expert and the layperson* is the most problematic territory for parents of and caregivers for the intellectually disabled. Family practitioners, along with nurses, can be especially effective allies of parents and caregivers in occupying a liminal, anomalous role in the context of modern medicine. Though family practitioners and nurses have been inculcated into the modern medical gaze and its esoteric technical language, their liminal role makes it easier for them to spot when the mantle of the expert is proving a barrier to engaging patients and caregivers. Since they have contact with patients over much longer periods of time, family practitioners and nurses have a vantage point from which the narratives about healthy states and episodes of sickness of the vulnerable are much more easily heard. Family practitioners and nurses thus possess a much greater capacity to help parents and caregivers see symptoms and developments better, as well as to empower them to play more constructive roles in the healthcare partnership.

Christians ought to consider what it would mean to add their voices as *advocates* for those who must negotiate the healthcare system alone. The CIPOLD report starkly illustrated how important it is that people become involved in advocacy for "the least of these" in medical contexts, not least to draw attention to the need for, and importance of, more collaborative health care. Outliers and their caregivers live under immense stress simply by being nonstandard. It is a travesty that Christians are not known for their work as buddies of disabled people negotiating modern care institutions. Those rare churches who have come alongside individuals and families, discerning the stresses of securing care for those with mental health issues and mental disabilities, serve God's redemptive embrace of those suffering under the glare of the gods of the age.[58] Such witnesses are all too rare, however, the Western church having largely internalized the normalizing gaze of modernity. Its professional theologians have fared little better, generally not being in possession of theologies supple and interested enough to take the full diversity of human bodies and minds seriously.[59]

At the heart of the problems of the field of health care today are *problems of communication*. Part 3 has drawn attention to the drastic impact of problems in communication on the day-to-day lives of people labeled disabled. Taking the time to hear is ultimately a matter of attending to bodies, of taking the creaturely tangibility of people seriously. Jesus' parable about the Samaritan's responsivity to the neighbor's vulnerable body foregrounds the moral centrality of attentiveness to bodies in time and place. Responding bodily to another body is a form of praise of the body's Creator and an agreement to be an agent of that body's Sustainer. If skillful health care is grounded in recognition of the importance of bodily particularity, it is intrinsically connected with forms of communication characterized by bilateral speech as well as partnership in diagnosis and treatment. The inequities that are evident in modern healthcare systems are ones that are susceptible to theological analysis because they are grounded in the goodness of creation, and intrinsically related to the problem of interhuman estrangement.

Only against the backdrop of human *estrangement from God* does interhuman estrangement become fully intelligible. The Christian doctrine of the *fall* helps explain why gaps and problems are endemic in interhuman communication, as well as the reflexive resistance that flares up when people feel they are not being listened to. Fear and uncertainty inevitably arise when people find themselves in an I-it relation with a "healthcare provider." The fall also helps to explicate why broken patterns of noncommunication become institutionalized. The constellation of institutionalized barriers to close listening has several unique components today: utilitarian economic rationality, the ideology of expertise, technological and algorithmic systems thinking, bureaucratic processes, and fears about legal threats, to name some of the most prominent. It is a theological claim to say that *compassionate attentive listening cuts against the powers that be in every age*.

The recognition and valuation of the diversity and particularity of creation grows from a theological hermeneutic of creaturely life with deeply political import. In lavishing full and conscientious love on one particular creature in creation, humans are given—whether parents, medical personnel, or farmers—special insights in the pathologies and relative faithfulness of the societies they inhabit. For those who grant that the issue at stake is how properly to care for created particularities, a proper *doctrine of creation* which valorizes diversity and attending to this diversity should play an important role in deciding how and why doctors and parents should converse and collaborate in the interests of any given individual. To affirm the created particularity of any given person bars caregivers, parents, or medics from claiming the exhaustive knowledge necessary for genuinely healing care.[60] By fully investing themselves in their vocation, they challenge those in contiguous vocations to face the ways society's self-understandings may constitute embodied rejections of the Creator.

A genuinely theological account of the quality of any *individual* creaturely life must not be disengaged from the richness of that person's life in *community*. Because those labeled mentally disabled today do not easily mask their loneliness, they announce the theological heart of the matter: human beings were made to be at home in reconciled community. Part 5 will elaborate what is entailed when Christians confess that the church is a community defined by its circulation of the *gifts of the Spirit*, in which people understand themselves as "the body of Christ and individually members of it." *In the church fullness of life is defined communally and communicatively*: "If one member suffers, all suffer together with it; if one member is honored, all rejoice together with it" (1 Cor 12:26, cf. Rom 12:15). Before engaging this peculiar togetherness of the church, part 4 lingers a bit longer with the theological reality of the fundamental problem of sin. The power of sin resides in the malformed love people have for habits that isolate them and alienate them from embracing their own particularity, and the particularity of others. Love of being isolated is not something easily remedied. Only a wonder can save us.

PART IV

THE EVERYDAYNESS OF MERCY AND WONDER

7

Health in a Fallen World

RESISTING WONDER

The desire to build societies that are progressively more humane for disabled people is one of modern Westerners' most closely held moral aspirations. It has only one devastating drawback: many of those whom progressive disability policies were meant to serve experience their deployment as a politics of humiliation.

> "Disability," marked from the get-go with that hissing "dis," is not a liberative identity. "Disability" is a disqualification, a sociocultural construction based in economics and couched in aesthetics and medicine that precedes one. To identify another as "disabled" is always already to submit that person to the politics of humiliation.[1]

That the very term disability can provoke such diametrically opposed assessments exposes the most fundamental, and difficult, questions any theological account of disability must face.

Part 4 addresses two of these root problems. In theological terms, disability discourse as it operates today is a law that can never justify, only condemn. A first clue that it is a condemning law is the unreality of its definitional baseline, the "normal" people who stand at its heart.[2] This spectral figure establishes "ability" as the orienting frame of reference. These are well-known critiques that have nevertheless done little to undermine the prereflexive assumptions held by most people in modern developed societies. For the masses, some human beings simply appear, indisputably, *as disabled*. Though the label "disability" has clear social utility in many practical contexts, a liberation is necessary from the reification of that practical usage into a concept of disability conceived as an ontological state. When disability is considered an ontological state, its use to designate those who have practical needs becomes an act of social othering. This deeper problem is one rooted in the sinful human heart, with its power to orient a hermeneutic stance in the world. We have come to the pivotal theological problematic presented by disability: *human beings need to be rescued from seeing themselves as fundamentally "able."* The Christian doctrine of sin names the impossibility of breaking this habit through sheer force of will.

What is often called "salvation" is another name for the working of God's mercy to break the power of sin. The theme of salvation leads into the other main theme of part 4, to be taken up in more detail in chapter 8: those who know themselves as having been recipients of divine mercy find their lives oriented as they respond to its appearance. Faith generates a theological hermeneutic for perceiving human life and bodies, discipleship being the sanctifying day-to-day work of responding to the divine claim.[3]

Disability is a phenomenon closely associated with a feeling of psychological shock. What is less clear is how those shocks are best named. They have been variously labeled "adjustments to reduced life chances," "identity transitions," or perhaps "failures to cope." The seriousness of a theological account of disability will be revealed by how directly this aspect of the disability experience is addressed. Facing sin is not only psychologically taxing, but theologically difficult as well, as one Irish priest discovered.

> Alan . . . is a young man in his late teens. He cannot speak, walk, or do anything at all for himself. His eyes never meet yours. He lives in a world of his own. Because he was relatively small and thin, carrying him was not too difficult. Until he chose not to co-operate. . . . This would often happen in the course of dressing or undressing him, making the task almost impossible. . . . Then I'd find myself boiling inside. Wanting to shake him, scream at him, or just throw him there! His going on strike, as it were, aroused in me the impulse to strike out at him. . . . This deeply wounded man who had been abandoned soon after birth, fatherless, motherless, belonging to nobody, ought to have aroused in me the deepest compassion and pity and love . . . but no. He revealed to me rather a darker self, that part which years of education and respectability had taught me to pack away carefully to the point that I had almost forgotten it existed. . . . My plan had been to be good to him. To give to him. Instead of that it was he who gave to me—a short, sharp lesson in the truth; the truth about myself. The hard and vulnerable truth;

> self-righteous, sinful, proud and not so graciously accepting the loss of youth and its powers.[4]

It is already a sign of having disempowered those perceived as disabled if such a story is heard to imply that people labeled disabled are free of the need for this same painful confrontation.

> Annette had learned to be helpless through years of being controlled by other people and through living the assigned role of "invalid." . . . Annette was bound by behaviour and thought patterns which made her unfree, that somewhere she had learned a script, which she lived, a script that told her she was of little value and no good at anything. Her true self was imprisoned. . . . I longed for her liberation . . . I cannot say when or how Annette started to choose differently. Annette's behaviour drove me "bananas" in those first few years. . . . but it taught me to confront my own baggage, to excavate some of the material in my own depths that caused me to be unfree. Over time it was clear to me that Annette and I were very alike—except that she, in her innocence and transparency, was unable to hide her faults, while I kept mine well hidden, even from myself.[5]

Disability precipitates crises of self-knowledge and brings sin to the surface. *Sin is an irreducible part of a theology of disability because theology has a concern with the misperceptions arising from living a lie in relation to one's self.*[6]

The Jewish theologian Franz Rosenzweig began just here, by emphasizing that God's merciful address *only* comes to people caught up in lies about themselves. Dietrich Bonhoeffer agrees: the condescending love of God in Christ Jesus is not addressed to people's "ideal" selves, the assumedly perfected sides of their personalities, but drives deep into their particularly configured fallen personas. In being confronted by God the agent is propelled beyond questions of *whether* or *how* God reclaims a sinful world into more personal questions about how the one who finds themselves so confronted should now *discern* and *respond to* God's ever-proximate working.[7] Brought face-to-face with their sin, human beings can begin to ask how God might be transforming them. It is important to explore these redemptive inversions of perception more closely, asking how the moment of conviction that calls for repentance comes alive in individuals so that they learn to welcome it, and even seek it, in the day-to-day.

Both Rosenzweig and Bonhoeffer assume that life with God is the healthiest possible state for human beings, a theme deeply woven through Scripture. The Old Testament traditions define human health with the term *shalom*, which is typically translated "peace" but primarily indicates the state of being in a right relationship with a personal God. This *shalom* is gifted by God and received by humans, who are brought into a state of security, friendship, prosperity, and justice. The New Testament depicts Israel's God arriving as shalom peace in the person of Jesus Christ, who liberates captives of all types and brings people into fullness of life. Being "himself our peace," Jesus' essential work is the rescuing of human beings out of a living death.[8]

From an Old Testament perspective, the twist in the story of Yahweh's peace arriving in Jesus is the appearance of the cross. Healing comes as human beings are incorporated into Jesus' *death*, which releases them from the living death of sin. As St. Paul puts in his letter to the Colossians, Jesus

> is the image of the invisible God, the firstborn of all creation; for in him all things in heaven and on earth were created . . . through him and for him . . . . he is the beginning, the firstborn from the dead, so that he might come to have first place in everything. . . . When you were buried with him in baptism, you were also raised with him through faith in the power of God, who raised him from the dead. And when you were dead in trespasses and the uncircumcision of your flesh, God made you alive together with him . . . So if you have been raised with Christ, seek the things that are above, where Christ is, seated at the right hand of God. Set your minds on things that are above, not on things that are on earth, for you have died, and your life is hidden with Christ in God. . . . You have stripped off the old self with its practices and have clothed yourselves with the new self, which is being renewed in knowledge according to the image of its creator. (Col 1:15, 16, 18; 2:12-13; 3:1-3, 9-10)

A complex web of theological linkages is set out here. Jesus Christ is called the image of God. He is also called the origin and end of creation. The ascended Christ is presented as drawing the gaze of Christians above their day-to-day lives, and that this looking up somehow leads to their receiving their own true and redeemed form from God. Furthermore, through mechanisms that are unspecified, Christians' alterations of daily practices are designated as the mechanism for their becoming living images of the Creator.[9]

On the surface Paul's rejoinder to Christians to set their minds on things above seems calculated to exacerbate dissatisfaction with their mundane lives. But both Paul and Bonhoeffer seem to think exactly the opposite.[10] For Bonhoeffer, these themes explicate how Jesus Christ draws creatures *into* rather than *out of* the world at the God-neighbor-creation intersection. "Today immensely important things will be decided by whether we Christians have strength enough to show the world that we are not dreamers and are not those who walk with their heads in the clouds, that we don't just let things come and go as they are, that our faith is really not the opium that lets us stay content in the midst of an unjust world, but that we, especially because we set our minds on things that are above, only *protest all the more tenaciously and resolutely on this earth*."[11]

I have introduced the theme of healing as an eschatological topic in chapter 3, and that theme will now be more closely investigated by asking how these complex theological affirmations situate a Christian understanding of health.[12] Christian theology is oriented by the premise that this bewildering set of considerations can be untangled only by those who gaze steadily on the One who is truly healthy, the sinless giver and saver of human life, Jesus Christ. As always, Jesus put the point much more pithily: "Healthy people don't need a physician" (Mark 2:17, ISV). The chapter will culminate in a brief reflection on how these claims position my own understanding of myself, God, and my son Adam. Adam, I will suggest, is the healthiest person I know in the way he reflects and disseminates the claim of the One truly healthy one, the One who lives at the heart of wonder.

Rosenzweig draws attention to wonder as an invitation to human beings to go deeper into life with God, other people, and all creation. In so doing he helps Christian theologians to appreciate a wider range of human experiences as means of Jesus Christ's appearing to claim enslaved and estranged human beings. Rosenzweig's theological reasoning thus resources Bonhoeffer's affirmation of the biblical promise that redemption is to receive fullness of life in *this* world—which the Christian understands as the truth of each person that is hidden in Jesus Christ. *Redemption is learning to receive the wonder of life, hearing the particular call that comes to each one in love.* When humans hear their names called out of love, the Christian tradition teaches them to hear it as an articulate claim of Jesus Christ, who is claiming them by name and *in this way* restoring them to their flourishing form as creatures. But an essential part of becoming liberated creatures is also to have been confronted with the sinful habits of evasion that are the infernal engine of human estrangement.

THE HEART OF WONDER

Franz Rosenzweig summarized his whole philosophy for common readers in the book he was working on when he died, *Understanding the Sick and the Healthy: A View of World, Man, and God*. Language of sickness, health, and paralysis recur in a book written during an illness so severe that he was often rendered sleepless by the cramping of his slowly decaying muscles. He had been stricken by the muscular degenerative disease amyotrophic lateral sclerosis (commonly known as Lou Gehrig's disease, or ALS) in earnest in his mid-thirties, which finally robbed him of his life at forty-three. With the ebbing of his voluntary muscle movement came the loss of the capacity to handwrite. He learned to type on a special typewriter. When he could no longer operate it, his wife Edith operated it for him. In the end he was reduced to having her recite letters of the alphabet until with minute gestures he indicated the letter he wanted.[13] An aphorism laboriously dictated in this manner near the end of his life summarizes his attitude toward his condition. "The sufferer alone is permitted to praise God in his works. But all men suffer."[14] Out of this debilitated state, the last message that this longstanding sufferer spent so much energy putting to paper comes as quite a surprise: he believed most physically healthy modern people are suffering from a mortal illness. That illness is an incapacity to appreciate and receive their creaturely lives with all their individual peculiarities—including their physical illnesses and incapacities.

Wonder and the wonderful are all around for Rosenzweig and should draw every human being deeper into engagement with their daily lives. The birth of a child is an obvious instance of the wonder of life, and this feeling of wonder helps to energize the hard work of parents to care for this often disruptive and frustrating new life. It is these processes of incorporating wonder through receptive action that Rosenzweig labels "living in the heart of wonder." Wonder lays its claim on people, demands they stay with its temporal unfolding. Post-Cartesian philosophers have made the mistake of responding by attempting to analyze and define what it "really" is. By searching for an essence, the living reality of the wonder of interpersonal relationships evaporates into ideas that are its ghostly mirror. Rosenzweig is disturbed by the rapidity with which the disease of detached observation has spread from professional philosophers to become the socialized norm of modern industrial societies. Its power is its promise to extract enduring and eternal moments from "mere" existence, and so escape the annihilation of individual meaning by time, finitude, and finally, death.[15]

Stalling in wonder is "the paralysis of artificial death," Rosenzweig suggests. What makes this paralysis "dead" is its power to cut the observer adrift from temporal progression. Wonder flares up in time, and attracting attention should then begin to draw people and reorient their action. In no longer looking for the living "heart of wonder," modern habits of mind become entrapped in modes of perception that do not pay the right types of attention. For temporal creatures, spotting the right moment to act is everything. The problem is that most modern people have been taught to look for eternal essences, not the happenings that matter.

It is useful to clarify why this apparently arcane philosophical problem is important for thinking about disability today. The dominant understandings of ethics in the contemporary Anglo-American context assume either that ethical claims are "personal beliefs" distinct from publicly provable facts or seeks to diffuse this subjectivization of ethics by making ethics a matter of universal duties and moral principles. Both types of view are organized by a fact-value distinction. By way of contrast, classical Greek thought not only had a much broader account of ethics but also assumed that a genuinely ethical life depended on a class of knowledge devalued by modern thought. The ancients assumed that real forms of practical knowledge were necessary for humans to act well. For them, knowing how to ride a bike or what an orange smells like is not simply *subjective* knowledge. Nor is riding a bike well a matter of knowing universal principles. It is possible to be certain about one's ability to ride a bike or capacity to recognize the smell of an orange even though it is difficult to prove this knowledge or describe it in words. Chapter 2 highlighted the importance of acknowledging kinesthetic intelligence when living with people with learning difficulties, most of their communication being bodily rather than verbal. People continually trust knowledge-how, not only for facilitating interactions with people who do not speak, but for all sorts of practical activities. Knowledge-how cannot be (as modern thought so often assumes) an inferior type of "merely subjective" knowledge. Knowledge-how is an intrinsic feature of acting in the world.[16]

If this knowledge-how is granted a substantive role in ethical thinking, the idea of wonder directing human action becomes far more intelligible. Again, the contrast with ancient thought is instructive. Greek philosophers of all stripes generally assumed that one might rightly claim to know that a genuine radiance or glory had manifest itself. The Greeks had no problem admitting that actions, events, objects, even people at times throw off an aura, a glow. They can be lit up from inside or light up things around them. It is possible for people to react well or badly to such showings. The Greeks admitted (as did patristic theologians like Augustine) the reality of an objective knowledge-how corresponding to the showing of a wonder, even though knowledge of this showing is of a type that cannot be argued for or defended in the manner of propositional knowledge. Wonder shocks, stings, and benumbs the one it befalls, an indubitably real experience. Wonder opens a fissure in an agent's certainty about the world by making a formerly hidden reality tangible. It can be cultivated and received, and so becomes a knowledge-how.[17]

Schooled in this more expansive ancient understanding of temporally saturated and agent-specific knowledge-how, Rosenzweig is attempting to direct attention to aspects of moral orientation that are ruled irrelevant in almost every domain of modern thought (often by applying the dismissive labels "anecdotal" or "subjective"). Such a dismissal substitutes mere formulas for a *life* that is saturated and oriented by a religious tradition. This is, for Rosenzweig, the "disease."

The cure, as Rosenzweig sees it, is for faith to become common sense. A proper relation to God is not dependent on having the right theory or intellectual conception of what God "really is." Nor is knowing God a matter of having a grasp of the essence of God, any more than a proper relation to other human beings or the world depends on having the right theoretical anthropology or cosmology. For him the central question of human life is not whether agents *know* things (that the world exists, for instance) but that they perceive and appropriately acknowledge the *right* things—such as that this person near me is in pain and needs consolation.[18]

Thus, for Rosenzweig, Judaism was not an *object* of study, but a *method* of studying all things, a way of exploring *life*.[19] To be Jewish is to insist that the concreteness of human life never be lost in thinking; to highlight the importance of the spoken word and dialogical relations, including gestures and other forms of communicative act; to emphasize the analytical importance of the experience of time and its rhythm and, in connection with it, the ability to wait; and finally the irreducible significance of the name, human and divine.[20] As time-saturated beings, the "highest," most profound, and momentous things in the lives of human beings are things that they *cannot* bring about, but which have to *come to* them and therefore which can only be awaited in readiness to receive them. Acknowledgement is something that can only be *enacted in a place and time*.[21]

All living is a responding to life known *as* something, avowing or receiving it under some name.[22] Naming is a primordial right of all human beings, and is constantly and forever exercised by every human: as Adam confronted things in creation and spoke names onto them, so also will his offspring (again this account includes gestures). Naming can express a gesture of grasping cooption when performed as an attempt to conjure the future, but it does not have to be, as Adam's naming in an unfallen creation suggests. After Eden, however, to name is to be constrained to embrace the historically congealed meanings of words, and because the created world always exceeds these names, social worlds are constantly adjusting their vocabulary.[23]

No human beings escape being embedded in linguistic relationships. *Someone's* names for things and events will be incorporated and shape individual's perceptions as they negotiate events and strive to integrate them into a coherent *life*. The only question is *which* language, *whose* story will provide the names that allow each person purchase on the events that befall them. To be part of a faith tradition is to have inherited names given to things by predecessors in that faith. By implication, the task of faith is the active work of appropriating within the smaller scenes of each person's lived experience God's words as the truth; about Godself, human beings and all creation.

The power of God's Word is the basis of these extravagant claims from Rosenzweig. Only sacred Scriptures purport to be words that can be trusted to be addressed to every human being.[24] Here Rosenzweig's account of Judaism converges with Christianity: both faith traditions endure in offering a particularly configured *way of life*. These ways of life do not maintain their vitality because followers adhere to a prescribed set of beliefs, rituals, or "rational" truths "liberated" from an archaic collection of stories.[25] Christianity and Judaism share a sense of both being traditions whose continuity is maintained by texts that each generation must find a way to inhabit.[26] Such inscripturated traditions are capable of being lived because their sacred texts point to a truth beyond those texts. Study of the scriptural text (*Gesetz*) brings it to life for the believer as something more than law—a bidding, a divine invitation (*Gebot*). Scriptures that speak of events long past in this way carry the youth of the world in teaching successive generations how to recognize the most determinative beginnings.

The commandments of the Torah derive their force by offering names for everyday life, not as a series of principles or theological doctrines about humanity, God, and the world. The irreducibly hermeneutic nature of living faith is killed when Scripture is read as presenting a set of generic rules or principles for living, placing the believer in a third-person relationship to God. Believers are being sensitized to the difference between responsibility to a relationship and living by a generic law in observing the ways that God's personal self-revelation in Scripture can be turned into a set of impersonal universal rules. To have seen how relationships can be turned into deadening rules is to be empowered to spot *a whole range of legal-social-symbolic imperatives that seek to govern human lives but differ in kind from God's inscripturated command, which is always the loving claim of personally invested divine mercy*.

The ethical potency of the theme of anomalous births, around which part 1 turned, now becomes more theologically intelligible. A child has been conceived and perhaps born. Everything turns on *what* this event will be named, how something that has befallen a person will be incorporated or resisted. The empirical scientists' narrative decrees it an accident, a random, morally meaningless glitch. Less often today the child will be perceived as a sign of the displeasure of God or of angry malevolent forces, so raising questions about who sinned—the disabled one or her parents. In such portent or punishment labeling, the new one is decreed an object to be feared and pitied. In some cultures, this will be tantamount to a pronouncement of the necessity that the new one be killed to protect the household or community. Yet the biblical traditions offer another word for the new one: "Behold, I do a new thing." Vast horizons of expectation are opened in each way of naming the scene of the new one's presence. Only the annunciative word of God, which resounds through the canonical Scriptures, is saturated by hope, a hope originating in a God who is love.

The ethical question is at root an existential question about who has given things their determinate names. The parents who name a child always attach hopes and dreams they desire to see fulfilled. Other voices also give names: customer, consumer, responsible citizen, taxpayer, subject of the law. "Through the voice of many callers, a single voice calls. Each call summons to the future. Who is the caller?"[27] The names each person owns for themselves will determine the form of life they will lead. Their lives will be shaped by the voices they believe call them to freedom.

Rosenzweig's pedagogical aim in this short introductory text is to draw attention to the internal connections between revelation, election, and the law. He wants to display God's commandments as an environment that sustains a living relationship between God and God's people as a vital experience. Drawing an analogy with marriage, Rosenzweig compares the Torah to a marriage certificate. Though the daily and even hourly reality of the living relationship of spouses is not publicly narratable, this living, hour-by-hour "knowing-how" is nevertheless the genuine substance of a living marriage, which is never reducible to the generic claim provable by a marriage certificate. The objectively present legal document is only a condition for a lived marriage to emerge that will remain vital only as the couple continue to call one another by name in trust. The heart of marriage can only be lived in the private rhythms of festive days and anniversaries.[28]

SIN AS CAPTIVITY TO GENERIC NORMS

To recap: God is never an essence or idea that can be extracted from events any more than human individuals or the world itself. God *is* to human beings *as* his name, and in revealing it has drawn a congregation together.[29] This offering of God's name forms a *people* into a kingdom bearing God's name, who have been called out from the patterns of a *world* organized by other name givers. God also summons individuals by name, bidding each take their place in the congregation. To be called by this God is to be released from having to secure a happy ending for history, to be allowed to be content to meet the demands of today. Today offers up claims enough to orient human action. This is what it looks like when human beings embrace the reality of being creatures who cannot leap out of time. It is not necessary to wait until the truth and the right action have risen from unfathomable depths. Every good work, every step needed into a flourishing life, is accessible in the present and the local, it "waits for him; it stands before his eyes, it is "in thy heart and in thy mouth," within grasping distance; "that thou mayest do it." In the same way as he has achieved certainty concerning the reality of the world and has found the courage to live his life, he must also have faith in Him who brought him into existence."[30]

This luminous vision of faith and hope flowing from its font in God's personal and communicative love exposes the hollowness of the peace that human beings in their estrangement have cobbled together according to their own lights. The imperative to be genuinely open to the stranger is not a generic ethical or legal demand. For the Scriptures to open up the neighbor as a limit who can be loved, the speaker of the law must speak into the eccentricities and perversities that characterize the everyday mental worlds of fallen human beings. Along with the biblical commandments, the ultimate stranger enters human life. This stranger who calls the sinner in love, paradoxically, leads the sinner to the strangest stranger, the lover of sin and isolation who lives in one's own breast. This sinful self who has irrationally enacted freedom has been hauled up short by the sound of their name being called out in love. The crushing revelation of the "monstrous" and "demonic" stranger who resides in one's breast, this stranger who seals sinners off in endless routines of escape from time and place, is an inescapable judgment that accompanies being liberated into ethical encounter in everyday life.[31]

Guilt enters the frame. It is embarrassing for people to be forced to face the false expectations that they have put on others, their demands about who their neighbor "should" be—embarrassing to the point of shame. An important moment in Israel's own telling of its story with God is indirectly invoked. Not two months out from having been miraculously, gloriously, liberated from their servitude in Egypt, "the whole congregation of the Israelites complained against Moses and Aaron in the wilderness. The Israelites said to them, 'If only we had died by the hand of the Lord in the land of Egypt, when we sat by the fleshpots and ate our fill of bread; for you have brought us out into this wilderness to kill this whole assembly with hunger'" (Exod 16:2-3). In the face of this severe provocation, the God who has rescued and called this people by name responds graciously. God's promise to Moses that the people will be given bread from heaven simultaneously reveals God's love and the shamefulness of Israel's forgetful defection from the glorious work of redemption so recently accomplished.[32]

The Israelites' turning in on themselves, even when faced with God's wondrous works of mercy, offers a paradigmatic exemplification of every sinner's constant need for liberation. The essential form of sin is captivity to the idea that satisfaction will be had in being somewhere else—if somehow reality can be bent to conform more closely to some imagined fantasy of normalcy. *Exile and captivity are not just geographical states. They are states of mind and heart, of practicalities and politics, of spirit and flesh*. A rescue is needed from this psychological exile. The biblical grammar of this rescue is forgiveness, the forgiveness that still calls people by their names even though they have refused to acknowledge their Creator. Scripture frames this merciful rescue not as a movement out of ordinary life into some space beyond it. Precisely the opposite. *Sinners need to be rescued from their fantasies about an exceptional "beyond" where all will be perfect within the terms of their imagination*. Despite their very real miraculous bodily liberation from captivity, the Israelites are depicted as remaining captive in their imaginations to Egypt's strictures and charms. This mental fixation on the past might be labeled "Egypt obsession." As destructive as the backward glance of Lot's wife, it is a fatal nostalgia that keeps people from recognizing what is most important in their present.[33] "Canaan obsession" is an equally tempting captivation by the idea that only in a promised future will a "real" life begin.

If human life is the gift of a good God, it is not in fact received with faith or integrity when the trials and discomforts of the present are evaded by imaginatively migrating to a place of happy resolution.[34] If in the biblical imagination real life *is* life with God, then to live it truly means not living in stylized futures or pasts, nor in imagined pictures of an alternative life, but in coming to terms with being creatures. The decisive liberation needed is from the captivity of minds and desires to the schemas of the age. What needs to be suspended to break this deadening cycle is the *enjoyment* of these dream images which sustain an active paralysis precisely because they seem so lively in the imagination. Rosenzweig has introduced a psychological element into the discussion of sin by highlighting the need for release from obsessions that do have certain adaptive functions and yet keep people from being open to the reality of their own lives.[35] God breaks in on this situation of inner estrangement by revealing them to be *alongside* human beings, *in* the world, and *with* God. This inbreaking comes as a word spoken in *love* that is *heard* calling to individuals by *name*. It is this call that overcomes people's distrust sufficiently for them to cease to try to control time and begin to learn to *wait*.[36]

If God is understood as nothing more than another entity in the cosmos, then all that can be done is to "believe in" or refuse to acknowledge such an entity. The person who merely acquiesces to "believing in" God as a culturally mediated expectation only deepens their enslavement to the laws of the generic social-symbolic order of the society they inhabit. Though a God understood in this way can only be discussed in the third person, a moral demand is presented within a universal law.[37] A real liberation requires God to show Godself as a "who," not an "it." A deadening enslavement to the symbolic laws that govern people's social worlds begins to loosen as the infinite difference between a *relation* and an *encounter* is tangibly experienced. It is one thing to acknowledge God's love rationally as the origin of a human being's existence, one's knowable "essence," and quite another to be exposed by the revelatory love of an eventful encounter in which one's own name is called in love. This is why the calling out in love by *persons* is needed to liberate human beings from their obsessions with "essences" and the laws of "things."[38] This claim that establishes Rosenzweig's work as irreducibly messianic in structure.

Human beings calling out to one another are different in a crucial way to God's calling to human beings, though the ambiguous relation Rosenzweig sets up between human and divine love is intentional. Human beings are only capable of calling another's name out of their own death-driven singularity. The address of revelatory love can only come to contingent and singular human beings who are malformed by their own self-oriented obsessions.[39] The first unique characteristic of the divine calling out to humans by their names is its capacity to expose this death drive.[40] Rosenzweig intentionally sets human-human and human-divine relations in an ambiguous relation with each other to make sure not to lose the mediated nature of revelation. It is through human words, spoken by human mouths, that God has chosen to reveal God's self—as the stories of the prophets, priests, and kings recounted in Scripture constantly emphasize.[41]

Only when God's revelatory encounter penetrates the agent's inner darkness is liberation effected. The internalized generic norms by which people are decreed to have fallen short are therefore exposed as a law that only condemns and cannot give life. The "I" who needs to hear themselves called out is thus in the same moment released by love and judged by it. To be called out to, in love, is at the same time to be put on display as a resistant, truculent, and misshapen agent who resists giving up closely held beliefs in some generic law of truth and rationality that is in fact a defense from reality and a captivity.[42]

One of the essential shocks of revelation is the exposure of the recipient's woundedness and love of being stuck. Each person's own forms of deadening imagination and routine do have their own distinct comforts. But they isolate. Amidst these isolating self-soothing comforts it is hard to admit to having settled for a loveless existence.[43] The pain of confrontation is the necessary cost of exit from the logic of sociosymbolic relations into the logic of ethical encounter, which for Rosenzweig is the decisive event of messianic divine love.[44] This divine call offers the sinner a foothold in truth, an exodus from Egypt obsession, which the Judeo-Christian tradition has called the kingdom of God. This opening is into the very heart of life in human beings' passion for what is singular about the other. This liberating call renders human lives genuinely habitable.

An elaborated account of the inner dynamics of God's work of claiming Israel underlies this account of the liberation of the individual.[45] The Jewish people provide the paradigm exemplification of the constitution of "undead" humanity by way of God's call: "There is no *essence*—that would be 'concept' of Judaism. There is only a 'Hear, O Israel.'"[46] Jewish history is never more than the history of the remnant of those "called out" and who have responded to this calling. In so responding, God's story is extended into the times and places in which their elected lives have taken place—as their stories become part of God's.[47]

The words and institutions provided by God to Israel continually open up a truly livable life. In the wilderness Israel is given form by God through temple, judges, and ordering in family groupings. But if God's glory does not dwell in the tabernacle, these institutional forms cannot sustain Israel on their own, being no substitutes for the real "place" where Israel can be at home: in relationship with God, a living part of God's redemptive story with the world. A long and arduous training will need to be undertaken to learn to find sustenance in living in relation with God, in letting God's words live within them. Only when they have learned to live as creatures, that is, as those who take their satisfaction from God and not from their material surroundings, will they be prepared to recognize health as life with God, "shalom" and bodily flourishing. Redemption is hungering and thirsting not only after rescue, but after this shalom life with this God, and so *God's* righteousness, justice, and compassion. This is the fullness of life for which human beings were created.

Rosenzweig offers an account of a messianic kingdom that is not entered by transcending social relations but in the dynamic interruption of the metaphysically reified loneliness of sinful individuals. With this interruption comes a new set of social relations. Ultimately, revelation for Rosenzweig is God's merciful assault on the fantasies (idols) that confine human energies in defensive forms of life, whether taking nostalgic, utopian, or self-soothing forms. It is these *fantasies* that cause human beings to overlook the actual *invitations* into their own lives, keeping them from being responsible to its own particularities and its own outbreaks of wonder. New life is born out of the deathly stasis sustained by the (unconscious) fantasies that entrap human beings in a distanced relation to their own lives, holding them back from embracing the renewal of their relations with others. They foreclose the openings that can only truly arise in the eventful space of encounter, as a rightly formed love of neighbor flows from an appreciation of God's prior gratuitous love.[48]

Sabbath celebration is for Rosenzweig the "holiday from the everyday" that suspends the daily fantasies that constrain people's capacities to hear and see the other. The collective celebration Sabbath revels in the new social order produced by divine speech. This speech neither transcends nor disparages temporality and emplacement but is God's condescension to human idiom and need. It thus reaches into human lives lived wholly on an immanent plane and in so doing brings them back to life.[49] The politics of his holiday from the everyday will be the topic of chapter 9.

IMAGING CHRIST, BECOMING A CREATURE

Very little separates Rosenzweig's theology from that of Dietrich Bonhoeffer.[50] For Bonhoeffer, any adequate account of creation must give due weight to the theological reality that creation can only be responded to and talked about by creatures who exist in the middle time between fall and the resurrection, who have been touched by the desire to be redeemed and yearn to experience it fully.[51]

The Paul of Colossians, Rosenzweig, and Bonhoeffer as we find him in *Creation and Fall*, converge in understanding the work of the messiah to be the establishment of life and liveliness at the heart of the estranged realities of concrete human existences. The God of Jesus Christ "does not will to be Lord of a dead, eternally unchangeable, subservient world, instead God wills to be Lord of life with its infinite variety of forms."[52] For Bonhoeffer, too, genuine gospel liveliness emerges from a direct challenge to the sterile repetition that is characteristic of living in the law of the generic.

The sterility of this law is definitively revealed in the resurrection of Jesus Christ, which continues to give life through the wonder of divine speech, "which creates that which lives out of what is dead—it is God's being able to raise up children to Abraham out of these stones, and calling Christ to rise up from the dead earth."[53] That true creaturely life lives from reliance on God's own speaking explains, for Bonhoeffer, why it is not nonsense to refer to living things as dead. Living things can be dead in the way Marxist or Darwinian materialism are dead: nothing in world occurrence is allowed to transcend the explanation that all that happens is caused by the force of material conditions. All such universalizing accounts of history and human activity, when lived into by human beings, produce routinized, hermetically sealed, and meaningless motion. Humans were not made to feel that the course of their life is determined by the immanent laws of their being; neither of nature nor historical sequence. Only human lives that have been rescued from entrapment in these natural and historical cycles can truly be called free.

Human beings were created to be free, but understood theologically, Bonhoeffer suggests, freedom is never a quality that humans possess, nor is it a skill or a thing:

> It is a relation and nothing else. To be more precise, freedom is a relation between two persons. Being free means "being-free-for-the-other" because I am bound to the other. Only by being in relation with the other am I free.[54]

In another striking convergence with Rosenzweig's account, Bonhoeffer, too, understands freedom as an event that befalls human beings only with and through another person. Bonhoeffer grounds this premise christologically, drawing on Paul in Colossians: the resurrection of Jesus Christ is a gratuitous offer of freedom to human beings. This true creaturely freedom can only appear as a paradox in a fallen world. The unfreedom seen as the rational and normal state of affairs in a fallen world hides the ways human beings are coerced by the norms that organize a given social order. Yet God is not determined by these laws of unfreedom, being genuinely free for relationship. Out of this freedom God is continually reestablishing the human desire and capacity for free interpersonal relationship. God patiently invites human beings into the realization that the laws of nature and culture do not decree their future, but the Lord of time. God must *create* free human beings by reordering their spirit and flesh. The unique work of Jesus Christ is visibly to manifest the grammar and aim of God's freeing individual human beings to image God. All other attempts at self-liberation generate new forms of bondage.[55]

Bonhoeffer is now positioned to clarify why the work and claim of Jesus Christ ties human beings to creation rather than detaching them and lifting them above it. The biblical creation story presents humans as creatures fallen out of touch with their true home in creation. Entrapped by the dynamics of their flight from God, they have become creatures ever more dissatisfied and uneasy with themselves and their limits. Bonhoeffer proposes that this state of unfreedom arises from the first couple's having lost the sense that the two trees in the Garden of Eden were created as perpetual reminders for the first couple that God is both the *boundary* and *limit* of their creaturely freedom. "You may freely eat of every tree of the garden; but of the tree of the knowledge of good and evil you shall not eat, for in the day that you eat of it you shall die" (Gen 2:16-17). The two trees are merciful reminders to human beings that remaining free creatures entails receiving the limits of existence as gift. In their original state this setting of a boundary ("you shall not eat") was perceptible as a grace, as an accessible and nonthreatening embodiment of a livable law. It asks only for Christians to live in a way that acknowledges their inability to exist outside of a temporally extended give-and-take with the God who is their source and sustainer.

Established as significant by the divine command attached to them, the two trees mutely transmit an address from beyond creation to Adam and Eve *through* embodied creatures. The trees have been positioned as the condition of human obedience and disobedience by God's word about them. God has offered in these bodies an "inner limit" releasing them from worry about the "outer limits" of their lives—threats outside the garden, their own deaths, or the severing of relationship with God and each other. The creaturely bodies of these trees, bound as they are to the divine word, offer everything the first couple needs to retain their true freedom, that is, to exercise freedom in awareness of their place in time and space with God and other creatures.[56] The trees protect genuine human freedom by resisting the movement of the heart's attention from the bodies at the center of God's care by beginning to define its essence or look for its boundaries. The essence of the fall is the reifying displacement of the first couple of a God with whom they had a temporally elaborated relationship in favor of a "being" who could be talked about and whose commands could be debated. Once God had been turned into an idea, it was inevitable that the first couple would hanker to take over some of his power as moral arbiter. This is the real defection from relationship with God, with the eating of the fruit only the consummation of their having walked away from relationship.[57]

Had they not defected from the word that holds God, creation, and humankind together, "this very revelation of the limit in bodily form, in the love he has for the other person, would have brought Adam an ever deeper knowledge of the grace of the Creator."[58] But in refusing relationship with their Creator they also reject the temporality and bodiliness of creaturely life and so give it up for the illusory dream of "the knowledge of good and evil"—the very eternal and enduring truth that Rosenzweig has called an escape from being a temporal creature. They remained free as long as they were content with this temporally elaborated relationship and received it as God's gift of presence.[59]

As God had promised, defection from receiving this word as gift is to die. For Bonhoeffer death here is not a metaphorical trope denoting more mundane realities like being "bored to death." This a death that has ontological depth and demands a view of humans as biological and spiritual entities. This death, as Bonhoeffer understands it, is not a simple opposite to biological life, but the perversion of human activity. The whole existence of this being becomes fixated on the preservation of their biological life. It is a spiritual death to be enslaved to the law of having one limited life that must be at all costs maximized. Life has become the rival commandment to God's commandment. To be obsessed with this false commandment to live is death. In repudiating the history of acts and responses which forms a temporally elaborated life with God, fallen humans are left only with their "bare" lives and the immanent laws that govern it.[60]

Having repudiated God's presence, fallen humans are condemned to make something of the limits of their naked biology, and to do so with no other imaginative resources than earth can supply. The ideas they come up with possess them, taking them away from the creaturely reality of the life that God has given them. In their repudiation of the divinely spoken inner limit, the first humans have given up their creatureliness. By aspiring to transcend immanent contingency, they have been utterly subsumed in it. This is the condition of those who wanted to be like God, who in their "not-wanting-to-be-a-creature" enact what Scripture decrees a living death.[61]

God has not been content to leave creatures in this estranged and fragmented state, however. The subjective "I" who has been severed from God and is in need of the Creator's life-giving address is not left bereft, because all humanity has been addressed "in Jesus Christ, in the cross, in the church."[62] This freeing address recapitulates the events of the first creation. In a strikingly new interpretation of the creation story, Bonhoeffer reads the designation of the woman as Adam's "helper," as a body who will replace the tree as Adam's way back into relation to the created realm (as she will for him). "The Creator knows that this free life as a creature can be borne within its limit only if it is love, and out of unfathomable mercy the Creator the helper who is a partner suitable for a human being."[63] By decreeing that the man and wife be faithful helpers to one another, another body is offered to the fallen human beings who will provide material resistance to their ideal imaginations, who will, in the most physical of ways, embody the limit who can be loved, and which will tie them back to the earth. The other is offered as a limit that is promising and merciful because *this* limit is one that can be loved.[64]

The provision of this embodied limit looks forward to the merciful Creator becoming the Redeemer who will make God's word present in creation, definitively in person, and in association with a tree. The concrete bodiliness of Jesus Christ challenges the public domain of generic symbolic systems in which "God" is an idea or metaphysical background for human events. Jesus calls people back into reality by binding himself to human beings, first in the church and then with neighbors of all sorts. This is what Bonhoeffer means with his often-misunderstood assertion that "there is no way back to the earth except via God and our brothers and sisters."[65] Because human beings are bodily creatures they are in fact related to the whole created world and to other bodies. To be a creature is to be dependent on and to depend on other creatures. But Bonhoeffer is not making the claim familiar in disability discussions—that disability is a reminder that everyone is dependent, a generic and impersonal claim.[66] As an impersonal generic claim, the universality of dependence implicates an almost infinite matrix of relations in which human life exists, dependence on physical laws like gravity, social laws like reciprocity, moral laws like truth telling.

Humans were not created to be *simply* bodies in such nearly infinite relations of dependence with other discrete created bodies and forces, Bonhoeffer insists. As the creation of humanity as man and woman in the image of God in the first account displays, human freedom "can be defined in simply no other way than in terms of the existence of human beings over-against-one-another, with-one-another, and in-dependence-upon-one-another."[67] And as the second creation account highlights, human beings live preeminently by God's Spirit, and it is the working of this Spirit which is the essence of human undeadness. *Freedom is not gained by admitting dependence. Freedom is received by concretely depending on God's enlivening Spirit.* And the Spirit of Jesus Christ ties human beings into loving relationships with other human beings. When individuals were yet dead in sin, trapped in a life rendered unfree in the routines of the laws of nature and history, Jesus Christ came to resurrect them through his Spirit.

> That is why where the original body in its created being has been destroyed, God enters it anew in Jesus Christ, and then, where this body too is broken, enters the forms of the sacrament of the body and blood. The body and blood of the Lord's Supper are the new realities of creation promised to fallen Adam. Because Adam is created as body, Adam is also redeemed as body [and God comes to Adam as body], in Jesus Christ and in the sacrament.[68]

True freedom is offered to human beings through relations with creaturely entities in time and space—through the incarnation and cross, through the sacraments, and through the neighbor. To hear God's call through these bodies is to come to understand the mechanisms of the divine work of freeing humans so that they can image God; to reenter the responsive life with an acting God who loves and can be loved in return without compulsion.

Human beings suffering their redemption are beings who are learning what it means to image God amidst their shame before others. It is shame that enflames the hate and desire to dominate others that express an "extreme lack of respect for things-as-they-are."[69] It is only because Jesus Christ is *above* these relations of living deadness, Bonhoeffer later explains,[70] that he can and must enter into the relations between creatures to challenge the obsessions that distort interpersonal relationships. This interruption reorients behavior by revealing that *the sheer "thereness" of the creaturely neighbor is good and loved even though fallen and therefore sometimes repellent to fallen human beings.* Being a recipient of gratuitous love frees human beings to receive even awkward others with gratitude because it is *through them that a way is offered back to living in truth.*[71] What God has done in Jesus Christ for all, and once for all, enters individual lives and remakes their patterns of relating to others in this gracious and personal confrontation of their projections onto others, projections that are inevitably framed in the idiom of the universal.

> Self-centered love constructs its own image of other persons, about what they are and what they should become. It takes the life of the other person into its own hands. Spiritual love recognizes the true image of the other person as seen from the perspective of Jesus Christ. It is the image Jesus Christ has formed and wants to form in all people.[72]

To confess the Christian God as Creator means then, concretely, to be liberated not to *transcend* creation, but to *receive one's true being in Christ* (from the Father's right hand) by learning what it means to be a creature, that is, to recognize and freely embrace loving relations with other persons as and where they are, with all their brokenness and angularity. For this to be enacted individuals will have to face and repent of the brokenness that bars their way to receiving the other, both divine and human. To receive another creature *in this way* is to image God's love through Jesus Christ. Only thus does a person discover their redeemed self that is hidden in Christ.

There are many points of overlap between Rosenzweig's account of undeadness and life in the heart of wonder and Bonhoeffer's account of creation in *Creation and Fall*: both emphasize the articulacy and centrality of God's speaking for theology and ethics; have a positive view of the connection of this living speech with command/Torah/law; see ethics as emerging out of everyday life; criticize generic/generalized ontologies in favor of an ontology of interpersonal encounter; and proffer an antimodern account of freedom as freedom-for-loving-relationship based on God's prior election and rescue.

This formal convergence yields a shared diagnosis of the predicament of faith in the modern world. First, a chief characteristic of the entrapment of contemporary life is its narrow account of human action. Some experiences (abilities) are taken to be more real and valuable than the rest of contingent temporality, which is perceived to be essentially meaningless. These obsessions displace any genuine seeking out and wondering at the given life that precedes, animates, and sustains our everyday existence. Second, they both resist the positioning of talk of God in the third person within conceptual frameworks that undermine more active accounts of hearing from and speaking to God that they see as irreducible responses to the entrapping and deadening obsessions with generic norms.

Rosenzweig's account also helps to clarify why Bonhoeffer's treatment in *Creation and Fall*, with its emphasis on God's address in Jesus Christ's cross and through the church, needs the supplement that he later develops in *Life Together* and *Ethics*. If the particularity of divine acts of "undeadening" is to be preserved, the stepping of Jesus Christ in the Spirit between human beings to reveal them as lovable in all their broken particularity must not be obscured as God's own articulate act. A wider range of human experiences become comprehensible as the means of Jesus Christ's appearing and claiming individuals if he is understood as the source of the many absolutely particular invitations to wonder that invite people into creaturely life, a life lived "in the heart of wonder." Rosenzweig thus offers a sympathetic way to fill out Bonhoeffer's allusion to the Christian's receiving of the life that is hidden in Jesus Christ. Human beings become the creatures they were created to be as the sinful habits of evasion that sustain their estrangement from others are confronted. In confessing, having been so confronted, they point the way for all humanity to learn to receive the wonder of life.

At the heart of their accounts lie the Sabbath celebration and Christian worship. In the space of worship, God's personal words are offered ever anew to the community in order that they might be received to reorient all of human living. As Rosenzweig helpfully highlights, when this gathered worship is conceived only as the gathering around a rule it can only be a law, another tragically demanding "relation" to which one is forced to accede. What brings this message to life as an event of interpersonal love is that the words at the heart of the gathering of those who have been called are received as a messianic and personal inbreaking. Worship invites ever anew the prayer "Thy kingdom come," and so flows out from worship to permeate everyday life.[73]

HEALTH AS HERALD OF THE KINGDOM

Taken together, Rosenzweig and Bonhoeffer offer a compelling conceptual explication of what is being said when Christians confess that to be saved is to be liberated to be free creatures. Being made free means continually being confronted with sin, and precisely so, invited into the kingdom of heaven. Here disability appears in a remarkably different light. Having, in chapter 8, articulated my worries and anxieties of living with autism, I will conclude this chapter by reflecting on the emotional realities of Adam's welcoming me through the gateway to the kingdom. If life in that kingdom is the shalom that is true health, Adam might well be the healthiest person I know. To indicate why I don't think the insights I will relate are unique, I will also draw in some testimonies of the assistánts and friends at L'Arche in Cork, Ireland.

Adam's *ability to live without worry about the future* is a constant convicting challenge. Things that would immediately worry me because of their future implications do not faze him in the least. His bodily carriage constantly communicates an absolute lack of dread of the future. The biblical language of wisdom allows this practical kinesthetic knowledge to be admitted as real knowledge.[74] By watching Adam live wholly in the present, I am provided with a potent witness to what it looks like for me as a Christian to confess that *wonder can only be lived in the present tense*. The judgment that accompanies this annunciation of good news is that my worries about an imagined future, driven as they are by my attempts to plan and order what I think should happen, are all too often symptoms of my having given in to temptation, becoming an enemy of Christ's rule.

Jesus says,

> No one can serve two masters; for a slave will either hate the one and love the other, or be devoted to the one and despise the other. . . . Therefore, I tell you, do not worry about your life, what you will eat or what you will drink, or about your body, what you will wear. Is not life more than food, and the body more than clothing? Look at the birds of the air; they neither sow nor reap nor gather into barns, and yet your heavenly Father feeds them. Are you not of more value than they? (Matt 6:24-26)

Second, there is *no gap at all between what Adam says and what he does*. His love is constantly displayed in the most intimate and physical gestures. When you are with him, you simply cannot wonder if he's lying or faking affection. He thus liberates everyone around him from suspiciously watching for signs of hidden motives, for other selves peeking out from behind masks. His body language is richly communicative, and what he says is absolutely coterminous with what he does. He communicates *with* his body *to* embodied beings: his hello meets others bodily where they say hello to him—by putting his hand on their mouth. His bodily comportment says in so many ways that he receives his body as a grace.[75] To be with him and to see how he experiences his body often jars in striking ways with the ways people unreflectively respond to his body as unsightly, unhealthy, disgusting, or ill. I am not alone in being helped across the threshold of grasping the meaning of unconditional acceptance by someone with learning difficulties, as one lawyer and mother relates.

> One summer, at a Faith and Light Summer Holiday, Anne taught me the true meaning of compassion. She cried a lot that week and I began by trying to make everything better for her. I failed miserably, nothing seemed to work. Then I began to feel frustrated, I really wanted her to enjoy this holiday. If Anne had been a friend whom society labels 'normal' she would have pretended she was happy, just to please me, but Anne would have none of that. Slowly I began to realise that I couldn't make it better, there was no solution to this problem. I simply knew that I should just walk quietly with her in whatever her pain was. And then we were both able to relax and be at peace in each other's company. We were friends. Prior to that holiday I thought I knew the meaning of compassion, but I merely knew a definition of the word. Anne taught me, at a heart level, the true meaning of compassion, a lesson that has had far-reaching consequences in my relationship with many people since.[76]

Jesus says,

> Do not swear by your head, for you cannot make one hair white or black. Let your word be "Yes, Yes" or "No, No"; anything more than this comes from the evil one. (Matt 5:36-37)

Third, Adam's levels of *emotional sensitivity* constantly astound me. When he is near arguing parents or squabbling siblings, he often suffers such immediate pain that he will break into tears as the pain and anxiety reverberate within him. He quite clearly comprehends the messages communicated through facial expressions, bodily comportment, and vocal intonations. Even more remarkably, this does not drive him to flee human contact. He constantly positions himself on the boundaries of ongoing social converse.

Neither a loner nor an attention seeker, with absolute innocence he gravitates to the force fields of human converse. Of late he has taken to wanting to sit where he can touch our pastor as he performs the liturgy—in stark distinction from a congregation clustering all too obviously in the back pews. At parties, in public places, the ways he positions himself is so far from normal social convention, and so revealing of social space, that it often reminds me of iron filings making visible previously unimagined magnetic fields. I can only wonder at his attention to fields of interpersonal communion of which I never even dreamed.

Timothy Kearney has been similarly struck by the empathetic engagement displayed by one L'Arche core member.

> Danny has shared with me [what it was like growing up and going to a special school] and being teased on your way there and back by "normal" children telling you that you're "a spastic" and that you're "mad." The pain of rejection in a world that values knowledge, power and social status, when you have few, if any, of these attributes and graces. Danny knows the reality of such pain. Just as Danny is intimately acquainted with the reality of his own hurt and anguish, which can propel him at times into outbursts of anger and violent temper tantrums, he is also sensitive to the pain of others. He is a man who has compassion for those who suffer. He often prays for those who are having "a hard time," including the homeless men and women—often refugees from Romania and elsewhere in Eastern Europe—whom he sees sleeping rough on Patrick's Street in Cork City. He is a peace-maker who abhors conflict and war in the world and, though from a nationalist background and culture, I have heard him pray for the family of a British soldier killed in Northern Ireland, that they be comforted in their pain and loss. He often prays for peace in the world. Whilst he loves flags and national emblems and is a passionate collector of same, he abhors borders, which divide human beings form each other. Though capable of anger and violence, Danny is a man capable of great gentleness, who loves children and who is naturally gifted with them. Danny is a person who is gifted in many ways on the level of the heart, and he has taught me much about what it means to be human.[77]

Kearney is assuming a Christology once made explicit by Jean Vanier in a talk to undergraduates at Harvard University.

> I told them that many of the people I was living with did not know how to read or write or even speak, and yet many of them had a deeper experience of Jesus than they, the students, had. I told them: "You are looking for a knowledge of Jesus whereas people with learning disabilities

> are seeking a presence of Jesus; their intellectual capacity for words and concepts is greatly limited, but their intuition, their sense of presence is greatly increased."[78]

The Apostle Paul teaches,

> God has so arranged the body, giving the greater honor to the inferior member, that there may be no dissension within the body, but the members may have the same care for one another. If one member suffers, all suffer together with it; if one member is honored, all rejoice together with it. (1 Cor 12:24-26)

This reference to rejoicing together brings me to a fourth and final observation—Adam's *enjoyment of many people* is constant. I personally have never once walked into the room after having been apart from him for any length of time and not received his own version of a smile and warm embrace. If the kingdom of heaven is a new social order whose characteristic is joy, I have most powerfully glimpsed what this might mean because I have lived with Adam.

Paul exhorts the Romans,

> Let us therefore no longer pass judgment on one another, but resolve instead never to put a stumbling block or hindrance in the way of another. . . . For the kingdom of God is not food and drink but righteousness and peace and joy in the Holy Spirit. (Rom 4:13, 16)

In sum, when I am with Adam I cannot for a second forget how different and beautiful the social order is to which he witnesses, in which we call to one another by name, without illusions or projections. Jesus often suggested that, were we all to live as Adam apparently lives, the kingdom would be present. Thus I hear transmitted through his life that first sermon of Jesus recounted by Mark: "Jesus came to Galilee, proclaiming the good news of God, and saying, 'The time is fulfilled, and the kingdom of God has come near; repent, and believe in the good news'" (Mark 1:14-15). This sermon interrupted the course of events in the first century in the Middle East as Mark expects it to interrupt the world of his readers. And it often interrupts me through the acts that Adam performs in which an alternative social comportment appears that is both extremely beautiful and a strikingly deep challenge to the social order of this fallen world. In this way his life *evokes* the almost unthinkable social dynamics to which Jesus pointed, and as he does so, he constantly *provokes* our world. Adam makes tangible, announcing in gesture and glance, an interpersonal order of relations that is the closest thing to a display of the peace between myself, God, and other people that I can imagine. When I "taste and see that the Lord is good," I do so *beside* Adam at the communion rail and in *dependence* on his constantly and gently reminding me in a thousand tangible ways of what the social order of the new kingdom that we eat and drink looks like.

An Irish priest nicely summarizes the location of this provocation within the biblical view of the world.

> For a number of years now I have heard the words of the prophets in the confused mumbling speech of the mentally handicapped. I have found the presence of God in the gentle presence of these people whose wounded nervous systems and peculiar limbs don't ever merit the headlines of even the local newspaper. The prophets of the Old Testament were all people of action. When God commanded them, they got to work, thundering out their charges against king or priest. But not all prophesying is thundering God's word or threatening his wrath. God can speak in silence. Elijah, one of those old prophets, learned this lesson on the mountain a long time ago:
>
> > "Go out and stand on the mountain before the Lord," he was told. "Then the Lord himself came by. Then came a mighty wind so strong it tore the mountains and shattered the rocks before the Lord. But the Lord was not in the wind. After the wind came an earthquake. But the Lord was not in the earthquake. After the earthquake came a fire. But the Lord was not in the fire. And after the fire came the sound of a gentle breeze. (1 Kings 19:10, 11, 13)
>
> Whenever we gather with the handicapped we are in the presence, I think of many gentle prophets. Sons and daughters called and marked by God for a special mission in life, and because of their handicap they speak to us every day in the quietness of their lives, if only we would listen.[79]

People like Adam help Christians to understand that the Christian faith is lived in the present. Because they (not unlike Jesus) live lives beyond what most people could have imagined, they demand the development of new forms of practical reasoning, of "knowing-how." And such knowing-how cannot be had without facing illusions.[80] Human hypocrisy needs the call of another to come to light, and when it does, it exposes the fears that drive it. It is God's mercy to expose these fears, to invite repentance, the painful and laborious work of giving them up. We will not succeed in being with those who are different from us, enjoying life with them and celebrating with them, unless these fears hiding in the heart are faced. None of this is sentimental, and none of it is easy. But it is the stuff of being a creature.

It is for all these reasons that it seems indisputable to me—certainly not hyperbole, a metaphor, or a father's special pleading, but a sheer descriptive statement—when I say that Adam is the healthiest person I know. As a baptized Christian who takes communion willingly and weekly, he displays a remarkable facility in living the life to which all those are called who are baptized into Christ's death. This is not to suggest that the cancer of soul Christians call original sin has no hold on him, but it seems not to entrap him so blatantly as it does myself and my other family members.

The short remainder of this chapter offers a diagnostic exercise to the reader. If the deepest problem of disability language is seductive power to assume *we are the nondisabled*, this is an extremely difficult problem to bring into view. The next paragraphs invite you to undertake your own critical self-evaluation. Pay special attention to your emotional reactions. Keep in mind the claims that have so far been made.

> *If* the kingdom of heaven is anything like Jesus teaches,
> *and* Adam displays in significant ways the tenor of this kingdom in his form of life,
> *and* if it is the state of our hearts out of which the social order of our world flows,
> *then*, to recognize the true health of those we call disabled, we will have to have our hearts assayed to see how deeply they welcome this kingdom. To genuinely receive the presence of another person means not to pity them, be repelled or frustrated by them, but to welcome them without regret.

Adam has Down syndrome. Hours after birth he contracted sepsis and came near death, at which point he experienced a significant brain injury. He did not walk until he was two and a half years old. He was not toilet trained until he was ten. To this day he does not speak and has various aversions to the textures of certain kinds of foods, traits that triggered his diagnosis with autism at age four. It is not clear how well he hears, and for years he wore hearing aids. He has had one perforated eardrum surgically repaired and the other one has been sometimes perforated for months, leaving his sinuses constantly draining through his left ear. At six months of age it had become clear that a pair of holes in his heart would need to be repaired and he underwent open heart surgery. He had second-degree burns on his chest and arm at four years of age after pulling a pot of boiling water from a kitchen counter. As he begins puberty he offers increasing but still quite limited help in dressing, feeding, and toileting himself.

Perhaps the most theologically unsettling feature of his story is his having contracted leukemia at eight years of age. He endured endless blood extractions in the course of his treatment, as well as countless lumbar punctures, eight months of intensive, and eighteen months of maintenance chemotherapy. Often during this process his mouth was ravaged with ulcers and sometimes he was so debilitated by the treatments that he could not walk. For years he has had problems with gastric reflux associated with low muscle tone in the pyloric sphincter, which often gives him heartburn that keeps him up at night, for which he takes daily medication. Nevertheless, one of his greatest joys is walking, which is why his development of a permanent degenerative condition in both of his eyes as a young teen is again particularly unsettling. The condition is called keratoconus and entails the breakdown of the collagen in the lenses of the eyes, leading to vision loss and eye pain. So far, thank God, only one eye has gone essentially blind, though its light sensitivity and fluctuating internal pressure often cause him pain.

This, I insist, is the healthiest person I know, which I assert neither because nor in spite of the regularity with which we take him to the doctor. He, his parents, and his doctors would of course be glad to be "beyond medicine," but by now it should be clear why it would be theologically inappropriate to perceive his life as determined in relation to the thickness of his medical files. Adam is more than his illnesses, as disability activists have been keen to emphasize in debates around definitions of health. In a physical sense, like many people with disabilities, he lives in a more precarious relation to the well-functioning of his body than do many, his genetic palette leaving him susceptible to secondary health challenges.[81] But his capacity to fight off disease is little different from others. It is entirely appropriate that these bodily peculiarities be recognized legally and medically. But a theological definition of health goes beyond this catalogue of bodily vulnerabilities in asking how people enact their creaturehood.

Adam lives with incredible grace and without worry for the morrow. He is a friend with time, his body, and the people with whom he shares his days. In theological terms, it is clear that he is content to be a creature. Grateful for the medicine which has kept him alive and which sometimes makes him more comfortable than he might otherwise have been, I am at the same time painfully aware of how his unselfconscious way of inhabiting time and place challenges the social conventions of his surrounding culture. The most significant way that he challenges contemporary culture is in drawing to the surface the prejudice that takes the claims of people with disabilities to value their lives, even to be glad of their disabilities, to be a rationalization of a difficult situation they would change if they could.[82]

None of this should be taken as a suggestion that Christians should not pray for healing. But it matters which healing is prayed for, and who is taken to need it. It is a lame and blind contemporary church that must ask whether it is acceptable to pray for healing. Jesus can still be affirmed as most definitely still wondrously at work ensuring that the past does not wholly determine the future. This includes the physical progression of bodily processes like disease. Christians can continue to hope for the healing that interrupts the bondage of sin to restore creatures to life. They do so fully aware that because all bodily occurrence must be interpreted, whether or not a healing has occurred will often not look the same to people with and without faith.

Christians can still pray to Jesus as healer because Jesus remains viscerally invested in bodies and in fullness of life, still being the merciful One whose ears are finely tuned to the distress cries of human beings.[83] Jesus is not shorn of his healing powers by modern people's belief that miracles have ceased. Neither is it necessary for Christians to affirm the modern view in an inverted form by making the question about prayer a debate about whether Jesus can contravene natural causality.[84] Hume's view of the miracle as a rupture of the natural order is also not Christian Scripture. That Christians will cry out to Jesus for healing is a constant assumption of the New Testament writers. Jesus is the healer whose work is to fulfill and restore all creation, and every human being with it.[85]

In taking such a position, Christians today join the Christians of the patristic era in affirming that the ongoing work of Christ the healer offers a hope that enlivens sufferers rather than guaranteeing to resolve any given case of suffering. This lack of guarantees is not threatening, however, because what Christians have to say about human bodies, their brokenness, and their healing, implicates more doctrines than creation. Christians will talk differently about bodies, about healing, and about the political power of the healings of Jesus when the center of gravity in a theological discussion of disability is shifted from creation and anthropology to eschatology and ecclesiology.

In sickness and in health, the fullness of life for the Christian cannot be separated from the strange joy of togetherness in the visible body of Christ.[86] By recognizing this, Christian boldness in praying for healing will never amount to a rejection of God's strange vocations. The Christian community lives in hope for miracles while remaining relatively agnostic about the shapes physical healing might take. Christians are emboldened in such prayers because they are *not* agnostic about their vocation to be part of Christ's kingdom.

8

Autism and Christian Hope

AUTISM AND THE REVELATORY CLAIM OF THE NEIGHBOR

Somehow a way must be found to wrench the idea of disability out of its etymological linkage with lack and brokenness. The truths it points to must be weaved into a more supple and encompassing account of human flourishing. In theological terms it is incorrect to say that human beings are flourishing as they were created to if not breathing the free atmosphere of a living, temporally extended interaction with God. As Frances Young has observed, this makes the appropriate starting point for contemporary theological thinking about disability its tendency to expose in quite precise ways human unfreedom and the routines that sustain it.

> Handicap is a kind of judgment. Clearly it is not some kind of punishment for sin. It is not usually anyone's fault. But it is a kind of judgment, a *krisis*, because it has that effect. Society is judged by the way it treats handicapped people and our society is ambiguous . . . handicap discriminates between those who rise to the occasion, and those who fail to do so. It discriminates between the good marriage and the shaky marriage, the stable family and the unstable family. It shows up people and their relationships and their values for what they are.[1]

This is eschatological thinking, ordered by hope for the redemptive reconfiguration of human lives by the involvement of a merciful God. Young invokes the New Testament language of *krisis*, which highlights Jesus' inauguration of a new age. The emergence of this new world reveals the corruptions of a fallen world by establishing an alternative time and a rival social world.[2] This chapter explains why the doctrine of the "last things" must be one of the first things accounted for in a theological account of disability, along with its cognate themes of revelation and pneumatology.

Because disability is a tear in the fabric of this age, it must be understood as both a judgment and invitation. Conditions such as autism reveal the truth of communities. The appearance of disability brings to the surface the capacity of individuals and social networks to affirm and support those who present special challenges with grace and genuine appreciation. It is indeed a "strange vocation" to live as a challenge to social norms, to be a living bearer of a *krisis* and judgment and call to responsibility to specific humans in specific historical circumstances, and with them whole social orders.[3]

Krisis is an irruption and a judgment. As such it is revelation from God. But earlier in a book about her life with her severely intellectually impaired son Arthur, Young expresses a much more conflicted sense of where such irruptions lead. What is clear is that disability judges and exposes people's fortitude and moral seriousness—or lack thereof. What is less clear is whether this destruction of the certainties of the age promise a better world to come—that is, healing. Young tells of a woman who believed she had been given a vision from the Virgin Mary of the precise date when the woman's daughter would be healed of her Down syndrome. The date came and went, and a new vision came with a new date. Young could not avoid seeing this as evidence that the woman had never really accepted her daughter, despite the woman's protest that she *had* accepted her daughter, just not her *condition*.[4] It was a conversation that made Young increasingly uncomfortable as the realization dawned that she might be infected with a more subtle form of the same disease.

> Part of me was as desperate as she was for a miracle, and our contacts made me aware of my own desperate desire to be left off the hook. I thought I had accepted Arthur; but I too had not accepted the situation fully. I could not make sense of it. Nor could I pray for a miracle with my mind convinced of its possibility. There was that desperate cry of the heart, but no faith that such a prayer could be answered. . . . I find it impossible to envisage what it would mean for him to be "healed," because what personality there is, is so much part of him *as he is*, with all his limitations. "Healed" would be a different person.[5]

Young's inner conflict is one familiar to anyone who has lived with or loved someone with disabilities, especially intellectual difficulties. Her case highlights how *theological images of disability and its healing are all ways of talking about the present*. Revelation is not primarily a matter of revealing something that will *one day* happen, but of what *is* happening. Hence the interconnection of eschatology, talk about the final resurrected state, and pneumatology, the present agency of the Holy Spirit initiating the new age that will culminate in the complete healing of heaven and earth. In New Testament terms, disability is the divinely initiated *krisis* that reveals *everyone's* human weakness, brokenness, and sin. And this exposure is an ineradicable aspect of being redeemed. "For he said to me, 'My power is made perfect in weakness.' Therefore I will boast all the more in my weakness, so that Christ's power might rest on me. . . . For when I am weak, then I am strong" (2 Cor 12:9-10).

Such a starting point is thoroughly theological. Different kinds of attention reveal different aspects of phenomena as well as situate different responses to them. Any adequate account of the historical endurance of Christianity must assume that the distinctive beliefs and practices of Christian faith do actually reveal features of existence that differ in substance from what is perceived and made tangible in other systems of thought or faith traditions.[6] It is easy to imagine a scientific expert on the cognitive psychology of autism who would be hopeless as a carer. This is easily imagined because different *types* of knowledge emerge from personally *engaged self-investment* as distinguished from the modern rationality that *studies* phenomena by way of disengaged description, however highly methodologically self-aware it might be. This chapter displays how theological claims direct attention to features of situations and relationships that other thought systems systematically overlook, or construe very differently.

Focusing on autism helpfully highlights the question pressed by a wide range of disabilities often lumped together under the heading of "learning difficulties" or "mental illnesses." What is meant by the term "healing" is certainly important for someone with a physical disability, as Young's story and struggles illustrate, but become almost unavoidable when people's minds are the locus of their condition.

Focusing this chapter on a condition located in the mind is not to equate mind and body or mind and brain. Although supposedly classic cases of autism may for complicated reasons be somewhat rare,[7] diagnoses of autism are routinely made without a clear understanding of all the etiology of the specific person's condition. Like other psychological conditions, any essentialist diagnosis is much more complicated to establish than is generally assumed.[8] Given Western medicine's rhetorical swaddling in the language of objective science, this makes it particularly ironic that, in practice, autism is now regularly deployed more as a label designating a package of therapies offered to certain children rather than an ascription of a rigorously researched and definitively understood neurological status. In a medical setting, diagnosis as the locating of traits corresponding to a syndrome is tied up with an offer of therapies, while diagnosis as a designation of the essence of a condition presumes a deep understanding of the phenomenon that often is not present to medical professionals, especially in the case of complex and diverse syndromes like autism.[9]

As a social activity diagnosis is clearly a political act and is consciously understood and deployed as such in the context of mental health diagnoses. To highlight diagnosis as a political act is not a claim that autism is simply a social construction, but to distinguish this social aspect of the process of diagnosis from a definitive pronouncement on the state of affairs understood in ontological or essentialist terms. Thus, in common usage, the label "autism" trades on a productive ambiguity—pronounced on the authority of science, its primary social role is to officially recognize worthy recipients of therapeutic resources.

Parents, or adults diagnosed later in life, often intuitively grasp the complexity of diagnosis. Some parents of autistic children find a sense of release in finding a label that explains their child's condition, while at the same time being very uneasy about the social coding that inevitably goes along with it.[10] The labels parents apply to children matter a great deal for how they learn to position themselves within their social worlds. A diagnosis of a learning disability at least promises the social support a child needs and deserves in order to reach their fullest potential. But to secure that treatment their parents and caregivers will not only need medical certification but will have to learn to describe them in the most negative possible light, as incapable, as falling short, as miles away from the goals of normalcy, and therefore in important respects, a burden to society. Bewilderingly, at that magical age when they become legal adults, the protocol is inverted: they (or others) will need to present themselves as capable of living on their own, of holding down a job, as capable of making a contribution to the productive work of society without demanding society make too many accommodations. Some will eventually internalize one or the other of these identities, to become permanently dependent, others permanently wed to the idea that they must succeed in the terms set by cultural norms if they are to be accepted. Parents and caregivers cannot evade a constant choice: whether to teach in any given moment conformity to the norms of society, or confidence to challenge those norms.

Caring for an autistic child is rife with social ambiguities that burst into view soon after diagnosis. The complexities compound as they spiral out into other domains of lived existence and produce emotional reactions. These social ambiguities and the emotions they evoke deserve closer attention. Mapping the emotional currents set up by a child medicine has labeled antisocial is a preparatory exercise exposing them to the cauterizing light of grace. It prepares the way for the repentance that leads to transformation, the enlightening release that comes with the discovery that much of the suffering supposedly arising from the condition of autism may be self-imposed or generated by frames of reference that make little theological sense.

Admitting our emotional reactions is a way of bringing to light what we really believe. I do so as a parent of Adam, who was diagnosed "on the autistic spectrum" at about four years old. While no textbook case (if there is one), he does exhibit some familiar symptoms, a narrowness of interest, limited social interactivity, and severely delayed and limited communicative skills. In the next section I account as honestly as I can my own reactions to living with autism, the hopes and fears evoked in the course of living with Adam. At times the testimony of others will be drawn in, as at least some of my reactions seem to be widely shared. Young is right—autism reveals the truth. But it may well be that the truth it reveals are attitudes and ideals in need of theological interrogation. I intend this to be robustly theological self-criticism: laying our affective lives bare is to expose to scrutiny the salvation we *actually* seek.[11]

AFFECTIVE RESPONSES TO AUTISM AS PRECURSORS OF THE KINGDOM

In my experience four negative and two positive emotions predominate in loving someone with autism: frustration, grief, longing, uncertainty, expectation, and enjoyment. Emotional reactions do develop over time, so this is a time-specific slice of a kaleidoscopic process. Others speak of denial, shock, guilt, and anger. My intention is not to give a comprehensive account of what all parents and caregivers might feel, but to give a more subtle and nuanced picture of the affective experience of one parent that prepares the ground for the theological reflections with which this chapter concludes.

Anyone who has come into contact with autism can immediately understand the problem of *frustration and embarrassment* in parenting a child with autism. Frustrations are of two main types. The first is linked to attitudes about space, place, and the ordering of materiality. Behaviors like repeatedly and compulsively slamming doors, blowing bubbles in puddles in the gutter and soaking clothing, or throwing food or objects down from tables violate expectations about the proper ordering and cleanliness of our material environment. Constant assaults on common expectations about an orderly home environment are frustrating. This frustration is exponentially compounded by the embarrassing or irritating social disapproval radiated in the gazes and gestures of others when the order of public space is likewise assaulted, when, for instance, items are unexpectedly flung down from store shelves. Modern developed societies are characterized by highly prescriptive expectations about comportment in physical space, and deeply ingrained policing procedures are constantly at work—to which the person with autism is oblivious and therefore constantly violates.

John Gillibrand encapsulates this experience. Notice that his frustration is primarily in relation to the tensions he must constantly negotiate in the fields of the public gaze.

> A few weeks after Adam's diagnoses, we went down to visit my parents-in-law in Cwmbran in South Whales. We went out for lunch, and took Adam with us. Adam was playing with a chair in the corner of the pub, lifting it up a few inches and dropping it back onto the stone floor. . . . people with autism often engage in repetitive and stereotypical behaviors, and we were only too glad that he was with us, engaged in such an activity, rather than running away. The person on the next table looked straight at Gill and said words which we had not heard before, but which are all too familiar to the parents and carers of people on the autistic spectrum: 'Can't you control your son?' Things have improved in terms of autism awareness even in this last ten years, but the words of Martin Lloyd Williams, an Anglican priest who is the father of a child with Down's syndrome, are still true, '*It is the common experience of people with disabilities and their parents or carers, that they are always being judged*. We know so many parents of children on the autistic spectrum who are thoroughly disapproved of because their children are perceived to be out of control.' [As a minister myself] I was thus *gradually being caught in a double difficulty: Being in the public gaze as a priest, but then having to respond to the not always kindly gaze with which the general public looks on those with disabilities*.[12]

Another layer of frustrations is more complex, in part because they spring from our highest aspirations for our children to join society, to have friends. We want our children to be polite, communicative, cooperative, and outgoing, and hence autistic behaviors appear to us to limit our child's life chances. Difficulties functioning as part of a group, difficulties cooperating with other children and obeying simple instructions all apparently leave the child socially isolated. Unreachable expectations from other parents, teachers, or caregivers who have no idea how to deal with such disruptive and antisocial behaviors compound this frustration. At home these frustrations are exacerbated by an awareness of the extra strains and limits a "less controllable" child puts on the family. These include the difficulty of finding competent respite caregivers and limiting the types of things a family can do together in public, at least in a public that does not understand these behaviors and often seems to have little empathetic interest in doing so.

Many of these same behaviors and dilemmas also generate feelings of *grief and fear*. An unawareness of social conventions about space is not only awkward and frustrating but also dangerous. Unawareness of the social organization of space also often appears a self-destructive behavior to a parent's eyes. Darting out into the street, eating things out of the toilet (including poisons) or off the floor, wandering off in crowded places are terrifying for parents and caregivers. The constant sense of danger and anxiety this creates is mirrored by grief at the actual or potential physical self-destructiveness that could well attend these behaviors. Unsanitary behaviors like seeking sensation through licking surfaces that quite evidently soothe the person with autism, come tinged with grief for a parent who feels responsible to protect a child from illness and social stigmatization. While a child might appear to greatly enjoy playing with and licking a wheel on a bicycle or pram, or the floor on a train, to take some examples, it is behavior that may and sometimes does lead to foreseeable consequences, such as virulent intestinal sickness. Grief wells up from the simple fact that life is so much more physically challenging. There is no easy way to watch those we love live with compulsions and pleasures that in the modern world, as currently organized, are patently self-destructive. The constant vigilance this demands is also wearing, the constant negotiation of the question of whether to divert attention from those "pleasures" or risk dealing with possible consequences later.

Grief, again, is also generated by the child's awkward ignorance of social context. An obsession with tipping over chairs or throwing things down from tables alienates a child from a group. Such a child may be watched as entertainment, or escaped as irritating, but it is very difficult to have them be part of a social group in any meaningful sense. This, like many of the emotions described above, are variants of the grief that any parent suffers in watching their child face social ostracization.

The grief associated with a child's failure to socialize with others is closely associated with our own *longings to connect or communicate* with our child. The reciprocated attention that emotionally buoys parents happens more rarely with an autistic child, and a parent cannot help but long for this contact. One mother of a severely autistic teenager told me of an unexpected joy amidst the horror of her teenage daughter's near-fatal sickness which momentarily liberated her from her severe touch aversion. The sickness made it possible for a mother to hold her daughter's hand, for the first time ever, and for this to be a genuine comfort to the daughter. Within such longing comes a heightened appreciation of the contact, whether physical, emotional, or intellectual, that may occasionally be made.

Uncertainty is not an emotion, but it is a cognitive state of confusion or lack of clarity that tends to generate the emotion of anxiety. In any case, it is the opposite of closure or certainty and the ability to put something out of one's mind associated with it. The ambiguities of diagnosis can cause moments of distrust or suspicion of medical judgments and second-guessing of treatment proposals or programs. These ambiguities also foster a gnawing sense that it is impossible rationally to determine whether one has "done enough" or "done the right things" as a parent. A chronic battle with uncertainty ensues about whether and how to respond to, treat, or properly ignore any given aspect of a condition one would dearly like to remedy, if not cure. Many of these layers are expressed in the confession of grief and perplexity that is the beating heart of Thomas Reynolds' book, *Vulnerable Communion*.

> Learning to love my son has meant putting aside presumptions about what love is, what counts for value in a person, what being human entails. This has not been easy. When there is struggle and pain in the process, I must confess my first impulse is to feel disappointed, cheated, even betrayed by life. Chris's presence ruptures my controlled, planned, and predictable world. I am inclined to think that somehow things have gone awry, pieces scattered in disarray, hopes deferred. Because of this, it is easy to feel a sense of failure, as if I am flawed in some basic way, have done something horrible to traumatize Chris, or have not done enough to help him accommodate to how a "normal" child should be, essentially fashioning him in my own ideal image. Indeed, I suffer. Encountering Chris exposes me to my own vulnerability. I am not in control, and I feel impoverished and insecure in his presence. In an effort to shun this sense of weakness, I am tempted to seek avenues of control and strength. I may push Chris away and reclaim security behind an air of parental authority or condescension, essentially shunning his weakness for my own benefit. But doing so makes him bear the burden of my projections. I thrust upon Chris my feelings of inadequacy and confusion, naming him their cause. He then becomes the "other," the one who suffers from disabilities.[13]

At the same time the sheer difference of some human lives can also be *exciting*. Life is not going to be as predictable and boring as it might have been! Parenting a child with special needs often generates a palpable sense that "real life has begun"—and it will be a life that will not conform to the familiar social scripts.[14] One mother calls her autistic son "'my unlikely ethnographer' as his rule breaking often revealed as much about the banality or stupidity of unwritten rules as it did about him not doing what he was told."[15] It can be exhilarating to be liberated from the triteness and tyranny of a normal life course into hope that the life that results will have its own special and unpredictable joys. But fantasies of upward mobility or dream vacations will also now have to be explicitly faced.

Tragically, this positive sense of expectation can be unexpectedly capsized by wider society's reactions to it. People on the autistic spectrum who are able to negotiate most social settings can dread the confusion in the faces of those around them who are startled and then threatened or discomforted upon realizing that they are dealing with someone whom they consider "different."[16] As a parent, one becomes sensitized to how people react to the unfamiliar, becoming a constant observer of human reactions. Most react in predictably self-protective or evasive ways. Some, delightfully, do not. One privilege of living with Adam is to meet remarkable people by virtue of this special person whom you accompany.[17]

If society throws up two faces, one unthreatened and open, one fearful and evasive, its roots are the same dynamics in the individual's soul. Battles are fought against selves that are repulsed by difference so that the selves at peace with it may come to the fore. Reynolds again:

> [Chris's] genuine otherness continually breaks through pity and astonishes me as something surprisingly precious in its own right. His is a young life seeking creatively to affirm itself, thwarted by conditions that he did not ask for and for which he is not responsible. This vulnerability rouses me to attend to him in ways that lure me outward beyond self-preoccupation; and the first taste of this conjures something akin to repentance. Confronted by Chris's vulnerability, I am humbled and brought to recognize how my own needs, expectations, and ideals have closed me in on myself and limited my capacity to be open toward him, to be there with and for him in *his* struggles as well as his joys.[18]

The sheer dynamism of these processes makes it harder to imagine who one might be after a decade or two living with this child. While for some these inner battles are anxiety inducing and need to be escaped, for others it is a release from a deadening sense that the rest of the story will unroll without surprises. This hope, however, can only follow the painful revealing and crushing of the illusion of being able to manage and control other people and the future. While having a child with special needs demands that others reshape their social habits, generating constant friction and annoyance, that same fact also gives birth to the hope that in having one's simplistic and socially accepted pictures of life demolished, one may become a person who is patient, flexible, and loving.

If frustration is the most obvious first experience of life with a child with autism, genuine *enjoyment* is also a constant companion. For some this sense of enjoyment may well be a very regular experience. As a busy academic, for instance, there are few things I find more enjoyable than being on the playground keeping a quiet eye out for potential disasters or taking long walks with a nonverbal teenager. I cherish the quiet forty-minute walk to church each Sunday morning, which helps me sift the sediments of my soul and allows Adam to be more settled for church upon arrival.

In joining him in such activities, Adam draws me into his time. His is a much slower time, which does not mean less full of joy or activity, but it is more spatially and conceptually limited and occupied in ways that are constantly cross-grained to expectation.[19] It takes time to learn his ways of behaving, what he enjoys, and how to help him enjoy things. Having invested in trying to understand his form of activity and slowing down to his rhythms, I learn to see how my presence is appreciated, and discover unexpected ways in which I appreciate his presence. This mutual enjoyment is doubly gratifying given its utter uniqueness and the time it has taken to develop. While Adam may not yet want to play ball, he is certainly pleased in his own way to have me present and pushing his swing. To see a child enjoying himself is gratifying no matter the child, and to learn what a child enjoys is similarly pleasing whether that be lying on the grass or writing a concerto.

To be an academic is to live in a world of clever people who value intelligence—but who are rarely able to even recognize Adam's intelligence. As Adam remakes me he invites me to become a different sort of academic. To the extent that I am remade I cannot but challenge the academy's presumptions about the value of intelligence. Adam's gratuitous gift to me is to enjoy me. His enjoyment invites me to spend my mornings, evenings, weekends, and holidays with someone who is easily dismissed by the intelligent, and this is a politically potent remaking. Adam is educating me in what intelligence is, and how different forms of intelligence found different sorts of community.

AUTISTIC IN THE RESURRECTION?

Conditions like autism reveal the cracks between reality and aspiration. In Christian theology the gap between what is and what should and will be is the subject of eschatology. Eschatology presses sharp questions about what constitutes healing, and pictures of healing configure how the tensions of living with autism will be perceived.

Eschatological expectation commonly takes two forms among Christians today. The first hews close to the familiar stereotype endlessly repeated in popular culture: heaven is that place where everyone becomes "normal" and everyone's bodies and minds are repristinated according to the Hollywood ideal. Everyone will be socially adept and well liked. Such images of heaven cannot but entrench stereotypes about disability as linked to sin or as a defect no one could reasonably desire to be eternally preserved. And they just as clearly undermine any real interest in embracing diversity in the present. This vision of resurrection entrenches common cultural stereotypes about human perfection that either marginalize or seek to remove the traits that are constitutive of the identities of people with all sorts of mental and physical disabilities, including autism.

Christian theologians interested in disability have tried to correct this view by recovering some sidelined strands of traditional Christian theology. Heaven is indeed a place where people's whole selves, including their bodies and minds, are perfected. The question is what *sort* of change this is.[20] Asking about change is but the reverse side of the question of the stability of identity. Too much change threatens the loss of being the same person. Evolving change can cross a line into replacement change, one person substituted for another.[21] Common views of the resurrection are characteristically modern in assuming that an individual's "self" is wholly individualized and somehow inside, or other than, the body. One important theological counterproposal draws a set of anthropological assumptions from patristic speculations about the resurrection. Resurrection is envisioned not as a point but a process, a gradual and eternal progress toward complete healing and redemption of body, mind, and self-identities.[22]

What the modern-normalizing and the progressivist views of resurrection both share is an anthropologically oriented definition of healing and redemption. Once anthropology has done most of the work of defining disability, it is almost inevitable that eschatological speculations become an arena in which Christians imagine what the "perfect" human might look like. This important intellectual work is therefore an indispensable part of any theologically sophisticated account of disability. It does not, however, exhaust Christian eschatology, and leaves several unresolved problems for a theology of disability.

To say that resurrection means slow perfection is not precisely the same thing as directly answering the question of in what the resurrection healing consists. If a Christian eschatology is grounded in anthropology, then it will allow questions to emerge about eschatology that reveal that it is anthropology, not eschatology, that is the dominating theme. One telling sign is whether or not the worry is admitted that in the resurrection people will be so changed that they will not recognize one another.[23] This worry assumes that in the resurrection people would be baffled and alienated by changes to the resurrected bodies and minds of those they love if these changes somehow take them beyond the identity that was theirs through their whole earthly existence.[24] This already betrays a deficient understanding of the kingdom of heaven which can only be entered by being born anew. The language of being "born again" is a confession that one has been drawn into a becoming and growing that can no longer claim to have perfect self-knowledge nor even knowledge of who one is destined to be.[25]

Hence the "recognition worry" garners its moral force from the claim that human beings will find their love for disabled people today undermined by the hope that they will be different and "better" in their future state.[26] It is important to be clear that these different eschatologies have direct implications for the hermeneutics of people labeled disabled. To love someone conceived as *temporarily* "defective" assumes that their "real" self has what is conceived as broken about them erased. When loving someone assumed to be *currently* "normal" reverses the problem—that they would be radically changed by being healed and restored seems unnecessary. A third view is a version of the holy-innocent tradition, understanding someone with severe cerebral palsy, for instance, to be innocent in their essence or soul and awaiting their release from their currently "broken" body or mind in the resurrection.

All three eschatologies read the resurrected body through a view of the created body. If in God's eyes every human being is to be known and loved as they are, as *neither* "defective" *nor* "normal," this must shape how the question is answered about whether the resurrection raises people as they are, or in a drastically altered form, or without change but to be slowly altered. It is actually the assumptions grounding the recognition worry that deserve querying. Those seen as disabled pose a sharp question: "*If you cannot love us today, what makes you think you would love us if we were different, healed, or better?*" To answer this question will demand that eschatology do more work shaping a theological anthropology and the moral psychology that goes with it.

The recognition worry also does not take sufficient account of how the epistemic and ecclesial implications of eschatology inform Christian anthropology. Focusing exclusively or primarily on the individual body as the locus of human identity betrays an insufficiently social definition of the human. Human beings are never explicable as bare monads. This phenomenological observation is heightened in Christian theology, which confesses that human redemption is into a redeemed *community*.[27] Individuals are destined to become stones in a living temple.[28] Discussions of eschatology that never transcend questions about the appearance and functioning of *bodies* in their resurrected form render it almost impossible to see how the resurrection's cutting edge is the renewal of *social* relations. The organization of theological thought about the resurrection around individual bodies lends undue prominence to questions that the New Testament intentionally defers. The Gospels emphasize especially clearly that the complete healing that will come to individual bodies in the resurrection is already present and beginning in important respects that demand notice today. The New Testament as a whole offers precious few examples that even hint at what it might mean to be healed fully at the end of time. Thus to focus on the complete healing of individual bodies as the core theme of eschatological thinking must downplay very real and widespread breaking of the unfreedom of sin to introduce people into redeemed communion that only occasionally is manifested in the healing of individual bodies. The mistake in such approaches is to configure their eschatological imagination around the very sorts of healing that appear more rarely in this time between the times—miraculous bodily healing.[29] The challenge of speaking theologically about the final healing of the body is one part of eschatology, but comes as a later step, not the first.[30]

When Christians have speculated about what it means to be perfected, bodily and morally, they rightly return to the biblical promise of resurrection in Christ. The Gospels do offer narratively couched speculations about the resurrected body. The Emmaus road story of Luke 24:13-35 depicts the resurrected Jesus' body as both so different and yet like his precrucifixion body that it takes some time for his disciples to recognize him. This depiction of Jesus' resurrection body is certainly evocative of some feature of post-resurrection life along with other Gospel pericopae, such as the depictions of Jesus' postresurrection eating and his invitation to Thomas to touch the wounds of his crucifixion (Luke 24:43; John 20:27). It is one thing for the Gospel writers to suggest that Jesus was resurrected with a body, and quite another to extrapolate that they would have wanted future believers to develop highly elaborate theories about the precise traits of all resurrected bodies. Following this route also means that the general anthropological relevance of a range of other texts will have to be explained, such as Jesus' resurrected body miraculously appearing with a ghostly visage, asking not to be touched, vanishing from sight, or walking through locked doors (Luke 24:36-37; John 20:17; Luke 24:31; John 20:19). Jesus was also transfigured (Mark 9:2-3; Matt 17:2

[28:3]), which the majority of patristic theologians see as the definitive display of the form of the resurrected body.[31]

The New Testament writers presume that "souls" and "identities" are not *other* than the body of the human being. Modern theologians have taken this point on board without thinking equally theologically about the idea of identity. Human beings were created to be conformed to Christ, and to be resurrected in this conformity to Christ. In this context "in Christ" is not an "ideal self" but a way of talking about the "marks of personal identity" that matter and will remain even when human beings are resurrected and perfected.[32] These marks may not cohere with the identity ascriptions that attached to the person during their lives on earth. What matters is that they indicate the role of this particular person in their own place, time, and body in God's redemptive story with the world. In this respect disabilities will almost certainly not be erased. They will be transformed in ways, as Francis Young rightly puts it, beyond imagination.

If eschatological description begins where the New Testament begins, then what is foregrounded instead is the new social order that is *already* being established. Part of what is exciting about this redeemed social order is that in it bodily differences already begin to find their prominence in other's eyes reduced. *Jesus' descriptions of the kingdom of heaven focused primarily on the renewal of human perception and relationships*. The Apostle Paul heightens Jesus' questions by intentionally limiting the role of anthropology in eschatological speculation.

> Someone may ask: How are dead people raised, and what sort of body do they have when they come? How foolish! What you sow must die before it is given new life; and what you sow is not the body that is to be, but only a bare grain, of wheat I dare say, or some other kind; it is God who gives it the sort of body that he has chosen for it, and for each kind of seed its own kind of body. . . . we are all going to be changed, instantly, in the twinkling of an eye, when the last trumpet sounds. The trumpet is going to sound, and then the dead will be raised imperishable, and we shall be changed, because this perishable nature of ours must put on imperishability, this mortal nature must put on immortality. (1 Cor 15:35-38, 52-53)

Paul seems to be simultaneously worried that the Corinthians are denying the resurrection as a bodily phenomenon and that they illegitimately hanker to understand in too great detail the forms of resurrected bodies. He replies that the resurrection is so transformative that it is counterproductive to speculate about the form of human resurrection bodies.

Given the limits of speculative anthropologies of the resurrected body as well as the foregrounding in the New Testament of knowing people "in Christ," it seems at least as plausible to note that in these stories, as throughout Jesus' life, the Gospel writers far more regularly emphasize Jesus' power to open eyes, first to who he is and then to all reality (Luke 24:30-35). The remainder of the Gospels seem to suggest that this opening of eyes and comprehensive reorientation is best understood as the inbreaking of the heavenly kingdom, an opening of heaven on earth (John 1:51). This inbreaking is a revelatory event marked by human perception being transformed so that it sees beyond surfaces, appearances, and preconceptions. The human gaze is not like a camera neutrally registering phenomena outside the body, but a physical gesture expressing the spiritual attitude of the person. This is why Jesus so intentionally founds his kingdom by calling forth a new gaze, by fostering a new way of looking on the world, explicitly rejecting a covetous gaze for a "generous gaze."[33] A generous gaze can acknowledge the good in the works of others and forgives what is not. It is not begrudging because it never loses sight of God's mercies as the source of all good (Mark 10:18). The gaze Jesus gives reaches out toward others without desiring to own or manipulate them but seeks their flourishing.

There is a direct correlation between the shape of the human gaze upon others and the God they believe beholds them—and for whose action they await. Jesus' foregrounding of the gaze draws from a deep well of the Old Testament expectation for God to enact mercy toward those who look to God.

> I lift my eyes to you, to you whose throne is in heaven.
> As the eyes of slaves look to the hand of their master,
> as the eyes of a maid look to the hand of her mistress,
> so our eyes look to the Lord our God,
> *till he shows us his mercy*. (Ps 123:1-2, NIV)

The emphasis Jesus lays on the gaze makes sense of Paul's lack of interest in encouraging the Corinthians' anthropologically focused speculations about the resurrection. For Paul, what is crucial about the person of Jesus Christ is his *contemporary* agency, the agency of the one whose appearance shines a blinding light that opens new perception, who shows himself when Paul is weak. *The New Testament's eschatology is not primarily concerned to establish an anthropological account of the resurrection, but to foster an embodied expectation that Jesus' heavenly kingdom of peace will arrive here and now*. Sight is only a root metaphor for a more fundamental resituating of our sensate relation to God, world, and the neighbor.

PERCEPTION, THE PRESENT, AND PRESENCE

Jesus' parable of the Good Samaritan in Luke 10 foregrounds the eschatological inversion of the human gaze. Jesus' interlocutor is presented as asking the wrong question, "*Who is* my neighbor?" a question assuming that it is *other* people who need to be categorized. To this misguided question Jesus responds by putting the attention on the perceiving and acting agent: "*To whom* have you been a neighbor?" The fundamental problem with a Christian eschatology organized by the objective of defining a theological anthropology is that it, too, easily tips into the register of defining and categorizing *neighbors*. Christian eschatology ought, rather, to engender critical scrutiny of the *agent's* action in the present. Christian love can be enacted without a comprehensive account of what is essentially human in the wide range of humanity. It is a work centered on the problem of not letting the neighbor's sin, hostility, awkwardness, or sheer unintelligibility excuse an escape from being responsive to them.[34]

The core question is *which* are the most pertinent eschatological motifs for a discussion of disability theology.[35] There has been a recurrent tendency in Western eschatologies to allow discussions of the perfection of resurrected bodies to precede and situate discussions of reconciled human relationships, which amounts to presenting eschatology as a doctrine of a *future* state with *implications* for the present.[36] The Gospels seem to approach from the other direction in assuming that our *bodies* will be included in the reconciliation of all creation in the ineffable way and to the extent that that this will be necessary for *interpersonal* reconciliation. *Resurrected bodies and intellects do and will make "sense" in the resurrection not because they stay the same, but because they are located in their rightful place in the peaceable communion of the body of Christ.*[37]

Christians confess they are not "other" than their bodies: humans are wholly bodily beings. Thus, anthropology is by no means unrelated to Christian eschatology. Christians should resist linking human identity to an imagined inner life in distinction from the body so characteristic of the post-Cartesian age. The question of resurrected bodies is an obvious place for this widespread mislocation of human identity to be addressed. The dominance of this Cartesian anthropology does help to explain the relative paucity of serious discussion of intellectual disability in disability theology, since moderns have real difficulties thinking of someone as a real person who is not self-conscious and rational. The liminality of autism in this respect, as a condition marked by a desire to *relate and reason differently*, exposes the weak point of anthropologies that separate the self from the body. Attempts to define persons with autism in terms of their self-image alone seem unable to do justice to the reality that such a description might accurately describe some people labeled autistic, but not many others (this is where the lack of a scientific account of its rooting in biology becomes philosophically interesting). What is present in every case are nonstandard approaches to relating to other persons and the material world. People with autism are not nonrelational, they relate differently to others and the world, they *sense* others and the world differently.

Ironically, many people referred to as high-functioning autistics, or who might be designated as having Asperger syndrome, are clearly self-conscious and in many cases conform quite closely to the Cartesian ideal. If Descartes insists that intellectual certainty is only achieved by abstracting from bodiliness (and with it, culture and the particularity of experience), then the very blindness to culture and social cues that often leads to a diagnosis of autism are hypermodern traits in their seeming conviction that social realities are not "real" because they are not concrete and testable. It is doubly ironic that post-Cartesian medicine has come to define autism as a case of individuals "opting out of" or being unable to access social intercourse.

Both sides of the polarity rest on a false division. If humans are irreducibly bodily and social beings, bodiliness and sociality cannot be opted out of. What autism reveals especially acutely is the shape of modern modes of perception. It presents moderns with a surprising fold of individual *social consciousness*, one that is liminal and perplexing in being a mirror image of the modern self-image. In its supposedly classic forms, autism is the state of Cartesian blindness to the empirically "unreal" enacted with absolute consistency. In a crucial sense autism is a mislabeling of an individual, since it only appears as a phenomenon through challenging *communities*. It is precisely this communal and cultural dimension of human life that high-modern thought sought to subtract from its definition of true knowledge.

But, as Steve Silberman discovered in writing his landmark history of autism, "The notion that the cure for the most disabling aspects of autism will never be found in a pill, but in supportive communities, is one that parents have been coming to on their own for generations."[38] Autism is revelatory in disturbing the anthropology of modern liberalism and with it is political order, in which it is assumed that the telos of human life is to be maximally self-possessed and individuated.[39] Many people with autism will face high hurdles to survival on their own as "autonomous individuals," not because they are *disconnected* from others, but because they are not tuned into the few levels of reality that modern liberal societies organize themselves around.

A genuinely Christian eschatology does not confine healing and redemption to the afterlife.[40] It was no accident that Jesus called the way of life he inaugurated the kingdom of heaven. To the limited extent that speculations about resurrected *bodies* may be necessary in Christian theology, they are elaborations of what Christians believe about redeemed *sociality*. Proceeding the other way around reproduces the most problematic aspects of the Western Christian tradition, its overweighting of creation in its definition of the human. The speculations of Western patristic theologians like as Tertullian and Augustine on the resurrection body signal the dangers of this doctrinal misweighting. Put more provocatively, if the crucial eschatological questions are really anthropological, then why do modern theologians not ask the real questions, as the Church Fathers do not shy from doing? These include whether the corpulent rise to heaven more slowly than the svelte,[41] what size the resurrected bodies of aborted and miscarried new ones will be,[42] whether or not all people will be resurrected in a uniform size[43] to an optimal age[44] or with or without their sexual characteristics.[45] Western patristic theologians also wrestle with whether the biblical promise that "not a hair will be lost" requires the restoration of hair and fingernail clippings[46] and applies to people who have been cannibalized.[47]

The main problem with such anthropological speculations is not their overdetermination by the doctrine of creation to the exclusion of Christology. Augustine, for instance, affirms that the measure of human perfection is the resurrected height, weight, and age of Jesus.[48] The problem is that the Christology and eschatology being assumed *are not social at their root, but individual and physical*. This problem leads almost inevitably into the generation of universal norms by which every human being must be measured and projecting commonsense views of human beings forward to define resurrected perfection.[49] In contrast, Jesus seems to think rather differently, that *eschatology's most prominent feature is its beginning in this age in the overturning and reformulation of human certainties and viewpoints. Eternity is a domain that reaches into and shakes up the present.*[50] To follow his lead is to escape the metaphysical quagmire of anthropological definition that always tends, in the end, to generate idealisms of human perfection and so us-them dichotomies.

AUTISM IN THE KINGDOM OF HEAVEN

In the Gospels Jesus is depicted as propounding a strongly eschatological ethic. The parable of the workers in the vineyard in Matthew 20 provides an obvious example. It begins, "For the kingdom of heaven is like a landowner who went out early in the morning to hire workers for his vineyard" (Matt 20:1, NIV). This opening line unambiguously signals that the topic of the parable is the forepresence of heaven in this world and its reconfiguration of human perception and social comportment. The plot is well known: at various points in the day the landowner keeps hiring additional day laborers, all of whom receive the same wage at the end of the day whether having worked all day or only an hour. Those who had worked all day began to grumble at the vineyard owner saying,

> "These men who were hired last worked only one hour," they said, "and you have made them equal to us who have borne the burden of the work and the heat of the day." But he answered one of them, "Friend, I am not being unfair to you. Didn't you agree to work for a denarius? Take your pay and go. I want to give the man who was hired last the same as I gave you. Don't I have the right to do what I want with my own money? Or are you envious because I am generous?"[51]

To the tale Jesus appends the enigmatic conclusion, "So the last will be first and the first will be last." The statement appears to be aimed at those who have, in this world, labored in faith and who look with envy on what has been given to others. But Jesus will have none of the Nietzschean *ressentiment* of the pious and self-concerned believer.[52] Such resentment embodies a forgetfulness of the radical equality of humanity before God, and that each person's vocation is not rightly oriented by desire for the reward that will one day be received. It is a privilege to be a worker in Christ's vineyard, in any capacity, to have been made a part of God's story with the world by being given work that serves and extends this life-giving kingdom.

The vineyard is a pregnant image in Scripture, primarily denoting the divine vineyard that is God's holy people.[53] Jesus is teaching that the dawning of heaven is not simply that humans are drawn into the labor of the church, but that as they do so they exhibit a very specific stance of faith within it—that the work they have been given is itself meaningful, and though laborious, will one day be consummated in a final rest with the whole people of God.

A theologically adequate account of "living with autism" is best located within this imagery of serving in God's vineyard. When the hour for payment comes, those who have worked all day betray their selfish reasons for working and their anxieties that their faith in the landowner will be let down. All along they have not understood the intrinsic value and meaning of their task but have done it only for the offered reward. Only at the end of the day has what was true all along become visible (1 Cor 3:12-15). That they have worked only in interest of reward is marked by their comparisons with others and the construction of hierarchies of relative worth.[54] The *krisis* that besets such judgments signals the working of the Spirit of Jesus Christ. If received repentantly and with gratitude, so too is the gift of a new perception of the social order. *This is a kingdom that can only appear in the present tense: where God is making all things new* (Isa 43:19; Rev 21:5).

To live with the challenges raised by autism is to be forced to learn to live in this peculiar present, to let go of the swarming fears about where this life is heading or whether life can go on as it is now for yet another year. Popular medical-related advertising and some medical professionals sometimes inflame these fears ("you need to do this now to avert that later, to listen to these experts to avoid disaster"[55]). Jesus' vineyard eschatology instead orients attention on present people and on the tasks of today as meaningful activities. In faith such works are enactments of hope that God will make them bear fruit in God's time. The ethical force of this vineyard eschatology emerges from this reorientation of perception. Human resurrection and healing does not exist hidden over the horizon of eternity. It is offered concretely in the given persons amongst whom human life must be lived. Loving them is a work of listening and obedience that disciplines believers, through which they discover their place in this world as a foretaste of the life of the world to come.

The parable also shows how one of the most obvious signs of being grasped by Jesus' kingdom of heaven is to be freed of anxieties about future reward and recognition. The church's gathered worship recalls and draws attention to this reality as a weekly foretaste and "theatre of heaven,"[56] an intensified reality that lets the comedy of day-to-day life appear as it really is. This perceptual gap looks very different from the side of the laws of this age, as the rabbis note: "from the perspective of the imperfect world, perfection appears deformed."[57] In worship Christians see how the powers that think they rule the world are really slaves and idolaters. They see that the laws of scarcity and normalization and social decorum and dog-eat-dog competition are all great and demonic illusions. The release is palpable, calling forth the Easter laughter of those who have just seen clearly the unreality of all they once believed controlled their lives.[58] In worship Christians bodily perform a recognition that they can know none of this on their own. To confess and celebrate the victory of the lamb constantly invites a translocation from the habits of this aeon into ones organized by another ethos, a renewal of human perception that reorients every sphere of life (Rom 12:2).

This proposal has a range of implications, not least for my life with Adam. It means to be set into perpetual conflict with my human tendencies to project my desires onto him, and to learn instead to be with him and listen to him responsively. If heaven is most fundamentally a healed and reconfigured social order, as the vineyard imagery presumes, communion with God and the saints being its essential feature,[59] I am sure that in heaven Adam and I will look back and have a good laugh at the absurd situations we have negotiated together. Theologically understood, this "imagination" is not a subjectivization of heaven, nor a psychological projection, but is the *actual reality of the kingdom of heaven*. When the "least" open us up, help us laugh, the light of the kingdom shines on us in our darkness. In Thomas Reynolds' words,

> Time and again, Chris's forgiveness and patience with me have become a sustaining grace. His humor and sense of irony about things help lighten my often overwrought solemnity and seriousness (we often joke together about our shortcomings). The paradox here is that, far from inhibiting my ability to attend to Chris, such openness actually works to establish a more *profound mutuality* that cultivates *compassionate regard* . . . a *relation to involvement*, of *empathetic attunement*.[60]

I want to suggest that this laughter is more than just a means creating empathy; it is an ontological reality, an eschatological reality, the laughter at the foot of the cross at the realization that the most powerful religious and political authorities have failed to stop this crucified healer.[61]

This insight is one of the more significant gifts of the Reformation to Western theology. At precisely this point Luther decisively broke with the more penitential tenor and sensibility of medieval theology. For Luther, joy and laughter were heralds of the redeemed state. When Abraham, to take one example, was told by God that his aged wife Sarah would bear him a child, Luther imagines that he first "wept for joy, until he finally regained his composure, as it were, and laughed when at last he felt this joy with a calm heart, a feeling which is a part of eternal life."[62] The laugher that Adam and I share is one infused by joy, a joy that ultimately flows from God's beneficence to us and the absurdity of our current lives. It is that *particular* joy that creates a *specific type* of togetherness and empathy.

To be liberated from the necessity to "control" or "manage" the other allows an approach to the other as an equal, with whom we will someday share some clear-eyed understanding about the ironies and farcical nature of this life. As Adam's parent, it is clear that those we meet who have this heaven's-eye view tend to have a special grace to accept Adam as he is. If the kingdom of God is characterized by this stance, much of the speculation about what he will be like in heaven can be seen as reproducing the prejudices that fuel injustice or inducing anxieties that undermine that freeing joy.

In other words, anthropologically ordered eschatological speculations are a temptation, not a solution to the pains of this life. Worries, anxieties, fears, struggles for definition—all threaten to take on a life of their own, to quench any existential sense of the intrinsic value of attending to and loving those who present special challenges. But it is precisely in the crucible of this struggle in faith *against ourselves*, our fears and false hopes, that marks the true church. Christians suffer from temptation only when they know it as a *temptation*. Only if they know enough of their own story in Christ, only if their false narratives have been sufficiently interrupted, can an existential struggle be recognized not just as a worry, but as a temptation. A temptation is an urge to not be faithful to the reality revealed in Jesus Christ. This renders temptation promising in that the suffering of temptation can be perceived as a sign and means of grace. The very uncertainty and turmoil associated with sinful weakness, loss, and confusion is self-inflicted. But to have this self-inflicted wounding revealed is a promise of its overcoming, and so offers the hope that is a sign of the presence of the true church.[63]

Daily life with Adam can proceed quite well without knowing what he will look like in heaven, what his body will be like, how well he will be able to speak, or of whether I will be able to recognize him in his redeemed state. What it does demand is a stance shaped by a constant awareness of our lives being lived out in the sight of God and in the company of the cloud of witnesses. In the eyes of those third parties, which the Spirit brings to life in us, Adam's real patience with me is exposed, and my real joy in him, even as it is at the same time a judgment on the fact that neither may be much in evidence in any given moment. Put in technical terms, an eschatology oriented by notions of past and future or by a strong interest in anthropological definition is less illuminative of the theologically crucial aspects of life together than an eschatology oriented by conceptions of sociality, vocation, and the real and effected transformation of perception.

A complete treatment of eschatology in its relation to disability would require not only this foregrounded emphasis on the subjective stance of eschatological faith, but also the development of important doctrinal and objective claims about what it is right to hope for in this life, in my case, for Adam. For instance, first, it is theologically warranted to hope for the realization of his *creaturely* givenness. It is therefore wholly appropriate to hope for a good ophthalmologist and glasses that fit and allow him to see, but I have suggested the reasons that, doctrinally speaking, this must be a second-order rather than a first-order question.

A formed hope for the *redeemed* community would also feature in a complete treatment of eschatology. I can hope for Adam to develop his own faith and to discover for himself how he might edify the church, and in and through it, the world.[64] As a baptized Christian he, too, needs a local church body that can carry him and listen for the Spirit's gifts through him and people like him. He is more than autistic, and the life of the church challenges the individualized and medicalized account of his life that assumes his most important need is for therapies that will solve his (individual) problems and deficiencies. What is lost in this approach is any envisioning and praising of communities that can recognize him as a conduit of the Spirit's gifts to the community, whether in a "leadership" role or not. Put more positively, it is important to ask whether a church that understands itself to be calling a fallen world into the new age of redemption can do so without not only allowing but valuing the unselfconscious expressions of "difference" from its various members. In such a church, individual differences can become a communal treasure to those communities who have become aware that embracing such internal differences is intrinsic to a plausible witness that can call other communities to be different.[65]

At the deepest level, and behind these more mundane hopes, I can hope to enjoy Adam. I hope that others, too, will enjoy him as he will be enjoyed in heaven. Such a hope expresses an eschatological and Spirit-gifted strength to love with the love that does not simply tolerate others but can say with unfeigned sincerity: "I'm glad you're here." *This* hope overleaps the paler belief that what "the disabled" bring to churches and individuals is a reminder of the dependence of every human being, or a sense of satisfaction of achieving inclusivity. Such a hope moves beyond the normal-disabled dichotomy in the prayer that our eyes will be opened to them, will see with eyes made to participate in divine vision: "the Lord does not see as mortals see; they look on the outward appearance, but the Lord looks on the heart" (1 Sam 16:7).

The challenge is to embrace the agonies that attend hearts being opened. The *krisis* provoked by disability with which this chapter opened now comes into greater theological focus. Strictly apocalyptic theologies emphasize the judgment that attends God's revelatory appearance in fallen societies. Theologies of annunciation position this judgement slightly differently, by highlighting a more positive emphasis on God's merciful claim. The issue at stake is how the continuity and temporal extension of divine revelation will be understood. How mercy and judgement are understood to relate to one another in God's self-revealing will deeply shape the believer's hermeneutic of disabling conditions as well as their hopes for healing.

The disabling condition of Frances Young's son Arthur originated in an accident due to a fallen world. To see his life this way makes clear sense, given that Arthur's brain was injured in a birth accident. Young understands God to have used Arthur's marred body and mind to expose the sin of society. *A victim of a broken and sinful world, Arthur evokes a divine judgement on that fallen world*. With this interpretation, Young locates the evil of his condition at the level of the individual biological body. In so doing she insulates God from the accusation of having directly caused evil or suffering. The cost, however, is to have located Arthur's life entirely within the domain of theodical thinking. Arthur is trapped in the question of why there is evil in the world at all if God is good.

I have *endeavored to present Adam as an agent of annunciation, perceiving him through a hermeneutics of divine mercy*. The mercy that is Adam's existence, including the state of his body and mind, does expose the sin of the world. But I have presented this divine judgment as the *effect* of God's merciful acts in the world, not a *separate* or *prior* operation. Adam is not an *occasion* for God to show mercy on a broken world, but a *vector* of the divine annunciation of mercy to the world—who in this appearance also reveals and judges my (as well as others') brokenness. Within this hermeneutic the sin and brokenness of the created order do not define Adam's being and life as a whole. The theological locus within which his true being is best understood is an eschatological ecclesiology.

An ecclesial framed eschatology allows me to remain agnostic about the causality of Adam's biological condition. I can affirm that his twenty-first chromosome probably would not have become conjoined in an unfallen world. But I can also affirm that the fact that every cell of his body has been impacted by this biological "fault" says very little about who he has been created to be. I can affirm both that he will be redeemed from pain in the resurrection, and that God has given him to his family, his church, and his nation just as he is. There is no other, better, or different Adam who was not affected by his genetic palette. Having been given him by God establishes my vocation as parent, engaging me in an extended work of responsibility and receipt. I have been presented with a limit I can love. With it comes divine confrontation and judgement of my habits as well as the habits of the world that live in me.

***

CODA: PART 4

Disability provokes painful confrontations with the false and denuding self-images people hold of themselves and others. Any adequate theological response to disability must go beyond defining what disability "is," to negotiate the psychological, spiritual, and interpersonal complexities involved in the revealing of sin. Such exposure is an invitation to repentance, a theme that has been almost entirely absent in theologies of disability to date. The absence of repentance is one of several breaks from the patristic tradition surveyed in part 1, in which repentance played a central role for understanding nonstandard lives.

Disability is not a medical condition, but a label attached to medically describable biophysiological conditions. That this label is not attached to every condition, and the conditions to which it is applied can change, highlights the social horizon within which decisions are made about what will be appropriately labeled a disability. In the final analysis, the conceptual and theological problem with disability is not the word, but the discomfort caused by the reality that the people to whom it is applied always exceed it. Disability activists have constantly emphasized how the very language of disability is a generic norm that inevitably smothers the interpersonal relationship that is essential for genuine human love and friendship. The language of disability thus produces problems that are simultaneously conceptual, linguistic, and political. Theological investigation of these dynamics has strongly repositioned the human phenomena to which the label "disability" is typically affixed. They can no longer be viewed as discreet entities in the world nor broken "parts" of a person. *Labeling something a disability is a response to, and intervention in, local configurations of interpersonal relations. A socially coded response is being made to a set of given features of a human body.*[66]

In occluding a wide series of invitations into interpersonal communion, the term "disability" provokes questions about how communion will be differently lived by the Christian community. The theological task remains to describe how the Christian tradition offers a rival understanding of the roles those called disabled in modern societies might play in God's own story of his people, as commemorated by and enacted in the worshiping community. At least as understood in the Bible, the Christian worshiping community is something more than a community of moral formation, though it certainly is that. It is a political reality in being constituted of individuals who have been formed into a body by being drawn into God's messianic new beginning. The messianic—and prophetic—character of God's merciful new beginning is always "militant" in initiating an alternative reality that challenges and displaces the regnant social orders of the age. To raise the specter that disability might be something much more, and different, than the medical diagnoses that have been attached to individuals presses sweeping questions about the regnant social order and intimates the need for massive cultural changes.[67] This is a challenge that cannot be avoided by Christians, because linguistically, politically, and theologically the very language of disability subverts attempts to take certain lives with the seriousness that they deserve, even at the level of basic social accommodation.

Several of the conventions of the contemporary disability discussion are decisively unsettled by this eschatological account of redeemed relationship. The most prominent is that "able" can be straightforwardly distinguished from the "dis," and that one's own position in this dichotomy is secure. But if at bottom some people are fundamentally experienced as different because disabled, a theology of disability highlights that the dominant frames of perception have positioned them as abnormal, as wrong. The widespread assumption that disability is a problem to be eradicated to the greatest extent possible must be recognized as wrongly abstracting disability from its social location and wrongly individuating it as the incapacity of specific individuals.

Theologically speaking, to experience someone as disabled is not to recognize, but to misrecognize them.[68] A theological repositioning of the human phenomena labeled disabilities allows Christians to move decisively beyond the powerful assumption that able-bodiedness is the starting point for the discussion of disability. Substantial intellectual and existential work will be required to unsettle the wider discourses that have so firmly positioned the discussion at the outset as not about "us," but about the people whose "lack" we need to accommodate. To understand how the redemptive inversion of perception works has entailed excavating precisely how this misrecognition becomes a "cult of normalcy"[69] sanctioned by vast cultural, political, and often religious forces, and internalized by individuals.

As creatures, human beings constantly receive their lives from others. A theological account of disability moves beyond descriptions of the *fact* of vulnerability (and with it, impairment), and towards a *moral* posture, an *ethos*, in which the vulnerable interdependency of human creatures is acknowledged and embraced. Beginning by asking about the temporal and mortal vulnerability that is in fact the condition of *all* creaturely life undermines the emphasis on *ability* as the measure of the human. This recognition defuses the negative valences attached to *dis*ability and hints at how weakness and vulnerability may have a secret power to open hearts to others.[70]

In the Christian theological tradition, norms of physical beauty and perfection have often been defined at the intersection of two claims: the confessions that to be redeemed is to be "conformed to Christ," and that humans are intended to be "raised in Christ," that is, destined for individual physical resurrection. To jettison either consideration is to exit the main stream of Christianity. The premise of both claims is that the beauty and perfection of the human, the human telos, is revealed in Jesus Christ, and is brought to life in individual human beings as they are redeemed in this life, a redemption to be completed in the eschaton. Both Christology and eschatology are not *primarily* doctrines about physical bodies, nor about the end of time (though they are also these). Christology and eschatology are doctrines explicating the dynamic working of the Trinitarian God to wondrously form human beings capable of interrelating as they were created to do.

The arc of a theological argument opened in the first chapter thus culminates in part 5. Drawing on the Gospel story of the Good Samaritan, part 1 elaborated the patristic wonder tradition as a theology of mediated divine mercy. God's mercy meets people by calling themselves out of their sinful routines of self-isolation through the bodies of other individual human beings. The discussion in part 3 of the manner in which autism reveals the importance of an existential openness toward community foregrounded an eschatological account of the kingdom of heaven derived from Jesus' parable of the vineyard. In part 4 the individual sinner's various mechanisms for resisting this approach of divine mercy through the invitation of other bodies was explored. The goal of God's merciful activity is to reclaim human beings by inviting them into redeemed community and so into an illusion-free clarity about creation. Part 5 develops this account of the ways of divine mercy by moving from person-to-person bilateral descriptions to a multi-polar account of the processes of ecclesial communion being created by the Holy Spirit. The creation of a redeemed community by the Spirit, with its own distinctive politics, cannot but challenge and displace the politics of liberal democracies, with their rooting in individual autonomy and agonistic struggle to secure one's own interests.

In Jesus Christ's assault on the Western status quo, those whose strange vocation it is to carry the label "disabled" once again appear in an indispensable role. This assault remakes what is typically considered the problem of disability. However difficult the issues may be, the problem of disability is not a conceptual one, defining its ontological status in debates about whether it is located in the body of individuals or in the prejudicial attitudes of society. Theologically understood, the problem of disability is being truly *present* with those who must carry the label "disabled." *This* problem leads to the animating heart of a theologically reconstituted account of disability.

PART V

BODY-LIFE AS THE COMMUNICATIVE LIFE OF THE WORSHIPING COMMUNITY

9

The Peculiar Togetherness of the Body of Christ

THEOLOGIZING INCLUSION

Modern Christians want to be inclusive. The Bible wants Christians to be members of one another. Christian theology offers a politics of *redeemed communion* that displaces the politics of both exclusion *and* inclusion.

The modern drive toward greater inclusivity stands in the long Christian tradition of resistance to behaviors, such as the violent and demeaning segregation characteristic of early modern theories and practices of disability. Yet the language of inclusion suffers from the same deficits as the earlier Christian model of "charity toward the unfortunate." Both presume a "we" positioned against a needy "them" whom "we" need to help become part of the social domain that "we" inhabit. An "othering" is the premise of the intention to then include those so othered into the very community who did the excluding in the first place.[1] The casualty of inclusion language is political self-awareness. In order for less domineering and more mutual forms of life to emerge, people's self-definitions, language usage, and the form of their relationships will all have to be fundamentally altered. A daunting proposition. What is clear is that nothing can happen until the patronizing certainty that "we" are the ones bearing the duty to include "them" is fundamentally destabilized—including for those who, feeling themselves outsiders, desperately want to join the "us."[2]

What is broken about contemporary forms of communion and communication only truly emerges into view when the grandness of this theological vision of redeemed communion is appreciated. St. Paul's famous discussion of the politics of the body of Christ in 1 Corinthians 12 is devoted to outlining this vision.

The subject of 1 Corinthians 12 is the renewal, healing, and opening of genuine communion with God and others called *church*. The chapter is focused on why the body of Christ is fundamentally a political entity that emerges from a distinctive manner of engaging interpersonal relations. Paul understands every member of the church as an active giver or conduit of divine love, a giving that is not reducible to any person's supposed physiological or intellectual deficiencies. He therefore offers a worked account of what it looks like to live together "beyond disability"—at least beyond the certainties about self and others derived from merely sociological or demographic descriptions, if not beyond bodily diversity.

Inclusion language is not traditionally Christian or even biblical. It originated within late-modern secular liberal, political, and educational philosophies.[3] Substantial criticisms have emerged out of disability studies of the intrinsic double binds characteristic of the ideas "inclusive society" and "inclusive schools." No satisfactory reply has yet emerged in education theory about how to avoid positioning some people as "in need of inclusion."[4] Nevertheless, in recent decades disability theologians have largely embraced the inclusion agenda.

Theological valorizations of inclusion regularly referenced 1 Corinthians 12. Many references are ad hoc and in passing.[5] Sometimes the chapter is cited as offering an essentially modern vision of inclusion suitable to motivate Christians to join the equality and inclusion movements, typically without any exegetical work showing the identity of ancient and modern views.[6] Sometimes single verses are picked out to a similar end, as supporting the claim that everyone is equal in the church,[7] or that every member of the church offers different yet essential contributions to the whole.[8] These treatments mount no challenge to secular inclusion accounts.

Despite this drumbeat of references to 1 Corinthians 12 in disability theology, no consensus reading has emerged. Those theologians who engage the chapter more substantively can read the chapter decidedly differently. Some take it to offer an ecclesial hermeneutics of vulnerability and weakness.[9] For others it provides a set of strict limits on the practice of labeling some Christians weak and vulnerable.[10] Rarely do these engagements exceed a paragraph or page in length, and the two extended treatments of the chapter in disability theology likewise offer markedly different readings.[11]

Jean Vanier has drawn on the chapter more deeply and systematically, his readings influencing several disability theologians to position the chapter as a treatise on the dynamics of a community of friendship.[12] God's befriending of human beings is taken to inspire Christians to greater levels of mutuality, recognition, and acceptance in their relations with other humans. This is a theologically serious step beyond advocacy and charity accounts of disability as well as the politics of inclusion. Yet a material hole remains at its center: it is not entirely clear how friendship works.

This disjointed conversation about 1 Corinthians 12 is valuable in having surfaced three exegetical questions of crucial significance for disability theology.[13] What is meant by "*weakness*" in the context of Paul's usage of the language of "weaker members"? The language of weakness clearly offers a point of contact with the phenomenon of disability, but just as obviously suffers from significant conceptual and contextual drawbacks. How does Paul understand the image of the human body to elucidate the *redeemed political dynamics* that are characteristic of the church? Different explanations here will have direct effects on how inclusion is understood to operate in practice. And what is meant by the claim that *each member brings gifts* to the whole *ecclesia*? A medical model of disability would seem to demand that these gifts be linked to people's physical or intellectual impairments. Theologies oriented by social models of disability will be attracted to ideas that disability is a matter of those who are "made weak" by society's disdain.

The apostle offers a single answer to all three questions. *The politics of the body of Christ arise from an economy of service to one another for mutual upbuilding*. In the hospitality of the Holy Spirit, Christians discover that they never escape the role of recipient. The Spirit thus upends widespread assumptions about who the "we" is and who needs to be "included." In the working of divine mercy that is the Holy Spirit, human beings receive their being in Christ from each other, in community.

ACTIVE GIFTS OF A LIVING SPIRIT

In 1 Corinthians 12 Paul is painting a picture of a functioning church, and therefore of genuinely redeemed human community. The overall flow of the chapter is best grasped by noting its unusually high number of references to divine action. God is described as energizing, giving gifts and honor as he wills, placing and appointing the church's members into their proper relationships. God is at work transforming individuals by restructuring the Corinthians' habits of relating to one another. By speaking of the church as a body, Paul draws attention to the priority of this divine organizing activity by way of an analogy with the human body, in which the organs and fluid flows of working of a human body in their concrete and non-rearrangeable order.

That the primary role of the Holy Spirit is to *open communication* is the premise of the first three verses of the chapter. The distinctive characteristic of the community formed in the Spirit of Jesus Christ is that it begins in a confession. No one can make this confession except those drawn by the Holy Spirit, the person of the Godhead tasked with opening "vertical" communication. The same divine person is also responsible for opening the "horizontal" communication that is the central concern of chapter 12. The Spirit brings Christ's body into existence by opening lively communicative connections between believers. The unique communicative configurations of this gathering *are* Christ's body, given and nonnegotiable.[14]

Verses 4-5 open the direct discussion of the gifts of the Spirit. Three terms are used to characterize what the Spirit gives to believers: "gifts," "services," and "activities."

> Now there are varieties of *gifts*, but the same Spirit; and there are varieties of *services*, but the same Lord; and there are varieties of *activities*, but it is the same God who activates all of them in everyone. To each is given the manifestation of the Spirit for the common good.

Paul is known for having given the language of *charismata* a uniquely precise definition and has been labeled the inventor of the Christian concept of the spiritual gift.[15] *Charisma* occurs only once in Scripture outside the Pauline corpus (1 Pet 4:10), and is used with extreme rarity before Paul. The term itself, *charis-ma*, derives from the term for "giving graciously."[16] As Paul is using the term in a historically novel manner, he offers three partial synonyms. The three expressions he offers provide a trifocal description of a single phenomenon. If a *gift* is not an *actually enacted* work of *service*, it cannot be associated with the Spirit of Christ at all.[17]

The first term, *diakonia*, literally translated "service," was as common and well understood in the first century as in contemporary usage of the term "deacon"—the ones charged with taking care of the practical matters of the church. The second term, *energema*, presents more difficulties. Based on the root *energia*, "power," *energema* is perhaps best translated as "efficient power."[18] The radiating light of the sun is an efficient power in being already underway and effectively warming the earth. This already working energy is to be distinguished from the vast reservoir of energy within the sun that might later radiate into the solar system. In calling the gifts of the Spirit *energema*, Paul is characterizing them as, by definition, "gifts *being* given." He is insisting on a point that is crucial for the whole chapter: spiritual gifts are never a potency that might *later* be discharged. *The gifts exist only as they are enacted.* Neither potentials nor capacities, spiritual gifts are always and only *acts*.[19]

The NRSV translation is thus conceptually unintelligible in speaking of a "variety of activities" that God "activates." The point is that God *has* given a *variety* of enacted powers and *is* working in everyone. For Paul the gifts are like the charge of static electricity that, unbeknownst to the individual believer, is gathering around him or her to be discharged toward other people in an act of service, at the time of the Holy Spirit's choosing. The non-negotiable for Paul is the claim that God is the source of the actual efficient powers visibly at work in all their variety in the Christian church.

In verse 7 Paul encapsulates the teleology of every *charisma* as "for the common good." Here the NRSV boldly uses a political coinage, "common good" to translate *sympheron*, "that which is useful." Having highlighted the political thrust of Paul's language here, rendering *phanerosis* as "manifestation" immediately blunts the point. For Paul, *phanerosis* emphasizes the *public* nature of the work of the Spirit,[20] and can be literally translated as "revelation."[21] The "spark" of service that passes between believers is essentially *revelatory*.

It is now clear that "every member" of the body is not merely a possessor of a portion of the respective gift allotted to him or her. The believer is only a *revealer* of the working of the Spirit to the body as a whole. No central agency is administering the Spirit. The Spirit alone chooses which gifts will be dispensed by any given part of the body. No human management or leadership is needed to make the body of Christ efficient. Since a revelation is never merely a deposit that can be known in advance, the enactment of a gift necessarily involves a moment of *discovery*. A revelation is an actual happening that generates a moment of recognition and reception. A *charisma* reveals the Holy Spirit to the body when the particular gift of the Spirit an individual brings is embraced. The Gospels also make it unambiguously clear that the physical conditions today called disabilities can play a role in this work of divine manifestation. John uses the same word Paul uses here when he quotes Jesus saying a given person "was born blind so that God's works might be revealed (manifested) in him" (John 9:3). This is the biblical basis of Augustine's insistence on strange Christian vocations.

Consider how young Christians discover their proper places and roles in the community. Perhaps someone in the community senses that giving a shy teenager some form of leadership role in a church's youth work might aid the discovery of her unique gift to the body. This invitation to serve becomes an encouragement for her to step forward to test whether the full *phanerosis* of the gift will appear. In a not dissimilar way, older Christians who may have been playing well-established roles in the community may find themselves asked to serve in quite unfamiliar capacities. In such cases the congregation will have to see whether they are prepared to have a new truth revealed, or whether these familiar faces will be forced to serve in the timeworn and expected ways.

The developmental fluidity of the gifts as Paul explicates them is implied in his refusal to ground his account in a doctrine of creation. When God is understood as a potential energizer of latent God-given but nevertheless human powers, the locus for explaining the gifts is shifted to God's *creative* act in a way that contradicts Paul's intentionally pneumatological description. It is to understand spiritual gifts as something someone "has" in the sense of physical capacities or known skills possessed by right of creaturely (bodily and mental) endowment. This creational reading of the gifts yields the familiar accounts of the "gift of disability" as a message about "dependence," or "need" arising from the biological state of human bodies. Infusion similarly undermines Paul's point by depicting Christians as being mysteriously *filled* with the gifts of the Holy Spirit, carried internally to be dispensed over time.

In taking such care to locate the *charismata* within the *ecclesia*, Paul insistently ties the gifts to the personal working of the Holy Spirit, and thus the theological discourses of pneumatology, revelation, and so eschatology. By insisting in verse 8 that the gifts come "through the Spirit" ("to one is given *through* the Spirit . . . and to another . . . *according to* the same Spirit"), Paul designates the Spirit as originator and giver of gifts that can only be understood as *spiritual* when enacted in such a way as to facilitate their bearer remaining inside (Greek: *en*) the reign of the Spirit and "in keeping" with the traditional witness of the particularity of the Spirit's ways. Because vocation of the Spirit is to reveal Father and Son, the Spirit's revealing may come unpredictably and surprisingly, and yet is never arbitrary.

By characterizing the spiritual gifts as efficient powers, Paul is insisting that there is no spiritual gift except one that actually happens. He seems to be flirting with occasionalism as well as denying the possibility of enduring gifts and so church offices. The *energema* dimension of spiritual gifts may in some cases be an occasional event passing between two people, perhaps a healer and one healed. But this bilateral account becomes multilateral as soon as we ask who is claiming that healing power. Because every gift is the work of the one Spirit of Christ, every gift is inextricably tied to the *whole* church. Paul presses this point with his use of the term *diakonia*: spiritual gifts are not an individual possession but are by *definition* service *to others*. To discharge a gift is to serve the Spirit's self-revelation *to others* in those gifts.

Grasping the intrinsic political horizon of the *charismata* explains why the subsequent development of official church offices does not contradict Paul's strict insistence that gifts are acts, and not formal roles. Formal procedures for recognizing and embracing the spiritual gifts given to the community have taken a variety of concrete forms over the centuries, from the mere grateful willingness of individual Christians to receive enacted *charismata* to more formal recognition procedures, such as fully institutionalized ecclesial offices. No office can displace the fundamental role of the gifts as *enacted* powers, however.[22] The office reveals nothing, only the activity of the officer—*energema*—reveals itself through the Spirit as the gift of service.[23]

THE SPIRIT GIVES TO EACH

The list of different charismata in verses 8-10 is punctuated by the unmistakably repetitious use of "to another," *allo*. Paul does not want his point to be missed: *individual gifts are always allocated to individuals*.

> To one is given through the Spirit the utterance of wisdom, and *to another* the utterance of knowledge according to the same Spirit, *to another* faith by the same Spirit, *to another* gifts of healing by the one Spirit, *to another* the working of miracles, to another prophecy, *to another* the discernment of spirits, *to another* various kinds of tongues, *to another* the interpretation of tongues. All these are activated by one and the same Spirit, who allots to each one individually just as the Spirit chooses.

In this translation the adverb *idia* is rendered "to each one individually," but is more literally translated "to each his or her *own*." *Idios* carries an unmistakably possessive overtone; something is first "mine" or "yours" *before* it can become "ours."[24] Although it is clear that the telos of each gift is what is "helpful to the body as a whole," the Spirit's gifts are always routed through gifts the Spirit gives through individual persons.

These spiritual gifts are allocated "just as the Spirit chooses." Invoking the Spirit's choice rules out any claim that gifts emanate from the skills of their recipients of the gifts—her desires or existing talents. Nor is the Holy Spirit a mere "atmosphere." Paul is insisting that it is the Spirit who chooses the allocation of the gifts to rule out the community's need as the engine of allocation. If need was the principle of the ordering of gifts people would need to be forced to fill roles in the church for which they do not feel gifted to ensure that the need is met. The uniqueness of each gift given through the individual does not, in the first instance, originate in skills everyone already knows they have (at work perhaps) but lies in the antecedent and distinct apportioning of individual gifts to individual persons. Paul states the end of the Spirit's allocation in verse 7: "To each [individual] is given the manifestation of the Spirit for the common good."

In sum, for Paul, the *charismata* are not skills or possessions. Neither are they single fixed social rules played by the giver. They are a "message" of service passing between two believers. In calling the gifts *energema*, Paul is distinguishing between potential power to act and acts actually enacted. Having previously used the example of the sun to illustrate this difference, a different image will help to clarify how the gifts circulate among people to bring to life a political body. Here the functioning of the nervous system is the most useful analog. The distinctive of a nerve cell is its capacity to both generate and hand on electric pulses. Nerve cells are specifically configured to sensitively receive and pass on very minute fluctuations of energy. The electric pulses initiated by any given cell have no "origin stamp" that would allow the origin of the pulse to be located in a specific cell once it arrives at the end of the long string of cells in a nerve fiber. What sets the cells that make up the nervous system apart from every other tissue in the body is this capacity to circulate electrical pulses. Nerve cells are identifiable in being united in this characteristic activity.

Gifts of service are the pulses of activity that hold a group of people together in a polity called church. Enacted works of service not only benefit the body but must be continually circulating if there is to be a body at all. The church only exists *as church* as long as the Spirit's gifts are being sensitively recognized and handed on. Far from being an occasional event, the revelatory discharge of gifts is therefore an extended reality, serving one another, being a work that is, by definition, extended in space and time. The body of Christ *is* a circulator of divine gifts, and if there is such a body it is because each member serves in a temporally extended manner the giving of the Trinitarian God to the church via each member. The individual believer is not *simply* an individual but a member who has and reciprocates charisma. Individuals are members of Christ's body *charismatically*.[25]

A PNEUMATOLOGICAL ECCLESIOLOGY

Paul now introduces in verses 12-13 the famous image of the church as the body of Christ to further clarify the political dynamics of the Spirit's knitting individual Christians into a dynamic whole.

> For just as the body is one and has many members, and all the members of the body, though many, are one body, so it is with Christ. For in the one Spirit we were all baptized into one body—Jews or Greeks, slaves or free—and we were all made to drink of one Spirit.

The originality of Paul's treatment here does not lie in his deployment of the image of the human body to explicate different patterns of political activity, which was a common ancient trope.[26] Attention can therefore be directed to which *type* of politics he intends to convey with it, which politics he is trying to *correct*. The Corinthians apparently think of the church as a negotiable social "arrangement" built up by ordering people according to a hierarchy of progress in wisdom. To displace this managerialist account, Paul introduces an image of the politics of the body gained from Israel's Scriptures and positioned within a Christian account of salvation history.

Individual organs are introduced by depicting them speaking to each other. Tales of conversations between individual body parts were standard fare in the ancient world.[27] Livy, a writer only two generations older than Paul, offers the best-known version of a fable supposedly told to subdue a rebellious crowd by the Roman senator Menenius Agrippa.

> In the days when man's members did not all agree among themselves, as is now the case, but had each its own ideas and a voice of its own, the other parts thought it unfair that they should have the worry and the trouble and the labor of providing everything for the belly, while the belly remained quietly in their midst with nothing to do but to enjoy the good things which they bestowed upon it. They therefore conspired together that the hands should carry no food to the mouth, nor the mouth accept anything that was given it, nor the teeth grind up what they received. While they sought in this angry spirit to starve the belly into submission, the members themselves and the whole body were reduced to the utmost weakness. Hence it became clear that even the belly had no idle task to perform, and was no more nourished than it nourished the rest, by giving out to all parts of the body that by which we live and thrive, when it has been divided equally amongst the veins and is enriched with digested food—that is, the blood. Drawing on a parallel from this to show how like was the internal dissension of the bodily members to the anger of the plebs against the Fathers, he [Menenius Agrippa] prevailed upon the minds of the hearers.[28]

Like Livy, Paul understands the utility of using the image of the body to dramatize a political conflict and to propose a resolution. The trick is to offer an account that directs attention to the aspects of a political situation that need to be addressed if political harmony is to be achieved. Both thinkers assume an ancient understanding of bodies as made up of discreet parts with their own integrity and even will. A modern understanding of the body as an assemblage of organ systems obscures the essential differentiation and discreteness ascribed to body parts by the ancients. Both writers take the human body to be an entity essentially similar to a political community in one essential respect: its discreet parts must be kept talking to one another and working to support one another.

By ending verse 12 with "so it is with Christ" Paul disrupts a straightforward political deployment of the image of the body.[29] The disruption has often been ignored to read "and so with Christ" as shorthand for "and so it is with Christ's body, that is, the church." In verse 13 Paul does point to baptism and perhaps Eucharist as the Christian's entry point "into one body"—a body that cannot but be Christ's. But leaping too quickly to the assumption that verses 12 and 13 supply the mental link between the physical body and the (community's) body of Christ misses the crucial theological point: the unnatural nature of the church. Aside from the many ways it might be compared to an organic body, in one essential sense the politics of the church cannot be compared to any other body—biological or political.

The Holy Spirit is this difference. Paul's fusion of pneumatological and ecclesiological discourses turns on the role played by the moment of intensified reality he associates with the revelatory capacity of the spiritual gifts. Paul presumes the Corinthian believers agree that their own bodily organs will scream in protest should an attempt be made to move them around inside the human body. They are to take from this the lesson that so, too, does God arrange the parts of the church in a given and nonnegotiable form.[30] Ontologically speaking Paul is not arguing from the doctrine of creation but from Christology. The bodily existence of human limbs and senses is not the datum on which the argument rests. The claim is far more challenging: *the Corinthians should understand their fellow congregants as parts of Christ's actual body* (*houtos ḳai ho ḳhristos*).

With this claim Paul inducts gentile believers into the dynamics of conflict resolution he sees as intrinsic to the covenant-shaped political regime presented in Israel's Torah. The covenant is the concrete and material embodiment of God's grace always on offer by God to Israel, written down for them to continually inspect and ponder. Israel knows in its bones that its members are part of a divinely assembled community of the faithful, a community that the individual can either embrace or reject, but to which some response must be made. In this manner the covenant became the *form* of, instead of a mere *means* or *feature* of, Israel's political existence. Paul is elaborating this covenant politics into a pneumatological ecclesiology.

The fact that in 1 Corinthians 3 Paul deploys different metaphors for the church, such as the activity of building, God's temple, or the organic life of plants, makes it clear enough that the natural wisdom of the physical body is not the only orienting guidepost for Paul's account of the body of Christ. Aspects of the operation of created bodies are being leveraged to highlight central features of the spiritual operation of the physical body of Christ. Seeing the features of bodies to which Paul is directing the reader's attention may well yield deeper insights into many other realities in this world, all of which have been composed by the one Creator. But each description ultimately aims to offer, in living color, this one entirely new thing: the christic body. This body is an earthly entity with describable boundaries—and so a *body*—but is at the same time *of Christ*, and so not exhaustively earthly.

The most striking divergence of the political form Paul is describing from Livy's account is the absence of any master organ. No heart or stomach in sight. As a result, the roles of "controller" or "reservoir" are banished from the politics of the church. No one can claim to receive and dispense the resources that keep the body alive, as the stomach does in Livy's parable, nor claim to control the whole body, as does Livy's head. Paul's body is one in which all the organs communicate directly with each other, a decentralized circulating nervous system wholly constituted by the ongoing activities of connection and service administered from "above" or "outside" the nexus of human interaction.[31]

Shifting the body metaphor from Menenius Agrippa's focus on the digestive system to the nervous system turns out to be of sweeping theological significance. The political life of the church as the christic body is characterized by ongoing direct sympathetic communication between all the members. This form of communication is much more immediate and diffused through the body than the political communication imagined as an interaction between organs by way of the digestive and circulatory systems. Menenius Agrippa's parable depicts political dissent as resolved, finally, by one party trying to break the other through a slow siege that wears resistant members down to produce conforming behavior. The body speaks to the head only to threaten it—the real politics begins with the coercive withdrawal of the stuff of life, food. Having no interest in coaching rulers how to coerce peace in the secular polis, Paul's goal is to explain what actually constitutes the church at its most fundamental level, holding it together as a political community. For him the politics of coercion is the betrayal of the church, a destructive politics antithetical to a politics of shalom. If the organs of a body are not talking, there is no real body, only people gathered on a battlefield.

The beating heart of his rival politics is presented later in the chapter: "If one member suffers, all suffer together with it; if one member is honored, all rejoice together with it" (1 Cor 12:26). Paul has deftly begun from the symptom—political conflict within the church—to bring Christians to attend to the root of the problem: the loss the sympathetic connection with other Christians that ensures they "may have the same care for one another" (1 Cor 12:25). The emphasis on keeping communication suggests Paul places a premium on the immediate effect that a suffering or dysfunctional member should evoke for the whole body.

If the sinew of the christic body is sympathetic connection, the gift of "faith" mentioned in verse 9 becomes especially interesting for a theological account of disability. Having said that gifts are enacted works of service, the gift of faith seems to fit oddly with Paul's own definition, since having faith must surely be the condition of having a relationship to Christ. The clue is Paul's earlier insistence that every gift of the Spirit is an act of service. Faith concerns more than the individuals own salvation but keeps faith for others. Jesus emphasizes this point in praising the faith of the friends who lowered the crippled man through a roof to bring him to Jesus.[32]

It is also unthinkable within the argument of 1 Corinthians as a whole that Paul is commending some believers for having a more "visible" faith. Such a claim would exacerbate the Corinthians' obvious temptations to religious heroism. Within his account the type of faith that can be called a spiritual gift is one that has a special sensitivity to those who are "drifting away" from the body, those slowly distancing themselves from the communicative nexus. To be gifted with the distinct *charism* of faith, as differentiated from the gift of faith in every Christian, is therefore to vicariously represent the single and foundational faith of the church by extending it in a special way to those who struggle with their faith. Faith is a spiritual gift when it opens other people to communicative communion.

What is distinct about this *charism* is its sensitivity to the dynamism that characterizes the rich ecology of types and levels of communicative connections in the body of Christ. It is easy to imagine people with learning difficulties being the *first* to register the distress or spiritual state of those around them. Adam is no doubt not alone in having a preternatural sensitivity to gesture and gaze as revealing of hearts.[33] By responding sensitively to those hearts, such believers enliven the whole body's empathetic connectivity. We can even say that this gifting is the paradigmatic gift in the church, since "Peaceable hearing is sensitive to soft voices."[34] What this insight reveals in turn is that every gift is a gift of healing (v. 9), in extending very specific and concrete invitations to congregants to once again cross the divides and wounds of sin into the vulnerable life of interdependence. Some may exhibit this gift so powerfully that the church asks them to pray over those congregants yearning for healing of body or spirit.[35]

To recap: in verses 4-13 of this chapter the apostle is conceiving the human body as, fundamentally, a medium of communication; a *medium* rather than a mere *instrument* of communication. The Spirit does not speak through the members of the church as a voice goes through a hollow pipe. Coming to know themselves as recipients of mercy changes believers from inside out, redirecting their affections and so their behavior, which in turn makes making God's mercy to others tangible through acts of service.[36] Paul's account of the politics of the church is fundamentally theological and does not rest on an account of biology or the body as imagined in modern medicine. The most important features of the body in Paul's account are its receptive and perceptive capacities, the senses that structure the communicative sphere as well as its limbs reaching out toward the outside world.[37] Paul's body is primarily one composed of skin, nerves, and limbs: the communicative body. Even the mention later of more or less "presentable" members (a reference to the pudenda) already presupposes the centrality of the communicative dimension of the body.[38] The remainder of the chapter is devoted to giving practical flesh to this theological account of the church's politics of peace.

EVERY BELIEVER IS INDISPENSABLE

The chief obstacle diverting readers from this train of reasoning appears in the next section (vv. 14-20), verse 15 particularly.

> Indeed, the body does not consist of one member but of many. If the foot would say, "Because I am not a hand, I do not belong to the body," that would not make it any less a part of the body. And if the ear would say, "Because I am not an eye, I do not belong to the body," that would not make it any less a part of the body. If the whole body were an eye, where would the hearing be? If the whole body were hearing, where would the sense of smell be? But as it is, God arranged the members in the body, each one of them, as he chose. If all were a single member, where would the body be? As it is, there are many members, yet one body.

Even one of the greatest Christian preachers of the fourth century got this one wrong, and in a way that has been repeated down through the centuries, to the detriment of those wearing outsider labels. John Chrysostom reads Paul's aim here as seeking to soothe "the feelings of one who has the inferior gift and is troubled by this."[39] To reduce envy and pride among Christians, Paul is supposedly reassuring the Corinthians that all spiritual gifts are equally valuable. The problem is that Chrysostom has displaced the question Paul wants his readers to ask, *"How, here and now, do I embrace the giving of the Spirit?"* with an identity question, "Which gift is *mine*?" or "What do *I get* from spiritual gifting?" *The quest to acquire and burnish an identity inevitably clashes with the aim to receive the Holy Spirit who fosters in believers "the same care for one another."*

Paul is also resisting the temptation to absorb the multitude of gifts into one single agency. "If the whole body were an eye, where would the hearing be? If the whole body were hearing, where would the sense of smell be?" (1 Cor 12:17). The question of absorption of the many into one is so fundamental for Paul that the continuing existence of the body itself depends on it. "If all were a single member, where would the body be?" (1 Cor 12:19). There are moments of need or peril in which the response of the body must be wholly animated by one sense or organ if it is to be responsive to its environment, as when someone flinches to avoid a flying projectile that the eye barely, but crucially, has registered. But such a momentary focusing of primacy of one agent in a community is very different from one agent claiming that they have the skill to do things that in fact require the cooperation of all the parts of the body.

The game of soccer illustrates his point. The aim of the game is attacking and scoring, but a team on which the strikers consider themselves the only "real" players would not just devalue others but is an abandonment of reality. Without a functioning defense and midfield, the striker is precisely nothing. He is a nonexistent reality since football is, by definition, a team sport. The social form called a team is made up of positions in the same way that Christians can only exist in the form of Christ's body. It will not do to read Paul as saying "midfielders are important too," or "every position is equally important." Both are true, but beside the point.

Verse 18 makes the formal point crystal clear. Rather than contradicting the problematic attitude "I do not belong" in order to correct it—"yes you do belong"—the problematic rationale underlying this attitude is brought out for critical examination. The literal translation of *etheto* would be "God *put into place* the members in the body, each one as he chose." The NRSV's translation of the verb here as "arranged" is misleading. The language of arrangement presupposes an initial putting into place followed by a process of reordering for maximal effect, as if God had given "gifts and talents" that can only coalesce into a vibrant church community once a good "leader" has arranged them. This common mistake not only boils down to the belief that the wholeness of the body depends on human beings tactfully arranging of what God has provided, but more problematically, inevitably demands that some believers end up being assumed to be not well endowed with divine gifting.

HONOR CODES AND UNPRESENTABLE MEMBERS

Verses 14-16 opened with limbs and organs speaking to their equals (hand to foot, ear to eye), and now verses 21-27 shifts to depict preeminent members "speaking down" to lesser members: "I have no need of you." The eye tells the hand that depends on it that it does not need it, and the head calls down to the members on the ground, the feet, calling them superfluous. Paul replies, "On the contrary, the members of the body that seem to be weaker are indispensable."

> The eye cannot say to the hand, "I have no need of you," nor again the head to the feet, "I have no need of you." On the contrary, the members of the body that seem to be weaker are indispensable, and those members of the body that we think less honorable we clothe with greater honor, and our less respectable members are treated with greater respect; whereas our more respectable members do not need this. But God has so arranged the body, giving the greater honor to the inferior member, that there may be no dissension within the body, but the members may have the same care for one another. If one member suffers, all suffer together with it; if one member is honored, all rejoice together with it. Now you are the body of Christ and individually members of it.

Paul's use in verse 22 of the expression "*seem* to be weaker" (*asthenestera*) emphasizes the conventional nature of all such hierarchical assessments. That his language of weakness concerns social ascriptions and does not suggest any ontological inferiority is indicated by his reiteration of the point in the expression *atimotera*, which the NRSV renders as "less honorable." In verse 24 the NRSV's rendering "inferior" is misleading in insinuating an ontological differentiation. The Greek is a comparative that literally means "more disgusting/despised." The passive construction *husteromeno* might best be translated as "disadvantaged" or "those who bring up the rear."

Far from claiming that there really are inferior or weaker members in the church, Paul is suggesting that the starting point for discerning the Spirit's gifts begins by becoming more aware of the codes of decency and honor that are inevitably present in every social grouping. Every human generation has its own code of honor and decency that ranks people, bodily functions, and even individual body parts as inferior and superior. Paul's train of reason is very close to the social model of disability here and suggests that he would have easily understood how the label "disabled" is one of many cultural routines in modernity that function to "other" or exclude some people.

Yet this proximity to modern accounts of the social origin of disadvantage ought not to obscure the different way it is constructed. Paul does not begin with a negation as does the social model of disability, which denies the physical account on which the medical model is premised. His account offers a contribution to disability theology in urging an awareness of social marginalization but without resorting to the main tool in modernity's political toolbox, the claim that, "We're all the same after all." For him awareness of social marginalization springs from God's work of composing the christic body, and in so doing "giving greater honor to the inferior member." A striking claim: *God* has given greater honor to the socially marginalized.

Those who think some gifts of the Spirit are inferior are being carefully positioned by Paul as guilty of conflating worldly assessments of stations and talents with the gifts of the Spirit. The believer who sees some gifts as inferior is no longer seeking a Christian discernment of the working of the Spirit and is instead viewing the church like any other human community, dependent on a good manager to arrange human talents assumed to already be known and understood.[40] Paul wants believers to be wholly invested in learning to pick up the crackling energy of the *charismata*. The receptivity required for discernment is only acquired, however, when the codes of social superiority and inferiority learned in the world are revealed as false social constructions. Empathetic practices of caring for one another are revelatory because they show that God has honored especially those who are dishonored in society with something that sustains the body. Some church members may indeed need support and accommodation of their physical or intellectual challenges understood in the functionalist terms of medical discourses. At the same time Paul insists that in the economy of the church's life, every person can serve in a manner that no incapacity can thwart.

It is especially important to get the reading of the "unpresentable" member right, since most of the theological debate about this passage centers on how to understand Paul's language here.[41] Being saturated by the Hebrew Scriptures, Paul instinctively connects the dynamics of shame that go with social exclusion to the story of their origin at the Fall. The first honor-decency scheme entered the world with the first couple's betrayal, according to the Genesis narrative. Mistrust toward God unleashes in Adam and Eve a mistrust of the goodness of creation, and they see that "they were naked." Repudiation of their relationship with God simultaneously ruptures their communication with other creatures, not only with one another, but also with their own bodies.

Sin is broken communication. Sin's entry is marked by the immediate birth of the shaming gaze. Those unworthy to be addressed are designated "shameful ones" on whom the sinner's own shame is then projected. God's first response to shame is to offer Adam and Eve covering for the parts of their own bodies that their feelings of shame had caused them to "other." God's cloaking the bodies of Adam and Eve is thus the first example of the divine mercy of "giving the greater honor to the inferior member." A redemptive intervention helps the first human couple to understand that the bodily parts of which they were now ashamed were parts that belonged to them, that they needed to own.

Every culture has its own enculturated rules of shame and pride over body parts. These can even include fantasies of cutting off some body parts and declaring "those" parts to be subhuman, or "not me."[42] Yet the very body parts that had become repellent and embarrassing to the newly fallen Adam and Eve are in fact critical in the sustenance of the human race. Sin produced shame and a disdainful gaze on those very parts that unite man and woman and connect generation to generation, "that part of the body which by its nature was most honorable and noble," Luther observes.[43] For Paul the social coding of individual and social bodies is simultaneously real, because enacting a repudiation of communication, and unreal in being revealed *as sin*, as a living anti-doxology, by the reconciling touch of Jesus Christ. Christians live "as if" because the hold of sin over them has been broken in their hastening toward the final overturning of whatever shame-based ideological constructions prey on people in their time and place.

With this argument Paul is retracing and concretizing one of the most striking characteristics of Jesus' earthly ministry, his subversive attitude toward human honor codes. Jesus proposed scandalous inversions of the seating order at a feast, redefined greatness as that service which allows others to grow rather than shrink in one's presence instead of lording over others, and blessed the persecuted, the sufferers of injustice, and the poor (Luke 14:7-14; Matt 23:11-12; 5:3-4, 10-12). Paul has made it plain from the first chapter of this letter that he considers himself to be carrying this teaching forward for the community that is Christ's body: "God chose what is foolish in the world to shame the wise, God chose what is weak in the world to shame the strong; God chose what is low and despised in the world, things that are not, to reduce to nothing things that are" (1 Cor 1:27-28).

Hence the insistence with which Paul strives to dissociate charisma and vocation from worldly status. If the temptation to rank spiritual gifts is to be overcome, Paul must totally break the link of spiritual gifting with social role ascriptions. The Corinthians are overrating some gifts, such as speaking in tongues or oratorical polish, not because they can weigh these gifts in themselves, but because they assume the spiritualists or the great rhetoricians are more valuable members of human society (see 1 Cor 1). The Christian church has been built from the beginning on a new and different "divine honor code" flowing from the subversive mission of Jesus.

Paul's contribution to the Christian understanding of the dynamics of Jesus' kingdom was in finding ways to simultaneously affirm and deny binaries like the normal-disabled binary. The importance of this move for theological accounts of disability cannot be overstated. Paul offers Christians a set of insights that allow terms like "disability" to be affirmed as categories necessary for the purposes of recognizing special needs in the context of secular government while at the same time denying that such a designation is a substantial theological category. Christians, Paul emphasizes, should live *hos me*—"as if . . . not":

> I mean, brothers and sisters, the appointed time has grown short; from now on, let even those who have wives be as though [*hos me*] they had none, and those who mourn as though [*hos me*] they were not mourning, and those who rejoice as though [*hos me*] they were not rejoicing, and those who buy as though [*hos me*] they had no possessions, and those who deal with the world as though [*hos me*] they had no dealings with it. For the present form of this world is passing away. (1 Cor 7:29-31)

For Paul, Christians can and must live within such polarities, and can affirm them for the purposes that they are fit but will only do so appropriately as long as they are aware they affirm them only *as if* they did not ultimately exist. Their ultimate reality is denied. *God may recognize lesser members, but God's view of who is lesser is emphatically not to be reduced to those whom human beings have socially marginalized*. This suspension of socially taken for granted categories was and remains politically revolutionary in deactivating the denial of capacity that is intrinsic to these public role ascriptions.[44] To deny that the outsiders *really are* outsiders is to expose the problematic status of shame and honor regimes. This application of Paul's thought is especially potent in relation to the language of disability. A *lack* of ability (*dis*ability) is the conceptual foundation of the term normalcy (*not* having a special lack) at the very same time that the lack is designated as a reduction of capacity in relation to the normal. To unhitch disability from such hierarchical social cues is to render it a very different entity. In Paul's eyes Jesus had inaugurated a social order that is, in crucial senses, "beyond" disability.

GIFTS OF THE POOR

The way in which the early church defined its stance toward the poorest of the poor, the class of beggars, was certainly an attempt to take Paul's account of the subversive political unity of Christ's body with full seriousness. From very early on Christians considered the poor as emblematic of the church's very existence, a badge of honor to be carried up front, for example, when a group of beggars was ostentatiously part of the traveling entourage of bishops.[45] John Chrysostom's sermon on these verses offers testimony to this alertness. Chrysostom preaches of beggars as "fixtures and splendid adornment at the doors of the sanctuary," without which the church "would not attain its full stature." The preacher is highly sensitive to Paul's agenda, even granting beggars their own embodied "proclamation" that appropriately seconds that of the preacher and even surpasses the preacher's eloquent voice in clarity and urgency. "While we preachers sit before you and recommend what will do you good, the one who sits before the doors of the church addresses you no less than we do, by his mere appearance, without saying a word."[46] Clearly Chrysostom considers the poor to offer a special gift and ministry to the church, granting those with no worldly power a voice of their own that the church needs to hear.

Chrysostom's fatal error is his equation of gift and social role. The sermon that Chrysostom understands Christian beggars to preach by their "mere appearance, without saying a word," assigns them the role of warning to the established members of church and society. "Man's life is a shifting and precarious thing . . . Our condition is like a swift river that never wants to stand still but always rushes downhill."[47] The assault here on the certainty of those who suppose themselves "normal," "able," and socially secure is theologically appropriate. The problem is that Chrysostom gets there by apparently ruling Christian beggars out as conduits of the much more diverse gifts Paul has enumerated. By reducing the supposed spiritual gifts of the poor to their ragged clothes, the gesture of the outstretched hand and their social location outside the church doors, Chrysostom reifies the poverty of the poor *as* their spiritual gift. He has locked them into the roles thrust upon them by the gaze of the "normal" masses. Their social disablement has been operationalized for theological ends.[48]

Few beggars appear in Western churches these days, which is not to suggest that churches have abandoned charity work on behalf of the poor. The poor, have, however, long ceased to be thought of as a visible badge of honor that the churches wish to keep as "fixtures and splendid adornment at the doors of the sanctuary." This train of argument offers us fresh purchase on Jean Vanier's stubborn adherence to the traditional linkage of the plight of the disabled with the plight of the poor. To call people labeled disabled "the poor" is appropriate to the extent that it is drawing attention to *socially constructed* inferiority. Every church would wish today to think of itself as having one or even two people with disabilities in their midst. Congregants are willing to make some adjustments to make the worship space physically accessible and to suffer some disturbances those members of the body might cause in the hour of worship. Unfortunately, the parallel with the poor also extends to the perception that what people with disabilities contribute to ecclesial life so often approximates Chrysostom's message. The focus remains precisely on their gestures, their lack, their occupying the social role of the outsider—the gift they bring to the body accordingly being reduced to their apparent poverty/disability. This baptizing of public social codes cannot be remedied by inverting it, simply by making the formerly marginalized the center of the community.[49] The problem is the lack of expectation that the Spirit's gifts will be given to the community from each member. The church will expect no gifts from those people whose contribution has already been predetermined as coming from the place of the social outsider.

Here the temptations of the charity model's positioning of disability lie extremely close. Exactly as with prayers for "the poor" as a class, Christian moral concern for people perceived as disabled can enact a failure of unity in presuming that what people in the class of "the disabled" need is to be "served." However pleasantly offered, such a gesture explicitly renders some "those who are not needed" in their own congregation. It shatters the unity to which the church is called as it prays that "we" will be one in Christ.[50] If the "we" who prays makes some in the congregation into a "them," the praying church has solidified the fractures in the body, as well as its unwillingness to know one another as a body that circulates acts of service among *all* its members.

Paul is asking Christians to look again. The gifts that those with disabilities reveal to the church may be manifold and are certainly not reducible to the "message" of their disability. The easy equation of gift with appearance deprives the church of the surprise, wonder, and discovery about what sort of gifts the Spirit might be attempting to give through the life of any individual member of the body of Christ. The gift that someone with a disability might bring to the Christian body cannot simply be said to rest with that individual (his or her disability), nor is it appropriate to say that it rests with those who receive it, as suggested in the patronizing gesture so common in liberal societies, whose manner of espousing equality amounts to the confession that "*even* the disabled should have a place."

Gifts need to be discovered "in between" the bearer and recipient. This in between is the particular theatre of operations of the Spirit who does not only *originate* the gifts but needs actively to *donate* them right into the middle of interpersonal relational space.[51]

Speaking testimonially as Adam's father, I can attest to having been confronted in particularly intense ways by the gifts that God gives through him. When I come home from a trip, to take one example, he beams with joy at the simple presence of his father, which makes me happy too. I have learned to forgo bringing him toys or other gifts from my travels, as they clearly add absolutely nothing to what is the greatest gift for him, the sheer presence of a formerly absent father. His delight is nothing more than the recovery of nervous connection.

In order to learn this, however, I had to admit my disappointment that Adam never really noticed presents. What I have discovered is a gift that is so rare that it needed some time fully to break through my much less rich, and conventional, vision of what our relationship should be. It took time to receive the relationship that exists with this other member of the christic body *as it actually is*. Being myself aware of the role of gift exchange as a mode of expressing care and affection, with all its complexities, I was not prepared to receive a relationship of such shocking simplicity, one which reveals the essence of Paul's definition of the church as characterized by empathetic communication.

To mark again the problematic twist in the well-begun analysis of Chrysostom, as a father I eventually learned to recognize the gift Adam had in store for me by relinquishing my immediate expectations that he should show some *extra* joy if I came with a toy. The arrival of the real gift, the experience of the purity of relationship, had to be patiently awaited. Until I was weaned off the cultural codes that led me to expect that a good father would bring home a gift and a good child would be excited to receive it, I was unable to really perceive the depth and purity of the "rejoicing together" that was already on offer from and through Adam. Nor could I ever have adduced in advance the mercy already being held out to me by examining the phenomenological configuration of his disability. He did not teach me that one day I will be "dependent." What I discovered was not good because he "taught me something." It is a theologically inflected and ecclesiological confession to suggest that it is through him that Christ is breaking and remaking me by embedding me more deeply in his body. In confronting me with the gift of presence through Adam, the Spirit had to reveal to me God's mercy in Adam's service of presence, even before I recognized it. When this service broke through on me, it could only levy a judgment on my previous view, my entanglement in ideals about the behaviors of gratitude to be expected from a child. Repenting of this isolating dream idol was the condition of letting the Spirit become a gentle teacher, teaching me to follow Adam's lead[52] This is but one concrete example of the sort of discovery Paul associates with the church's fundamental task of recognizing and embracing the Spirit's gifts.

If such testimonies are plausible examples of how God's "giving the greater honor to the inferior member" might look in our world,[53] Paul's next move in verses 24-26 will make much more sense. Again, he draws on an image of the nervous system, this time the way the whole body is immediately jolted by a pain in a single part. The church's sympathetic connection allows the members of the Christian body to suffer and rejoice together: "If one member suffers, all suffer together with it; if one member is honored, all rejoice together with it."[54]

Relinquishing the status markers that are everything to competitive and pecking order–attuned humans is the condition for the gifts God gives to become visible (Mark 10:26-31 and par.). The gift given by the disabled person, the poor person, the recovering addict, all those of low esteem *to the world*, emerges only through the *spiritual discernment* that is utterly certain that in the places where the eyes of fallen humanity expects nothing there is a *charisma* to be received. This is not to erase people's legitimate needs, but to treat it "as if"—taking it only as seriously as necessary without allowing it to constrain our expectations of what the Spirit might be bringing into the world through them. The inability to grasp this point is the fundamental problem of the modern church.

It is important not to end with a story from the family domain, because the Spirit's gifts are to his family *as* church. And the Spirit serves the church through Adam entirely independent of his parents' intervention. Adam does not "sit at the doors" of the church, preaching with his need and dependence. Ours is a large cathedral church, laid out along the traditional Western pattern of the cross. Upon entering the church one is faced with a long nave filled with wooden pews; beyond that, a long set of choir stalls, and even beyond that, the communion table. In the middle is the crossing, flanked by a pulpit on one side and a lectern on the other. Much of the liturgical action takes place in the crossing, where our priest Isaac Poobalon speaks and sings, stands and kneels, for most of the first half of the service.

For years the Brock family has occupied a pew near the front of the congregation, in part so that Adam can hear the "action," but originally to be near an exit. In the course of his thirteenth year Adam decided that he wanted to sit with Isaac in the crossing. On Pentecost Sunday he got up and sat on the ground next to Isaac, taking off his shoes and socks and staying within arm's reach of his presiding minister. The habit has continued from that day forward.

As parents we had (have!) to resist the urge to force him back to "his" seat with the congregation. We have had to negotiate a running inner war with our own expectations about the behavior of children in church, which include squirming under our inner monologues about the gaze of other congregants and choir members. But encouraged by his minister (and here I use the pronoun intentionally), we have let him continue to pursue expressing his membership in the body in his own way. We would need to think about how, or if, we should guide him toward occupying this highly visible space in a contributory manner.

Adam's insistence on being right next to the minister has changed the tone of church in ways we could never have anticipated. A choir used to "performing" has been forced to ask what it means to have Adam humming between them and the congregation. A "flagship" church has had to ask what it means to have a teenager who walks into the center of the church, takes off his shoes and socks, and then sits "stimming" (rocking back and forth, often swinging something repetitively in his hands and gutturally vocalizing) literally at the feet of the presiding priest. Speaking for myself, one aspect of the Spirit's gift through Adam is to liberate the congregation from any pretention that we are a church devoted to presenting a culturally and aesthetically flawless performance, or that we are not a church for everyone. His lively presence disturbs many common expectations about the behavior of young people in church, as his godfather observed in a letter to him for his confirmation, a few weeks from his fifteenth birthday.

> I only wish I could be there to witness your becoming a stalwart of the church. I put the matter that way because confirmation means the church will depend on you to be fully embodied in Christ. There matters are tricky because you have for some time represented Christ for the church through your dancing. Some may say that is a strange description of your presence at worship. You just cannot be still. But I have always thought when I have been with you in worship that you are dancing to the music God's angels make as they glorify God. My hunch is you were granted the grace to be closer to those wonderful creatures than those of us who are identified as normal and grown up. So on this wonderful day dance for the gathered body of believers because we all need the joy that animates your movements.[55]

It is theologically important to admit that the mediator of this liberation in our church is a person who carries the label "inferior" in his day-to-day life.

He embodies a life that most of the congregation, were they honest with themselves, would be ashamed to have to live. But in *not* being at all ashamed in this way, by being unselfconsciously present in joy among those who (whether admitted or not) feel themselves to be capable and "doing church properly," the Spirit, through Adam, invites this congregation to engage with a person and hold more loosely to their ideals of performance and aesthetic purity.

A church that treats some as continual recipients, and never givers of gifts, enacts a forgetfulness that Christians are Gentiles. Christians have been grafted onto the true vine, and so are beggars themselves, the unsightly ones being added to Israel. Mediated by Adam's body, the Spirit is inviting the congregation into communion—as tangibly as the bread and wine given for us that consummates our communion with the person of Jesus Christ. Thanks be to God, the church never escapes the Spirit, who continually and mercifully reveals that our genetic, physical, mental, national, and religious status is not all there is to us.

10

A Remarkable Stroke in a Strange and Remarkable War

THE PROPHETIC PUBLIC PRESENCE OF THE MENTALLY DISABLED

Most modern Westerners think of themselves as responsive to the needs of those they see as disabled, despite the evidence of widespread inhospitality.[1] This inhospitality can take the form of arrangements of public space that exclude, coercive cultural expectations about how it should be inhabited, and legal constructions that stabilize such inhospitalities. Churches can be equally inhospitable. People who bear the label "disabled"—especially those called intellectually disabled—are buffeted daily by disparaging comments, the stares of strangers, and the shrinking of their social worlds as those around them refuse to enter into meaningful friendship. But the God of the crucified Christ has promised vigorously to contest this denuding and isolating lack of communion. The promise of the God of mercy is relentlessly to set upon this inhospitality and break it open.

For some this bold claim is less objectionable in a more modest form, as a confession that God has used one person labeled disabled to break open my own inhospitality. I conclude by offering a few glimpses of that process, ones I hope others might find to resonate with their own experience. Attempting to put these glimpses to words is also a testimony to how the Christian church has had a decisive role in preparing me for the radical shift in life trajectory that has come with being wondrously wounded by the experience of disability.

I grew up in a Christian home on a dead-end street. Just around the corner was what we used to call a "home" for the mentally disabled, which occupied a repurposed residential house. I have only the thinnest residue of childhood memories of its handful of residents, who didn't seem to get out much, certainly not as far as the large yard around the house. My memories are more of gestures than faces, of shapes rather than personalities. It was impolite to stare at the small clusters of awkward forms who occasionally shuffled single file past the entrance of our dead-end street, accompanied by a single bored-looking carer. I cannot recall the faces or races of these spectral and discomforting figures, despite living in a context saturated with racial codings. These fleeting memories are most recognizable by the feeling of foreboding that accompanies them. The appearance of these habitants was the appearance of a portent, the appearance of a strange and unmentionable tragedy lurking at the edges of the polite, public world. Having been born at the tail end of the long era of hiding such lives away in large institutions, only through such spectral public glimpses could I know that such people even existed.[2] The emptying of the large asylums had begun, even if social expectations about the mentally disabled among the general populace remained essentially unchanged. The "handicapped" should live in "homes" and attend their own special schools. They never appeared in church.

How Adam has changed me. I live today an inverted version of my childhood. I almost never attend church without Adam, a bearer of the label "intellectually disabled." He has attended a school with mainstream children and is in principle welcome in every public space modern society has to offer. His peculiar combination of Down syndrome and autistic tendencies has left him largely nonverbal, sometimes unresponsive to verbal commands, and capable of defiance when he understands them. Along with a warm and open personality came for many years a fascination with throwing or pushing objects off of tables and playful slaps at the passersby who might be in arm's reach—behaviors precisely calibrated to expose the inhospitality of a modern world supposing itself to have opened its arms wide for disabled people.

DISABLED AT PUB AND POOL

The British family pub is an intentionally hospitable public space, a place to relax and enjoy a nonthreatening convivial atmosphere. Translated into North American terms, it is a cross between a coffee shop and a diner. These are public venues of the service economy, designed to make a profit, but intentionally configured to be inviting to families. Our family was out for a Friday evening meal, feeling celebratory and relaxed.

Before ordering our food, I took Adam (at that time four years old) and our other son Caleb (then two years old) to wash their hands in the men's room. After washing Adam, I was ten seconds into Caleb's wash when I saw Adam fishing the suspiciously candylike sanitizer balls out of a urinal. The viscous surface material from the balls had coated his fingers within seconds. Before I could stop him, to my horror, he was rubbing his eyes.

Immediately he began to cry and then to scream, and my forcing him to wash his hands and face in the sink only made him scream louder. All eyes were on the three of us as we emerged hurriedly from the men's room, Adam's frantic howling rising above the music of the jukebox. We met Stephanie at the table, whose nursing training immediately kicked in. The exact makeup of the sanitizer balls needed to be discovered, and quickly. With Adam howling at the top of his lungs a manager was not slow in arriving, soon disappearing again into his backroom office, visibly rattled by the turn of events. Reappearing a few minutes later he offered a glass of milk (unsolicited) while thumbing his folder of emergency procedures. The toilet sanitizers, he said, were made of a very strong base that needed immediate neutralization. Adam would need to be taken to the emergency room. The manager gave us the number of a cab company, and we decided a crying and hungry two-year-old would not help us negotiate the emergency room with a four-year-old in very loud agony. Stephanie shouldered the burden of a few grueling few hours holding Adam down as his eyes were bathed in a neutralizing solution intended to protect them from permanent damage (though he did have burned and red irises for several days afterward).

Contemporary law ensures that business establishments are at least wheelchair accessible. These legal frameworks are conceived with physical disabilities in mind. They are therefore not necessarily organized to ward off the very different hazards that can emerge when someone like Adam enters the space. In this case the proprietors may not have easily foreseen that the sanitary balls could became a hazard, though they may have been legally liable for it. The manager clearly felt the pressure of this potential legal liability, soon documenting what had happened in writing. The manager was friendly and helpful, whether from fear of legal repercussions or genuine concern, which we certainly appreciated. In the end we were left with the financial costs of the taxi ride. The more taxing cost was the unwelcome emotional shock of going for a happy family outing and ending up with no dinner and several hours with a screaming child in the emergency room.

Nor is domestic space free of many of the same dangers. A child who repetitively slams doors, throws things, or flushes things down the toilet is bound to find trouble at home. Nor is the family home sealed off from the public. Adam once badly burned himself pulling down a cup of boiling water in the kitchen and did so within arm's reach of a family friend. The friendship later frayed to a breaking point under this person's crippling guilt at not having stopped him in time. This time the hospital stay took a week.

The most disconcerting threats in public spaces, however, are not rooted in the arrangement of space, but in the attitudes of the people who populate it. It was a beautiful summer afternoon, and Adam and I spent a pleasant few hours swimming, talking, and playing with other swimmers at a pool on the campus of a major private university in the southern United States. This particular pool presented one physical barrier for Adam: it had no steps or shallow area in which he could splash or paddle on his own. Unable to swim at the time, if he were to enter the water, he had to be held. He also found it fun to be placed on the ladder to climb out and be caught as he jumped back in. A workable, if tiring and energy-intensive routine, having the decided benefit of wearing him out for a good night's sleep. The main drawback of the situation was Adam's passion for throwing things into the water, the lid to the skimmer, swim floats, sandals—whatever was near enough to the pool to be grabbed and thrown in before we managed to swim over and stop him. Objects several feet away from the pool's edge presented no danger, as his gestures telegraphed his urge to throw something in plenty of time to intercept him. The physical arrangement of the pool did, however, leave us with the nagging worry that one day he might be that one step ahead of us with something in hand that shouldn't go in the pool.

Adam and I were feeling particularly buoyant on the day I have in mind, it being the first time Adam's joy in throwing things into the pool had made him some playmates. A group of five children discovered that if they sat on the edge of the pool he would invariably push them in. They spent a merry half hour jumping out of the pool, only to be pushed into the water in rapid succession by an industrious and constantly grinning Adam. As this game wound down, I took Adam and moved twenty yards to the other side of the pool to talk to a friend. He wanted to sit and rock at the side of the pool (such forms of self-soothing are common among people with autism, and are also called "stimming"). The geometry of the situation made me nervous. Ten feet away an undergraduate had decided to stand in the pool and read, her book on the pool's edge and a bag next to her. Would it be best to move Adam? Cut the conversation short? Move to the other side of the pool? Warn the student that Adam liked throwing things in the pool? Hope for the best? Not being able to see what was in the bag, and assuming that the student would grab it if Adam attempted to pick it up, I decided to stay as close as I could and to hope for the best. Better not to interrupt the student.

Wrong decision. Adam dashed for the bag, and because it was so close to the water, with a flick of the wrist its light canvas was floating on the surface of the pool. The student made no attempt to reach for the bag when Adam picked it up, apparently not having noticed the game he had previously been playing with the children at the other end of the pool. Adam deftly flicked the bag into the pool and the student just as quickly snatched it out. She then fished out a phone in a carrying case, which looked damp on its surface, but happily, worked just fine. Apologies all around, smiles, no harm done.

Having spent the better part of the afternoon at the pool, this unpleasant turn of events suggested it was time to go. I changed Adam out of his swim nappy and began herding him toward the car. Running to catch up with us and now clearly in a panic, the student explained that she had discovered some worrying glitches, though the phone was by no means debilitated. Apologizing again, I handed her my business card, promising to cover any costs that might arise and asked for her to keep me up to date about the unfolding health of the device.

Within hours I received an e-mail explaining that because the dunking had clearly caused some effect on the phone, I owed her $399 plus tax. I responded that it was perhaps worth turning it off and giving it a day or two and some standard drying procedures to let it dry out. To my great surprise, the next day I received an e-mail sent from the very phone in question saying that the dealer had informed her that any wetting of the phone voided its warranty. I therefore owed her an entirely new phone. A series of negotiations ensued about how much loss the invalidation of a warranty was worth, which it soon became apparent she interpreted as attempts to escape financial responsibility. Believing that I was shirking my responsibilities for Adam's actions, a police report was filed and a threat to sue was issued if she had not been paid in full by a specified date. Frantic at our apparent absconding, she contacted all authorities who would listen to her story at the university, some who wrote me wry e-mails seeking a resolution to an absurd situation, some who wrote kind and concerned e-mails, and one moralizing and condescending e-mail from the vice principal of student affairs, who reminded me that as an academic, I had a responsibility to set an example for students. Pay up immediately, he warned.

The episode was a telling one in so clearly displaying what is counted as justice in public space. Justice meant protecting individual property rights. Neither the student nor the moralizing vice principal had the slightest interest in acknowledging the reality that the decisive actions were taken by a child with little awareness of common social rules and who at the time did not take verbal direction in any meaningful sense. Any acknowledgment of Adam's condition, or that the student might have also had some role to play in the events that unfolded, had been coded from the beginning as an intentional diminishment of the student's property rights. *Legal rights functioned not to bind all of us to Adam but to protect us from him. Legal rights were assumed to stand between us and him.*[3] Disability never appeared in the stories the student told the police and vice principal of the injustice she had suffered. For her, protecting her rights was totally unrelated to any questions about taking responsibility for supporting a child with special needs.

Universities generally pride themselves in being the most accessible and equitable of public spaces. It is entirely appropriate that universities are configured to serve adults. Within such an institution, however, a staff and student pool might be considered one of the few places genuinely open to a child with disability. Adam had not damaged a book in the library, nor had he spilled a coffee on a computer in the refectory. We knew better than to venture taking him into those spaces. What we could imagine is that in an "enlightened" public space like a civically progressive university, a lifeguard tempted to ban Adam from the pool for having thrown something into it would be rebuffed. At least the lifeguard's superiors would be aware of the legal liability that such a ban would court.

On this day it was not deficits in the physical environment that rendered the pool threatening (though they did make the situation more precarious). What ruined the day was the myopia of acquisitive individualism and its capacity to blot out any awareness that public space is always *shared*. It is very difficult to entice students to an elite university without playing on their drive to acquire precious goods for themselves in the process. If they have made financial sacrifices to do so, their sense of entitlement is sure to be strengthened. Performance pressures do not sit easily with an ethos of accessibility. Even a university explicitly committed to producing "moral" and "civically engaged" students cannot guarantee this will have the effect of opening students' eyes to the marginalized in our societies, as it clearly had not in this case. Even volunteering for public service can become something done to complete a well-rounded curriculum vitae.[4]

At our final face-to-face meeting to hand over a check and discuss what had transpired, the student in question told us that she was "not a bad person" and was involved in voluntary service in a nearby socially deprived area. Nevertheless, we never really enjoyed the pool after the incident. We took to driving a bit further away, so Adam could paddle at a small rocky river's edge. Not only could he sit on his own in the shallow water there, but it was also populated by people of lower socioeconomic status who we experienced as less socially threatening. Whether through active support or evasive inattention, the antiempathic tendencies we felt so strongly in at least one student were echoed and even reinforced by some of the academics who run universities. Theoretical awareness of the importance of accessibility is all too easily submerged by the much stronger currents of justice conceived as the protection of individual property rights. Perhaps the riverside offers better accessibly experiences than the university. At least there are no academics there.

Once again Adam and I were left at the end of a trajectory beginning with the expectation of enjoying a public environment, followed by complications and threats, and ending with bailiffs at the door, further threats, and personal cost ($427 to be exact), as well as the acute sense that any welcome extended to Adam and people like him was, in reality, highly conditional.

At the height of the fraught discussions associated with the pool incident, we talked to a lawyer at the local autism advocacy center. She told us of the plight of an older autistic boy with balance problems. While at school, and in a special education class, he lost his balance on the stairs. Instinctively reaching out for support, he caught the necklace of his teacher, breaking it. The teacher sued his family for damages.

Such stories reveal the absurdities that can issue from modern liberal accounts of rights. Within modern liberal democracies, disability access and personal property rights are often positioned as competitors. Even in the public space that is school, even within spaces especially configured to host those with special needs, the actors who inhabit it can render it threatening. And they are within their legal rights. In modern liberal societies, legal rights do stand between people. An ethos of shared care and responsibility has to fit around it. Modern liberal societies position the disabled and those who care for them as legally liable for infractions of cultural expectations about behavior in public spaces. Little wonder that public space feels so threatening for those who do not or cannot conform to precise social norms.[5] Public space in Western secular societies is covered by the most tenuous veneer of empathy and shared responsibility. On its own terms political liberalism is incapable of fostering hospitality to people who do not conform, or who have demanding special needs. Since the practical challenges presented by such lives are not easily acknowledged within the norms of liberal secular society, the claim that such lives have intrinsic value rings hollow.[6]

CHURCH AS PRACTICE GROUND FOR LISTENING

Every public space in Western society is susceptible to becoming inhospitable when the actors who inhabit it treat the challenges of disability as "their" and not "our" problem. This raises the question of where hospitable empathy might be learned. Public spaces organized with the aim of making a profit or educating students appear to have no *intrinsic* connection with fostering attitudes of welcome to all types of people. There must be "dark publics" not immediately visible in the popular consciousness in which people can be freed into the genuine welcome of those with disabilities that alone can make public space truly accessible. Liberal societies rely on communities where people are learning to trust one another and learn the practices of mutually serving one another.[7]

It is true that the familiarity bred of casual interactions in the many public spaces in liberal societies can, on occasion, generate the personal bonds that open people's arms to welcome those labeled disabled. Such a welcome is, however, not guaranteed to rub off on others. It is possible to have a favorite "other" without developing any fondness for the outsider class to which they belong. In addition, such individual goodwill bears no inner relation to the notions of justice or the configuration of public space in our liberal societies, oriented as they most often are for profit making, personal entertainment, or consumption.

At least one space in liberal society exists solely to foster a more receptive openness to others, a greater willingness to hear, and in which taking responsibility for one another defines its social form. This place is the church. Adam loves church. When he was young he refused to go to the nursery until he had attended the main service, insisting on sitting in the front row, as close as possible to the piano.

One church we attended had a sanctuary with a door opening directly onto stage center.[8] One Sunday, having already attended the first service and then nursery for the following hour, Adam managed to get away from us long enough to make his way through the door at the front of the sanctuary. The congregation was already well into its first hymn. It was a dramatic stage entrance, the door very visibly swinging wide open as Adam ran onto the platform a few steps ahead of his jogging father. Chasing him into the stage, as I swooped him up I chanced to glance at the congregation. I was stunned by the realization that every single eye in the congregation was on us. In that split second, I saw Adam framed by a congregation singing praises to God. That wall of eyes, of love and of course mirth, showed me the welcoming gaze that is the essence of the communion of saints. I had run through a door into literally another time.[9] In this alternative time all those gathered find their ethos of capitalist liberal individualism challenged and reshaped as they learn what it means to be a body, a community of praise.

The church serves liberal societies as a dark public holding open an alternative time, eschatological time. As a community of eschatological gratitude, it offers an alternative to those many publics that train citizens in acquisitiveness and litigiousness, and to protect themselves and their rights against others. And it does so without appeal to the tenets of secular citizenship. It remains to be seen if attempts to generate this welcome out of the rituals of liberal democracy will effectively form hospitable citizens.[10] What is clear is that over many centuries the church's liturgy, with the scriptural word at its center, has been a domain where a time opens up in which the pitting of individual property rights against the claims and needs of those called disabled is not only impossible, but exposed as absurd.

In this assembly the experience of social marginalization is reversed. Those who have been bent low by work and social opprobrium for six days can walk proudly upright on the seventh. The experience of being irradiated by the eternal light offers them a new perception of their humanity. When people begin to experience this seventh day as real life, the machinations of sinful political communion suddenly appear for what they are, a comedic parody. What has been assumed for six days to be real is revealed as unreal, an embodied retreat from worship and its eschatological reality.[11] The time of this eon is exposed and judged in the creation and renewal of these opened eyes. The kingdom of heaven is truly present when the time and space of Christ's rule become tangible. An eschatological question mark, a parenthetical "as if" is laid against every ascription of outsider status.

Modern people are constantly updating of the nomenclature of disability. This is one sign of an ongoing sense of ticklish discomfort about "them."[12] What secular liberalism cannot admit is that this is the discomfort of a wound barely scarred over. The pushing of vulnerable lives to the margins of cultural space projects modern people's rejection of their own vulnerability. If this cultural default is to be reversed, more will be needed than the regular destigmatization of the language of disability. Places are needed to learn firsthand the practicalities of living with difference that is not existentially experienced as unsettling "otherness." A body is needed where human beings can discover themselves as members of one another.

The church is conspicuously powerless to open up this eschatological communion on its own. The rarity of churches that genuinely welcome people labeled disabled is a symptom of the fatal transition Jesus warned against, in which his kingdom is turned into "religion."[13] Many and gut wrenching are the stories of parents being told in so many words (or actions) that their children are not part of "us," that "the program" cannot accommodate people with their challenges, of communion and fellowship being denied to those who cannot understand, and with those presumed not able to comprehend and so maybe even incapable of (or not in need of) being saved.

The ethos of secular public space can be reproduced in churches, when, to take one example, "difficult" children are assumed to be the sole responsibility of parents. It is no wonder that pastors of Christian churches often believe they have no disabled people in them,[14] or that parents who are told to "be responsible" and look after their "own" children often find it easiest to do so at home, abandoning such churches altogether.[15] Our own experience is that in the vast majority of the churches we have visited, the only workable option is to keep Adam with us. Unwelcoming churches are a provocation to the God of mercy, the God of liberation. That churches and parachurch organizations have sprung up who hear the call of congregants with special needs is a hopeful sign that God has not abandoned the Western church, despite the resistance of believers.[16]

A theological account of how public space becomes truly accessible must explain how Jesus Christ actively engages and confronts not only the world, but a church that should know better. In doing so it must go beyond the limited moral injunction that motivates liberal societies, to be tolerant of all people. Liberal tolerance does not go so far as asking people to enter relations of mutual service with people labeled disabled, but leaves them as recipients of our good intentions and responsible behavior. Liberal tolerance assumes that those labeled disabled should be expected to make no contribution to the generation of a truly accessible public space because, in effect, they are assumed not to be "real" democratic citizens.[17]

Sometimes Adam overturns this whole equation. Disability advocates have highlighted the importance of activism that challenges barriers to accessibility through legal means. But Adam, I believe, has sometimes served an assault on contemporary habits of inhabiting public space of an entirely different kind.

PUBLIC BEGGARS AND DANCERS

One Saturday morning around Christmas time we heard music from a street performer's accordion wafting through a busy shopping area in Aberdeen. Knowing Adam's love for music, I let him find his way to it. Soon he was dancing with utter abandon, obviously filled with joy, and totally unconcerned with the gazes his nonstandard dancing was attracting. Though a cold day, we stood and danced for some time with the shoppers streaming by. It was quickly apparent that Adam's embodiment of joy was radiating out to give a new tenor to this busy public space. A few people would scurry by without a glance. Most would smile as they passed. Many would pause for a moment to watch, with obvious pleasure. Adam was unconcerned with these gazes, abandoning himself to the folk music that so attracted him.

In between songs I discovered that the young musician was from Romania and unemployed. Between Adam and this legal alien something was happening that broke through the logic of a public space organized for commerce and duly inhabited by shoppers bent on efficiencies and exchange. This was no grand act, nor was it a powerful incursion into normal patterns of this public space, but it was undeniably real. The situation was captivating, impossible for most to ignore. Somehow Adam's joy and lack of shame were resonating with the bravery of a social outsider willing to play what most would hear as "primitive" music, for pennies, in the legal borderlands of public space. Such music, especially when combined with a tip jar, tends to tempt Western Europeans to xenophobia, reminding them as it does of the "immigration problem."[18]

Between them was emerging what I as a theologian can only call an assault of grace. The two of them were combining to give something to all who passed by, something they did not merit or expect. They were breaking open the shell of acquisitive busyness that captures this space in a particularly all-encompassing manner at this time of year.

There may well be many ways to explain this incursion. Academics from the humanities and social sciences could no doubt describe it in their own illuminating terms. But only theology is concerned with the ultimate source of hospitality, the sheer inexplicability of human hospitable activity.[19] In Christian theology, such a scene appears in its truth as an incursion of the prophetic Christ. The name of Jesus was not explicitly pronounced. But undeniably, an incursion had happened into normal habits of that public space. The incipient antagonisms, the discomforted and disapproving gazes would normally be attracted by a "disabled boy" and a "begging immigrant" had somehow been broken, turned over.

The prophets of Israel longed for just such an assault. Isaiah depicts the suffering servant as an object of hope precisely because he is not put off by Israel's unfaithful lives and worship. This promised one is the messiah in mercilessly attacking sin, unexpectedly setting upon the chosen people and the nations alike.

> I was ready to be sought out by those who did not ask,
>   to be found by those who did not seek me.
> I said, "Here I am, here I am,"
>   to a nation that did not call on my name.
> I held out my hands all day long
>   to a rebellious people,
> who walk in a way that is not good,
>   following their own devices. (Isa 65:1-2)

The earliest Christians immediately recognized that this assault had taken place in the work of Jesus Christ. They also recognized that the kingdom he inaugurated had drawn them into this assault of grace. They were in for an extended discipleship in militancy.[20] And in Jesus' assault those most despised by the powerful were to have pride of place. "God chose what is foolish in the world to shame the wise; God chose what is weak in the world to shame the strong; God chose what is low and despised in the world, things that are not, to reduce to nothing things that are, so that no one might boast in the presence of God. He is the source of your life in Christ Jesus, who became for us wisdom from God, and righteousness and sanctification and redemption" (1 Cor 1:27-30). God's special honor for the weaker member.

In the worshiping life of Jesus Christ's body everyone is invited to learn to recognize the distinctive ways of this jealously unique God. The God who is the origin of the church's liturgy must continue to reveal God's power *as* the power of powerlessness.[21] The ways of the Trinitarian God are thus the measure against which the church's liturgies are to be assessed and reshaped. Jesus Christ has promised to announce himself in that space too. It is a work of annunciation that presses back against the sinful human temptation of believers to transform Jesus Christ's ways into the liturgies of this aeon that seek strength, prowess, and possession. Adam's stimming, dancing, and lying on the floor at the center of worship serve the Spirit's work of reminding a church also often absorbed in its pictures of decorum and performance that it, too, is a servant not of institutional order, but of a God lowered into the messiness of human life. The "shaping" and "training" that takes place through such divine irruptions in Christian worship continually invites Christians to let themselves be made vulnerable to a God who captures humans and is never captured (Ps 68:18; Eph 4:8; 2 Cor 2:14).

WELCOMING THE ASSAULT OF THE PROPHETIC CHRIST

It is not Adam's radiation of infectious joy that establishes it as having to do with Jesus. What most obviously marked this event as having the character of divine presence was the way two outsiders, who typically make people uncomfortable by challenging the smooth operation of various social expectations, effortlessly commandeered and controlled space. This was accomplished without intent or manipulation. Simply by gratuitously being themselves together, they served the reversal of normal ethical polarization of a public space. By radiating music and joy they set upon all around them, joyfully demoralizing and disarming the habits of productive-and-consumptive, efficient-and-boundary-keeping, security-and-property-conscious humanity.[22] In incursions like these, Adam joins those who might be termed "angelic" bearers of witness. These messengers are not dependent beings crying out for care, but collaborators with the prophetic Christ announcing his love.[23]

Having endured two world wars and in the middle of an increasingly Cold War, Karl Barth was tired of the language of military assault. Repulsed at a church that had reveled in martial exploits, he turned the language of assault around to draw attention to the aggressive destructiveness of human folly and sin. Assault language is not to be given up by the Christian, he suggests, because human sin is not some harmless metaphysical taint. More education will not eradicate it. Sin is a blinding, anti-doxological self-absorption lived out in the active crushing of actual human beings. Jesus Christ announces himself by assaulting these activities that demean human life. The mercy of Jesus Christ is focused with great intensity on ending this violence against the weakest.[24]

> It is a remarkable stroke in a strange and remarkable war. For the attack is that of the love of the Father and the Son. It is the attack of the grace of God. It is the attack of His affirmation of the world, of his generous self-giving to it, His intervention for its salvation, of His pleading and guaranteeing of its life. This is what the Prophet Jesus proclaims to the whole world and to all people.[25]

In revealing the gap between the claim to be hospitable and a lived inhospitality, Jesus' prophetic work is the salvation of human beings. Those who believe themselves hospitable cannot but find the revelation that they are not offensive. It is equally inflammatory to call holding one's self aloof from others a self-alienation.[26] Multiple psychological defenses and self-comforting routines prop up the moral self-satisfaction characteristic of this alienation. Jesus Christ alone is capable of opening a rift between the enculturated routines that grow out of human beings curved in on themselves and the time of the kingdom. This is the sole aim of his prophetic work.[27]

As liberator, Jesus' interventions may be unpredictable, but they can never be absent, for he is true to his nature as revealed on the cross. Language of divine assault is important for Barth in highlighting the priority of God's merciful activity and tying it firmly to Jesus' positive ethos of constructive welcome. Jesus' assault is a war to end all wars—and precisely so is a hopeful breach of the liberal order that encourages us to figure *ourselves* as life-giving warriors securing our borders and eradicating the threats of cancer, autism, birth defects, and terrorist alike.[28] Militant language preserves the ethical bite and political force of the gospel.

In breaking the stronghold of sin, the Spirit of Jesus Christ reaches into history to create humans whose traits cannot be explained by the normal course of historical cause and effect. Genuinely grateful and welcoming human beings are raised up out of the living death of entrenched habits of ingratitude by the address of Jesus Christ. These are the grounds for hope that Jesus' assault will crack open the shells of self-protection built against those labeled disabled in both the church and the world. *Jesus' "assault" is not against humanity, but in the most fundamental sense creates humanity. Jesus' work is to bring into being human beings who do not stave off and resist the demands of others but receive them as an offer of new life.*

Hence the conclusion of Jesus' parable of the vineyard, suggests Maureen Springer: "the last will be first, and the first last" (Matt 20:16; cf. 19:30):

> His kingdom is not an otherworldly domain of future happiness for good people. It's a real, boots-on-the-ground, right-now kingdom happening around us. What if "the least" are actually powerful commandos making inroads for their leader in enemy territory? . . . To crack a cold heart, to train it in love, is the most liberating service any person can do for another. These gifts do not show up on an ultrasound. They aren't measured by tests, and they aren't included in studies on compassionate euthanasia.[29]

Astonished by, gathered by, praising, and placing its hope in Jesus Christ, the church is that community gathered by the good Neighbor who makes believers into a single communion of good and grateful neighbors. Bringing fullness of life, Jesus Christ's healing peace quietly but gloriously enters the world—one pool, pub, hospital visit, and street corner at a time.

***

CODA: PART 5

I might have chosen any number of stories to highlight Adam's role as a servant of the revelatory annunciation of peace. A last vignette underlines the fittingness of this annunciation being called an "assault of grace." Again, the setting is a public space, this time a crowded sidewalk on the main street in the middle of Aberdeen. An obviously inebriated man is confronting people on the busy sidewalk, shouting into each recoiling face in turn, "Come on, want to fight?" Adam is not spared the challenge, offered with the same aggression that is setting the teeth on edge of everyone within earshot. Without hesitation, Adam reaches up, placing his hand flat across the mouth of the angry man towering over him (Hello!). This hurting man's aggressive mask immediately crumbled at a personal touch suffused with kindness.[30]

Such events are not out of the ordinary. And they demand interpretation. Something is being shown here that can be ignored and explained away or received with wonder. Those who dare to respond to this wonder gain a knowledge-how that leads into a wholly different life. This was the central message of the Greek philosopher who most attracted the Christians of the patristic era. Socrates understood himself as a servant of the gods' exposure of the hypocritical illusions of his fellow citizens. He doggedly challenged these illusions one interpersonal interaction at a time, in the streets, marketplaces, and workshops of Athens.[31] He ignored the disgusted and mocking stares that followed him, along with the taunts that he was ignorant and ugly. Writing nothing, he was a living and constant challenge to the superficialities that passed for the wisdom of his age. But having one's illusions punctured evokes shame, and shame evokes anger, and anger evokes the desire to kill. At his trial Socrates responded to this anger by highlighting that he had been given to the city for its own good.

> So, men of Athens, I'm far from pleading in my own defense now, as might be supposed. Instead, I'm pleading in yours, so that you don't commit a great wrong against the god's gift to you by condemning me.... For, even if it seems ridiculous to say so, I've literally been attached to the city, as if to a large thoroughbred horse that was somewhat sluggish because of its size and needed to be awakened by some sort of gadfly. It's as just such a gadfly, it seems to me, that the god has attached me to the city—one that awakens, persuades, and reproaches each and every one of you and never stops alighting everywhere on you the whole day. You won't easily find another like that, gentlemen. . . . you might easily kill

> me. Then you might spend the rest of your lives asleep, unless the god, in his compassion for you, were to send you someone else.[32]

Out of compassion the gods gave Socrates to Athens. Out of mercy the Creator gave the church to the world. *The crucified God stings both awake by giving strange vocations*.

As the early Christians saw it, Socrates was luring the Athenians toward the God they did not yet know.[33] The early Christians also saw Socrates as a precursor to Christ because his life shared the fate of the prophets: misunderstanding, persecution, and finally fatal resistance from the very ones to whom he was sent. Like Socrates and Jesus, many of those labeled disabled today are unjustly threatened with marginalization or death for outraging the distorted moral, religions, and political sensibilities of their age. Such people are liable to termination not for anything they have *done*, but for who they *are*.[34]

Some Christians today have begun to appreciate how much the gifts of the Spirit in those who carry the label "disabled" exceed their all too visible neediness, dependence, and vulnerability. They dare to hope for a church that longs to receive the spiritual gifts that people like Adam bring into its body, despite their inability verbally to articulate their joy and pain. Christians dare hope that the challenge of lives like his will not be erased or hidden away for the impiety of challenging us all to slow down, to notice our reliance on others, to become aware of bodily communication, to love and become interreliant. Christians praise the God of annunciation and mercy for sending such gadflies to sting us awake.

Perhaps I was wrong to worry at the outset of this book that "using" Adam to talk about disability might negatively impact him in the way the martyrdom of Christian parents affected their children in the first Christian centuries. Perhaps it is *Adam* who is the provocateur revealing the resistance of the church and world to lives like his, and is drawing *us* in. Or perhaps each of us has been given our own strange vocations in service of the merciful assault of Jesus Christ on the sin of the world. In a church born from this mercy, we might well discover that Jesus Christ is making humans of us all.

Notes

Preface

1 Franz Rosenzweig, cited in Nahum N. Glatzer, ed., *Franz Rosenzweig: His Life and Thought*, 2nd ed. (New York: Schocken, 1961), 97, emphasis in original, translation altered for gender inclusivity.

2 Throughout this book I will be unapologetically concentrating on the Western experience of disability, as the questions raised in this one sociocultural domain are more than sufficient for a single volume.

3 "Disability is not just an individual experience—it is, at least in part, socially and theologically constructed, and thus any reflection on disability should similarly be understood as necessarily more than any single individual's perspective." Deborah Beth Creamer, *Disability and Christian Theology: Embodied Limits and Constructive Possibilities* (New York: Oxford University Press, 2009), 8. "People who really care about the mentally handicapped never run out of things to say, since they do not write 'about' the mentally handicapped precisely because they do not view the mentally handicapped as just another 'subject.' They write for and in some sense with the mentally handicapped." Stanley Hauerwas, "Timeful Friends: Living with the Handicapped," in *Sanctify Them in the Truth: Holiness Exemplified* (Nashville: Abingdon, 1999), 144.

4 Isaiah 52–53; Dietrich Bonhoeffer, *Ethics*, ed. Clifford Green, Dietrich Bonhoeffer Works 6 (Minneapolis: Fortress, 2005), 258.

5 This starting point performs a movement that Hans Reinders has described from a theoretical perspective as an essential passage of the disability experience. "The issue of making sense of disability . . . is ultimately about what kind of space one believes the universe to be." Hans S. Reinders, *Disability, Providence, and Ethics*: *Bridging Gaps, Transforming Lives* (Waco, Tex.: Baylor University Press, 2014), 3. To cast this book as a conversion narrative highlights the role of subjectivity in reality accounts, and owes much to the long tradition originating with Augustine. J. M. Coetzee, "Confession and Double Thoughts: Tolstoy, Rousseau, Dostoyevsky (1985)," in *Doubling the Point: Essays and Interviews*, ed. David Atwell (Cambridge, Mass.: Harvard University Press, 1992), 251–93. Augustine

understood his conversion as a retracing of the journey of the prodigal son, a movement toward Christ out of the womb from which every human being is born—the fallen city of man. Augustine, "Exposition of Psalm 138," *Expositions of the Psalms (Enarrationes in Psalmos) 121–150*, Works of St. Augustine, vol. 3/20, trans. Maria Boulding (New York: New City Press, 2004), 259–64, 270.

By taking myself and my own transformation as part of the subject of this book I am trying to take the next step in disability theology, refusing to study "them" (people with disabilities) or "it" (disability), but us-with-supposed-others. This deeper engagement with the methodological assumptions of the Christian theological tradition can help us to think more deeply about the theological implications of the authorial positionality assumed by theologians concerned with disability. The methodological development this starting point presumes is highlighted by comparison with Amos Yong's positioning of his own work as an attempt "to make sense of the life of my [Down syndrome] brother within its wider ecclesial, social political, economic, cosmic, and finally theological contexts." Amos Yong, *Theology and Down Syndrome: Reimagining Disability in Late Modernity* (Waco, Tex.: Baylor University Press, 2007), 293.

6 The practice of telling stories to establish the moral authority of the speaker, inherited from both liberation theologies and identity politics, needlessly narrows the discussion and excludes important voices. Creamer, *Disability and Christian Theology*, 5–8. The self-described nondisabled philosopher Licia Carlson, like many others, is "not entirely personally distant from the issue" and yet "fervently believes that the philosophical questions that emerge in connection with intellectual disability are matters that not only are worthy of scholarly interest but speak to the deepest problems of exclusion, oppression, and dehumanization; and that one's proximity to persons with intellectual disabilities should be neither assumed as a basis for participation in this conversation nor grounds for disqualification when speaking philosophically about this topic." Licia Carlson, *The Faces of Intellectual Disability: Philosophical Reflections* (Bloomington: Indiana University Press, 2010), 2–3.

Some will see this work as methodologically closest to autoethnography. The label is apt if understood as defined by Stacy Simplican: as a practice of including stories within academic analysis with the intent of frustrating and disrupting a wide range of expectations about the able-disabled binary. Stacy Clifford Simplican, *The Capacity Contract: Intellectual Disability and the Question of Citizenship* (Minneapolis: University of Minnesota Press, 2015), 14–16, 103–4.

7 Jay Timothy Dolmage has cataloged the pitfalls of narration that all too easily draw on standard (and mostly demeaning) narrative positionings of nonstandard human lives. Jay Timothy Dolmage, *Disability Rhetoric* (Syracuse: Syracuse University Press, 2014), 31–61. The methodological double bind faced by theologians attempting to write about disability is incisively described by Peter Capretto: "Whenever theologians speak of disability, they are not speaking of an *object* of study, but rather a personal experience with disability: the subjective or first-person experience, as well as dyadic relations. Operationalizing cardiovascular health in terms of cholesterol levels may be a simple and understandable decision; experience, disabled or otherwise, is another matter entirely." Peter Capretto, "On Not Operationalizing Disability in Theology," *Journal of the American Academy of Religion* 85, no. 4 (2017): 889–919, quotation from 903 (emphasis in original).

Olivia Bustion has recently excoriated John Gillibrand as an example of academic theologians having "projected their own fantasies unto their nonspeaking autistic children, turning them into symbols of divine ineffability." Olivia Bustion, "Autism and Christianity: An Ethnographic Intervention," *Journal of the American Academy of Religion* 85, no. 3 (2017): 653–81, quotation from 654. Among theological analysts of disability, Stanley Hauerwas has most outspokenly worried about this dynamic. See the chapter "Timeful Friends," in his *Sanctify them in the Truth*, 143–56.

It is arguably not academics but novelists who have most deeply engaged with these problem of speaking about very different others. Carson McCullers' 1940 novel, *The Heart Is a Lonely Hunter* (London: Penguin, 2008), 204, strikes at the heart of the problem: "The thing that mattered was the way Blount and Mick made of him a sort of home-made God. Owing to the fact he was a mute they were able to give him all the qualities they wanted him to have. Yes. But how could such a strange thing come about? And why?" McCullers explores the question of why projections arise by following the life course of someone verbally unable to speak, highlighting issues of communication between people with and without learning impairments that have long fascinated novelists. Michael Bérubé, *The Secret Life of Stories: From Don Quixote to Harry Potter, How Understanding Intellectual Disability Transforms the Way We Read* (New York: New York University Press, 2016).

The facts of my biography make these particularly tricky questions for me as a writer on disability. The most obvious and important issue to be negotiated involves the entirely appropriate demand of disability activists that they get to speak for themselves. I will need to address this dilemma while remaining palpably aware that not every disability is visible, or at least visible to the untrained eye. People whose disabilities are apparently written in publicly legible ways on their bodies may experience disability very differently from those whose inner pains, compulsions, and mental impairments reveal themselves far more subtly and intermittently. Gender-related themes will also appear in some of the narratives I will relate: it makes a difference that I am a man and Adam a boy. Were I a woman and he a girl, or an adult male, some very different dynamics would enter the scene. Similarly, my story is inevitably implicated in complex racial problematics. (Gender themes will be especially prominent in ch. 4, and those of race in ch. 10.)

All I can do in response to these limitations is to admit that I feel compelled to write about what I have understood Adam to reveal about God and the world. This is not anyone else's vocation, but it is mine. To be as transparent about these problems of representation as I can, I will attempt not to hide the limits and particularities of my own creaturely location. I will consider myself to have succeeded if my descriptions of others allow the limits of my own voice and perception to appear, not only in relation to Adam, but in relation to other people with disabilities as well as the women and people of other social groupings whose experiences clearly differ from my own.

8 Michael Bérubé, "Family Values," in *Mental Retardation in America: A Historical Reader*, ed. Steven Noll and James W. Trent Jr. (New York: New York University Press, 2004), 494–500.

9 Drawing overly strong distinctions between congenital and acquired disabilities is a theological mistake. Those who suffer acquired disabilities will no doubt be more acutely *aware* that they could only arise in a fallen creation in which human beings and the material world do not work in the way God intended. But even if it is harder to see, the very same is true of congenital conditions. The only *theological* difference between an acquired and a congenital condition is a *pastoral* one—that some people find themselves

having involuntarily to make the difficult passage from one state of life to a radically different one with a rapidity that is painful.

The passage from one bodily or mental state into another very different one is one most people must undergo, at least those who reach middle and old age. It can even be experienced by people with congenital conditions upon becoming aware of the ways in which their bodily capacities differ from others. I can add little on the problems associated with coming to terms with an acquired disability than Shane Clifton and John Swinton have recently done. Shane Clifton, *Crippled Grace: Disability, Virtue Ethics, and the Good Life* (Waco, Tex.: Baylor University Press, 2018); John Swinton, *Dementia: Living in the Memories of God* (Grand Rapids: Eerdmans, 2012).

My purpose in concentrating on congenital disabilities in this book is to insist that these pastoral problems, as pressing as they are, must not completely overshadow a central theological problem for a theological account of disability: that those who wrestle with *either* congenital *or* acquired disabilities must eventually come to terms with the reality that God has allowed (if not caused) their lives to become what they have. More abstract questions about the impact of the fall on individual human lives must eventually give way to an existential question with momentous theological import: "Surely there is a true need for understanding, but understanding does not necessarily take the form of *explanation*; it might also take the form of *discovery*. Instead of asking why God allowed this to happen, we can also ask, 'where is God present in all of this, and how?' In many ways, Scripture testifies that God will not forsake 'the work that his hand has begun' [Ps 138:8], so why not ask what it means, in this connection, that he remains faithful to his creation?" Reinders, *Disability, Providence, and Ethics*, 159–60. In the end, one of the most difficult aspects of conversion is having our sense of what counts as a tragedy be challenged, and one of the most difficult aspects of negotiating healthcare contexts is conflicts over what constitutes a tragic situation or life.

10 Eva Feder Kittay's best-known contribution to disability studies is to have deployed a characteristically feminist concern to make a nongendered point in political philosophy about the social location of care for people with disabilities. The western default assumption has long been that the sort of care that disabled people need falls squarely in the domain of "women's work." Michael Fine, "Eva Feder Kittay: Dependency Work and the Social Division of Care," in *The Palgrave Handbook of Social Theory in Health, Illness and Medicine*, ed. Fran Collyer (New York: Palgrave Macmillan, 2015), 628–43.

11 Martyrdom of young mothers was particularly disruptive in this regard and was praised by patristic Christians for the special fortitude it showed in forsaking father and mother and children for the sake of the kingdom. Brent D. Shaw, "The Passion of Perpetua," *Past & Present* 139 (May 1993): 3–45. The martyrdom of Christian parents deeply shaped the early generations of Christians, most famously Origen, whose father was martyred when he was seventeen. Joseph W. Trigg, *Origen* (London: Routledge, 1998), 4–5; Peter Brown, *The Body and Society: Men, Women, and Sexual Renunciation in Early Christianity* (London: Faber and Faber, 1990), 160–61.

12 "Ignoring disability means ignoring life; it is the precursor to isolation and powerlessness." Nancy Eiesland, *The Disabled God: Toward a Liberatory Theology of Disability* (Nashville: Abingdon, 1994), 13.

13 Henceforth he will be called "Israel," which means "soldier or struggler for God."

14 In the Gen 33 scene of Jacob's reunion with Esau, Jacob along with all his family and herds bow before Esau seven times and call him "Lord" five times. Jonathan Sacks

suggests that this oddly over-the-top obeisance indicates that Jacob has finally embraced the place God has had all along for him in his divine purposes. Close attention to the story reveals that Isaac has given *both* of his sons blessings befitting their characters. Esau was an earthy man, whose blessing was to have the power and success such talents can achieve in the political realm. Jacob was to be the carrier of the covenant (Gen 28:1-4). "Jacob's blessing had nothing to do with wealth or power. It had to do with the children he would teach to be heirs of the covenant, and the land where his descendants would seek to create a society based on the covenant of law and love. To receive that blessing . . . *he had to be himself*, not a man of nature but one whose ears were attuned to a voice beyond nature, the call of God to live for something other than wealth or power, namely, for the human spirit as the breath of God and human dignity as the image of God." Jonathan Sacks, *Not in My Name: Confronting Religious Violence* (London: Hodder & Stoughton, 2015), 137.

15 On the theological import of the humanly visible side of the wrestling of faith see Paul G. Tyson, "The Wounds of Faith and Medicine, and the Balm of Paradox," *Christian Bioethics* 20, no. 3 (2014): 330–58.

For Martin Luther, Jacob's example displays the quintessence of Christian faith and the icon of the struggle to receive the identity that is ours in Christ. This story, Luther argues, "should be set before the church with special care. For we are reminded that in our life we should prepare ourselves in the same manner and learn to recognize the church of God in that picture of Jacob's struggle. For God hides the church and also our salvation under a dark and horrible cover, to which we must become accustomed so that we do not despair or fall into unbelief even in the greatest dangers and adversities which our thrown in our way. . . For Paul says in Col 3:3: 'Your life is hid with Christ in God.' This is the sum and substance of this example." Martin Luther, *Lectures on Genesis: Chapters 31–37*, ed. Jaroslav Pelikan and Hilton C. Oswald, Luther's Works 6 (St. Louis: Concordia, 1970), 146–47.

Late in life Frances Young also came to view her struggles as a theologian and mother of a child with severe disabilities through the lens of Jacob's struggle. "I could not let the matter rest. I had to go on wrestling. I will always be marked by the struggle. But it is through it that I have seen God, like Jacob, and like him, found my vocation. I too demanded a blessing before I would let go, and I have received it." *Face to Face: A Narrative Essay in the Theology of Suffering* (Edinburgh: T&T Clark, 1990), 68.

16 Some of this earlier material appeared as: Brian Brock and Stephanie Brock, "The Disabled in the New World of Genetic Testing: A Snapshot of Shifting Landscapes," in *Theology, Disability and the New Genetics: Why Science Needs the Church*, ed. John Swinton and Brian Brock (London: T&T Clark, 2007), 29–43; Brian Brock, "Autism, Care, and Christian Hope," *The Journal of Religion, Disability and Health* 13, no. 1 (2009): 7–28; Brian Brock, "Praise: The Prophetic Public Presence of the Mentally Disabled," in *Blackwell Companion to Christian Ethics*, 2nd ed., ed. Stanley Hauerwas and Sam Wells (Oxford: Wiley-Blackwell, 2011), 139–51; Brian Brock, "Theologizing Inclusion: 1 Corinthians 12 and the Politics of the Body of Christ," *The Journal of Religion, Disability and Health* 15, no. 4 (2011): 351–76; Brian Brock, "Quality of Life and the Statistical Outlier: On Caring in an Industrialized Age," *The Journal of Disability & Religion* 18, no. 4 (2014): 318–39; Brian Brock, "Supererogation and the Riskyness of Human Vulnerability," in *The Paradox of Disability: Responses to Jean Vanier and L'Arche Communities from Theology and the Sciences*, ed. Hans Reinders (Grand Rapids:

Eerdmans, 2010), 127–39; Brian Brock, "Menschliche Freiheit in der Medizinethik," in *Gezwungene Freiheit? Personale Freiheit in pluralistichen Gesellschaften*, 2nd ed., ed. Markus Mühling (Göttingen: Vandenhoeck & Ruprecht, 2009) 222–43; Brian Brock, "Looking at 'Us,' Attending to 'Them,' Seeking the Divine: Revisiting *Disability in the Christian Tradition*," *The Journal of Religion, Disability and Health* 17, no. 3, Special Issue on *Disability in the Christian Tradition* (2013): 327–37; Brian Brock, "Mercy, Compassion and the Flesh: On the Inbreaking of Divine Mercy," in *Mercy: Theories, Concepts, Practices*, ed. Hans Schaeffer, Gerard den Hertog, and Stefan Paas (Zürich: Lit Verlag, 2018), 31–49; Brian Brock, "Health in a Fallen World: Meditations on the Healthiest Guy I Know," in *Jesus der Heiler und die Gesundheitsgesellschaft: Interdisziplinäre und Internationale Perspectiven*, ed. Martin Wendte (Leipzig: Evangelische Verlagsanstalt, 2018), 117–44.

Introduction: Disability as a Matter of the Heart

1 "First, changing the environment so that the wheelchair user has more accessibility avoids the interpersonal component of ableism in that it promotes everyone's accessibility and requires very little behavioral modifications of the abled. Indeed, the abled need not sacrifice any of their own privilege in their support of ramps. But confronting the problem of anxiety [that arises when engaging with people with profound intellectual impairments] forces us to rethink the ways in which we engage (or fail to engage) across radical differences in cognitive capacities. Promoting inclusion may not be so easy—it may in fact be discombobulating, as dominant norms of interaction are likely to be upended, ignored, and challenged." Simplican, *Capacity Contract*, 90.

2 John Lewis, "Student Attitudes toward Impairment and Accessibility: An Evaluation of Awareness Training for Urban Planning Students," *Vocations and Learning* 2 (2009): 109–25; Simplican, *Capacity Contract*, 90.

3 This description of the heart as the orienting point of the human being is drawn from biblical anthropology, in which it is assumed that the affections of the heart orient perception and direct action. Bernd Wannenwetsch, "Plurale Sinnlichkeit: Glaubenswahrnehmung im Zeitalter virtueller Realität," *Neue Zeitschrift für Systematische Theologie und Religionsphilosphie* 42 (2000): 299–315. I have also drawn on Jean Vanier's reflections on the role of the heart for thinking about and living with disability, an account that is strongly inflected by French psychoanalytic thought. See Jean Vanier, *Becoming Human* (New York: Paulist, 1998), 85–93; and Henri-Jacques Stiker, *A History of Disability*, trans. William Sayers (Ann Arbor: University of Michigan Press, 1999), viii, 1–4.

4 I am by no means suggesting that I have somehow escaped the need to be challenged in this manner. I, too, am part of this world and resist the discomfort associated with the overturning of my pictures of the successful, beautiful, and disciplined human form. For example: if I as an author write for the highly literate, the academic audience, how am I not perpetuating the very exclusions of some human beings from life together that I wholeheartedly wish to overturn? The academy is certainly one of many in contemporary society in which people with disabilities, especially the learning impaired, are often excluded and demeaned. I was sensitized to the importance of this criticism by Amy Laura Hall's "A Ravishing and Restful Sight: Seeing with Julian of Norwich," in *Disability in the Christian Tradition: A Reader*, ed. Brian Brock and John Swinton (Grand Rapids: Eerdmans, 2012), 153–54.

5 Rosemarie Garland-Thomson, *Extraordinary Bodies: Figuring Physical Disability in America* (New York: Columbia University Press, 1996), 13–14.

6 Writing allowed him to externalize his own hopes and examine their fittingness to local context in searching "for a description in which every word would be linked to my life, which I could draw to my heart and which would transport me out of myself." Quoted in Franz Kafka, *Collected Stories*, trans. Willa and Edwin Muir, ed. Gabriel Josipovici (New York: Alfred A Knopf, 1993), xvii. These dynamics led Kafka to understand his writing as the essence of his vocation. He "adapted and reworked what he encountered, both inwardly and outwardly. He had no choice—hence the impression that he had a calling, in a sense very different from that of all other authors in his milieu" Reiner Stach, *Kafka: The Decisive Years*, trans. Shelley Frisch (Princeton: Princeton University Press, 2005), 4.

7 "Augustine's search for God is self-interested, in the sense that he finds his own self a source of intense theological interest as a knowing person who is comprehensively known by God." Geoffrey Rees, *The Romance of Innocent Sexuality* (Eugene, Ore.: Cascade, 2011), 164–65. My reading of Augustine and his place in the Western literary tradition are usefully encapsulated in Samantha Thompson, "The *Confessions* of Saint Augustine: Accessory to Grace," in *Autobiography as Philosophy: The Philosophical Uses of Self-Presentation*, ed. Thomas Mathein and D. G. Wright (Abingdon, U.K.: Routledge, 2006), 31–63; Charles T. Mathewes, "Book One: The Presumptuousness of Autobiographies and the Paradoxes of Beginning," in *A Reader's Companion to Augustine's Confessions*, ed. Kim Paffenroth and Robert Peter Kennedy (Louisville: Westminster John Knox, 2003), 7–24.

8 Adeodatus, I quail to note, died at sixteen years old, not long after having been baptized with his father. "Augustine, the sometimes professor of rhetoric, surpassingly eloquent on almost any subject, surpasses himself here with the excruciating eloquence of his silence in relation to a death that he merely mentions in an aside [in the *Confessions*] and not again." Michael Banner, *The Ethics of Everyday Life: Moral Theology, Social Anthropology, and the Imagination of the Human* (Oxford: Oxford University Press, 2014), 41.

9 Inspired by Augustine's example, the sixteenth-century Augustinian monk Martin Luther thought the idea all the way through that the term "God" is unthinkable without entering a conversation with the person it names. Because conversation is always necessarily in one's own voice, theological language must not drift far from context and biography. The legal training of his contemporary John Calvin offers an example of a theological voice much closer to most modern Christian theological writing in rigorously screening out any reference to his own life and converse with God.

10 The manner in which I have been presenting Adam to this point has been schooled by the witness of Jean Vanier. He invariably refers to the core members at L'Arche by their given names to highlight the dangers inherent in labeling people according to their medical or psychological diagnoses. This practice of naming points to a key theme of this book: that a robustly Christian view of disability should undermine contemporary habits of narrating disability within center and periphery frameworks. What really is the difference, Vanier presses us, between thinking "about" disability or disabled people, and being concretely in communion with a person whose personhood seems so different than mine? What does it mean to receive *every* human life as a work of God?

11 Augustine, *Confessions*, trans. Henry Chadwick (Oxford: Oxford University Press, 1991), 10.12.30.

12 Judith Butler, *Precarious Life: The Powers of Mourning and Violence* (London: Verso, 2006), 23. If I were to speak and write as an academic as if Adam and his Creator were

not definitive factors organizing my sense of what I am saying when I utter the word "I," especially were I to write about disability, I would indeed be wide open to the accusation that I am tacitly supporting the very cultural trajectories that attempt to ignore and hide away lives like his. I thus take my task as an author and an academic to refuse to speak as if I have not been drastically changed by Adam, as if he had not become part of me. With this comes a commitment to unhand the temptation to use the life of the mind and my academic training to protect myself from the vulnerability entailed in bringing this aspect of my life, and our lives together, into the public domain. Put more precisely, I understand the most important theological claims that I will be making to be intelligible because they have been situated as statements about how I understand my life with *both* God and Adam.

13 There are good moral grounds both to abandon the term "disability" and to insist that it be retained as a legal and political lifeline that allows real people access to the support provisions that they so desperately need. The knot cannot be untangled without questioning the certainties of *both* the medical model of disability (which the definition of disability to concepts of disease and disorder) and the social model (in which disability is essentially a social construction). Carlson, *The Faces of Intellectual Disability*, 86–91.

14 Only a smattering of complaints can be found in Kafka's letters and diaries about the disastrous public policies of his government, the rampant nationalism and anti-Semitism of the time, or the crushing economic hardship everyone was experiencing. What obsessed Kafka was the weight of the morally disapproving gaze and his own struggle to root its internalized forms out of his soul. Reiner Stach, *Kafka: The Years of Insight*, trans. Shelley Frisch (Princeton: Princeton University Press, 2013), 80–81.

Few moments in recent decades have been so revealing of the moral location of disabled lives in the contemporary Unites States than the newly elected president Donald Trump's casual mimed mockery of the physically impaired reporter Serge Kovaleski. Sharon V. Betcher has acutely described the violence of this gesture as expressing a regnant "politics of humiliation." "Crippling Donald Trump's 'Crippled America,'" in *Faith and Resistance in the Age of Trump*, ed. Miguel A. De La Torre (Maryknoll: Orbis, 2017), 137–45. Trump continually and casually slights even people that he intends to honor, as when he told gathered Paralympians at the White House that they were "incredible and so inspiring" if "a little tough to watch." D. Parvaz, "In Cringe-Worthy Speech, Trump Tells Paralympians They Were 'Tough to Watch,'" *Think Progress*, April 28, 2018. That such a politician could be elected by Christian voters, who have also failed to excoriate his mockery of nonstandard human beings, gives some sense of the scale of the problem of hearts hardened to those labeled disabled in the contemporary United States.

15 There are inherent risks in taking the memory of a gaze as data for analysis, given the notorious susceptibility of memory to being shaped by the emotional investments of the agent. Nevertheless, sometimes a gaze or gesture seems so obviously revealing of truth that it cannot be escaped. Before such revealing gazes and gestures, "we are reduced to the testimony of our own senses concerning which we wonder, confronting this isolated and incoherent memory, if we were not the victim of some illusion; so that these attitudes, the only ones of any importance, often leave us with some doubts." Marcel Proust, *Swann's Way*, trans. Lydia Davis (London: Penguin, 2003), 128.

Such epistemic doubts also destabilize the majority's incredulity that they have projected violent gazes and gestures. Precisely because most "non-disabled people are pretty personally invested in being non-disabled, it is easy to confuse the view from normal for the view from nowhere. And then it's uniquely the minority voices which we single out as biased or lacking objectivity." Elizabeth Barnes, *The Minority Body: A Theory of Disability* (Oxford: Oxford University Press, 2016), ix.

16 Parents who have undergone the death of a child speak in just these terms. "This condition progresses rapidly and most children with [spinal muscular atrophy] die at around the age of 6 months. It is a terrible condition. But Daniel—typical of SMA children—was very bright in the eyes, very mentally alert, and profoundly relationally aware. He is our first born, a beautiful child, and a great joy to our hearts. Daniel, via the mystery of love, to this day is part of the very fibre of our lives and even the grief we bear from his death is precious to us for it is a part of who we, as spiritual and relation beings bonded to our son, are." Tyson, "Wounds of Faith and Medicine," 333.

The theme of this book, however, is not the bonds that transcend death, but a confrontation in love with a living God in the face of a living person. "Face to face with God, the problems do not disappear, but they do appear different." Young, *Face to Face*, 92.

17 On being "abled" by others, see Eiesland, *Disabled God*, 38, 103.

The church is notorious among people labeled disabled for the ferociousness of its judgmental gaze, as the Archbishop of Canterbury's daughter and sufferer of chronic fatigue syndrome Katherine Welby has observed. "'You can feel quite uncomfortable [in church], like people are looking at you, like you're not paying attention or not engaging properly.' She says more flexibility and acceptance is needed. 'If someone goes in and the first week they're there they get tutted at, then they're not going to come back.'" Beth Rose, "Archbishop Justin Welby: I Don't Pray for My Daughter's Disability," BBC News, July 6, 2018.

18 Butler, *Precarious Life*, 25.

19 Martin Pistorius, with Megan Lloyd Davies, *Ghost Boy* (London: Simon & Schuster, 2011), 101–2.

20 Quoted in Stach, *Years of Insight*, 419.

21 Eiesland drew heavily on liberation and correlationist theological frameworks as she sought a Christian theology more open to the whole breadth of the human condition. My divergence with Eiesland is in how the Christian tradition is assessed. We agree, as Hans Reinders has pithily put it, that theology's responsibility "is to clean up its own mess." *Disability, Providence, and Ethics*, 10. But unlike her I will undertake this critical work, not by stripping out problematic aspects of historical Christian faith, but instead attempting to display the rounded fullness I have found constantly present in the broad Christian tradition of thinking about the human. To take this approach demands being constantly on guard against extremes: either assuming Christians have always been resistant to what they took to be disabled lives or falling into nostalgia about a supposedly pristine past in which Christians loved everyone without regard. The task of Christians today is to face our tradition as a work of repenting of the sin that has so obviously been carried by malformed theological ideas and church practices over the centuries.

22 Timothy J. Basselin, *Flannery O'Connor: Writing a Theology of Disabled Humanity* (Waco, Tex.: Baylor University Press, 2013); Glatzer, *Franz Rosenzweig*, 138–42.

23 Social constructivist models of disability typically assume that social justice is best achieved by eliminating the category of disability—to see people as people, in all their diversity. At the same time, much of the energy of discourse comes from the sense of moral injustice that rankles at the plight of people called disabled today, and who grasp the power of the term "disability" to undermine and reshape the moral and legal status quo.

"What is interesting, worthwhile, useful, etc. about disability as a category is . . . that it's a social category people have found useful when organizing themselves in a civil rights struggle. It's a social category that people have used to explain what their experiences of social oppression have in common, and it's a social category people have used to group themselves together to work for progress and change. The social category of disability is philosophically interesting, that is, because of the disability rights movement." Barnes, *Minority Body*, 41–42.

24 My discussions of the gaze throughout this book draw on and are in tacit dialogue with the feminist critique of the depredations of the male gaze, African American critiques of the positioning power of the white gaze, and gay and queer theorists' explorations of the moral opprobrium promulgated by the heteronormative gaze. In all these discourses "gaze" stands for a way of looking at the world that disseminates subtle but powerful normative judgments.

Chapter 1: Wonders from Jesus to Augustine

1 It is perhaps more accurate to say that Augustine's question has much in common with human beings in almost every time and culture. "Stone Age cave drawings, for example, record monstrous births, while prehistoric gravesites evince elaborate ritual sacrifices of such bodies. Clay tablets at the Assyrian city of Nineveh describe in detail sixty-two of what we would now call congenital abnormalities, along with their prophetic meanings. Aristotle, Cicero, Pliny, Augustine, Bacon, and Montaigne account for such disruptions of the seemingly natural order in their interpretative schemata. For these fathers of Western thought, the differently formed body is most often evidence of God's deign, divine wrath, or Nature's abundance, but it is always an interpretative occasion." See Rosemarie Garland-Thomson's introduction entitled "From Wonder to Error—A Genealogy of Freak Discourse in Modernity," in *Freakery: Cultural Spectacles of the Extraordinary Body*, ed. Rosemarie Garland-Thomson (New York: New York University Press, 1996), 1–22, quotation from 1.

In directly addressing the problem of anomalous births, Augustine is deploying Christian theology to parse one of the perennial problems of human kinship formation (Banner, *Ethics of Everyday Life*, ch. 2). Contemporary prenatal testing practices are directly and intentionally configured to reshape these processes and do so in ways that position the anomalous new one as a problem. Lisa M. Mitchell and Eugenia Georges, "Cross-Cultural Cyborgs: Greek and Canadian Women's Discourses on Fetal Ultrasound," *Feminist Studies* 23, no. 2 (1997): 373–401. Kinship-formation processes are deeply intertwined with typologies for classifying "good" and "problematic" newborns and continues to have life and death stakes implications in both Western and non-Western contexts. Jónína Einarsdóttir, "The Classification of Newborn Children: Consequences for Survival," in *Disabled People and the Right to Life: The Protection and Violation of Disabled People's Most Basic Human Rights*, ed. Luke Clements and Janet Read (London: Routledge, 2008), 249–64. Mary Douglas discusses the hermeneutical questions at stake with reference to the Nuer tribe of the Sudan, who spoke of anatomically anomalous babies as baby hippopotami born to humans, and who restore social order by leaving the child in the river. Mary Douglas *Purity and Danger: An Analysis of Pollution and Taboo* (London: Routledge Classics, 2002), 47–50.

2 Along with the various myths circulating in the ancient world, Augustine has Gen 6:1-4 in mind here. Though offensive to contemporary sensibilities, Augustine's use of the

language of "monster" to describe the anomalous human form was utterly conventional. *Monstrum* or *monstra* indicated any break with the natural order, which could be regarded as unnatural (as in modern usage), but also an omen or portent. Paul Murgatroyd surveys the wider landscape in *Mythical Monsters in Classical Literature* (London: Duckworth, 2007). It would be counterproductive to obscure Augustine's terminology with a more politically correct translation, not least because this chapter will attempt to show where his language is pushing beyond convention and where it is not—and more importantly, the direction of travel of these changes. In *Abnormal: Lectures at the Collège de France, 1974–1975*, trans. Graham Burchell, ed. Valerio Marchetti and Vanonela Salomoni (London: Verso, 2016), Michel Foucault offers a penetrating discussion of the theological and legal issues which swirled around the term "monster" from ancient to early modern contexts, which includes a biopolitical account of the transformation of descriptions of "monsters" from a designation relating to bodies into our modern usage as a category of particularly antisocial behavior (63–75).

3 Augustine, *The City of God against the Pagans*, ed. and trans. R. W. Dyson (Cambridge: Cambridge University Press, 1998), 16.8. Augustine is assuming ontological stability in making this argument: human beings cannot turn into nonhumans and vice versa, a view that held throughout the medieval period, though increasingly complex theories were developed to account for the illusion that they might (visible, for instance, in Luther's assumptions about nonhuman babies). Augustine did not oppose all metamorphosis and was undisturbed with the changing of rods into snakes in Exod 7. It is important to be clear that an author's sensibility about the possibility of metamorphosis in creation in general is distinguishable from his or her beliefs about the possibility of animal-human transformations. Caroline Walker Bynum, *Metamorphosis and Identity* (New York: Zone Books, 2001), 82.

4 Augustine, *City of God* 16.7. Augustine's strategy here is incredibly prescient. "The presence of the anomalous human body, at once familiar and alien, has unfolded as well within the collective cultural consciousness into fanciful hybrids such as centaurs, griffins, satyrs, minotaurs, sphinxes, mermaids, and cyclopses—all figures that are perhaps the mythical explanations for the starling bodies whose curious lineaments gesture toward other modes of being and confuse comforting distinctions between what is human and what is not. What seems clearest in all this . . . is that the extraordinary body is fundamental to the narratives by which we make sense of ourselves and our world." Garland-Thomson, "Introduction: From Wonder to Error," 1.

5 Augustine, *City of God* 16.8. Augustine is keen in this passage to emphasize that this is not a claim he makes from second hand knowledge, continuing, "There is at Hippo Zaritus a man who has crescent-shaped feet with only two toes on each; and his hands are similar. If there were any race with these features, it would be added to our list of the curiosities and wonders of nature. But are we for this reason to deny that this man is descended from that one man who was created in the beginning? . . . Again, though they are rare, it is difficult to find times when there have been no *androgyni*, also called hermaphrodites: persons who embody the characteristics of both sexes so completely that it is uncertain whether they should be called male or female. However, the prevailing habit of speech has named them according to the superior sex, that is, the male." Augustine, *City of God* 16.8. This last comment also highlights Augustine's prioritization of the male gaze, in conformity with Greco-Roman philosophy. Augustine's lack of awareness

of it provides another barrier to contemporary readers sensitized to both feminist and disability concerns.

6 Augustine, *City of God* 16.8.

7 Augustine, *City of God* 16.8. This question was still alive and well in Christendom one thousand years after Augustine. John Locke discusses anomalous births in *An Essay Concerning Human Understanding*, ed. Peter H. Nidditch (Oxford: Oxford University Press, 1975), and concludes very differently from Augustine. To be *born* from a human and to have a human *shape* is no guarantee of being human: a human *mind* is required. What he calls "changelings" and "idiots" are in Locke's scheme marginally human at best, and so are excluded from the kingdom of heaven and secular political life. *Essay Concerning Human Understanding* 4.4.13–14.

8 "Moreover, the explanation which is given of monstrous human births among us can also be given in the case of some of these monstrous races." Augustine, *City of God* 16.8.

9 For this quotation only I have used the Walsh and Monahan translation: Augustine, *City of God: Books VIII–XVI*, trans. Gerald G. Walsh and Grace Monahan (Washington, D.C.: Catholic University of America Press, 1952), 16.8. Chapter 2 will trace how the wonder tradition was subsumed in early modernity into the naturalistic pathology narrative. That discussion is worth mentioning in the context of Augustine's approach to conjoined twins. The modern genre of the Siamese-twin separation documentary is best read as a restoration of the ancient wonder tradition, as well as the tradition of making a public spectacle of "monstrous births" with a new twist:

> It seems worth asking how, in the postmodern milieu of media images and simulations, this line of development from the freak as a sign or augury to the freak as sickness is complicated, perhaps even folded back upon itself. Contemporary representations of conjoined twins pathologize them, to be sure; yet deviant corporeality remains uncannily portentous, even if what it provides comes in the form of a profoundly secular revelation: through it, we witness the advent of a world of fully instrumentalized bodies, a "high-tech" place of "postmodern plasticity" where there will be no morphology, no matter how malformed, that cannot be altered and normalized. Under these spectacularized conditions, we are not so much looking at conjoined twins as peering in awe at the expensive expertise that will transform us by transforming them. (David L. Clark and Catherine Myser, "Being Humaned: Medical Documentaries and the Hyperrealization of Conjoined Twins," in Garland-Thomson, *Freakery*, 338–55, quotation from 352.)

10 Sharon V. Betcher, "Disability and the Terror of the Miracle of Tradition," in *Miracles Revisited: New Testament Miracle Stories and Their Concepts of Reality*, ed. Stefan Alkier and Annette Weissenrieder (Berlin: Walter de Gruyter, 2013), 161–82.

11 Simplican, *Capacity Contract*, ch. 2.

12 Dariusz Karłowicz, *The Archparadox of Death: Martyrdom as a Philosophical Category* (Frankfurt am Main: Peter Lang, 2016), 216–25.

13 Betcher, "Disability and the Terror," 167–69.

14 Isaiah 53:3; Betcher, "Disability and the Terror," 171. No modern Christian has plumbed the connections between the grotesqueness of Jesus and disability better than Flannery O'Connor. See Basselin, *Flannery O'Connor*.

15 This formulation is intended to resist the reading of Christianity offered by the masters of suspicion—Nietzsche, Marx, and Freud—who established the now dominant view

that Christianity was attractive through the centuries for offering suffers a piety that buffered their earthly deprivations.

16 Betcher, "Disability and the Terror," 175.

17 Betcher's work helpfully displays how a return to the biblical narratives and early church history offers a much deeper challenge to the ethos of our time and at the same time expands the scope of contemporary disability discussions. It is also suggestive in its fleeting appeal to the theological messianic adventus tradition as a more promising approach in disability theology: "miracle need not be aversive to bodies differently abled; the miracle tradition need not be the terror it has been to persons living with disabilities . . . the miraculous might better be related to "the Christian-advental imagination" and its "sudden flashing" or "opening up . . . of the new world." Betcher, "Disability and the Terror," 179, quoting Ernst Bloch, *The Principle of Hope*, 3 vols., trans. Neville Plaice, Stephen Plaice, and Paul Knight (Cambridge, Mass.: MIT Press, 1986).

18 Thomas F. Mathews, *The Clash of the Gods: A Reinterpretation of Early Christian Art*, rev. ed. (Princeton: Princeton University Press, 1993).

19 Both Betcher and Mathews emphasize that to the Christians of the patristic era, "miracles are the core, the mainstay of Christian imagery" and are "repeated to the point of saturation." Mathews, *Clash of the Gods*, 5–11, 65.

20 Luke 9:1-43; 13:31-32; C. Kavin Rowe, *World Upside Down: Reading Acts in the Graeco-Roman Age* (Oxford: Oxford University Press, 2010), ch. 4.

21 Jan-Olav Henriksen and Karl Olav Sandnes, *Jesus as Healer: A Gospel for the Body* (Grand Rapids: Eerdmans, 2016), 97–109.

22 Mathews, *Clash of the Gods*, 66–67. Whether or not Jesus is labeled a "magician" turns on how best to designate the "wand" or "staff" that recurs in early Christian art to indicate Jesus' working of miracles. As Jefferson Lee points out, Mathews overstretches his argument by equating the presence of the wand with magic since, "'Magic' and 'magician' were terms of slander and ridicule in late antiquity and early Christians would not likely have associated their savior with such a negative designation. Moreover . . . there are no artistic renderings of magicians in existence from late antiquity. Additionally, no magician in late antiquity ever used a wand. Magicians relied upon the proper vocalization and physical execution mandated by the spell in order to procure the desired effect, not the use of an external tool like a wand." Jefferson Lee, "The Staff of Jesus in Early Christian Art," *Religion and the Arts* 14, no. 3 (2010): 221–51, quotation from 223. Lee substantiates that patristic theologians saw the staff as a visual linking of Jesus with Moses, who is often depicted in Scripture doing wonders by way of his staff. The salient point remains: Jesus' miracle working was considered an indispensable aspect of his person to the earliest Christians.

23 Mathews, *Clash of the Gods*, 72, 76–77.

24 Michael Banner, "Children and Commodities: A Commentary on Mantegna's *Adoration of the Magi*," Paper presented at the Research Seminar in Theological Ethics, University of Aberdeen (2018).

25 Mathews, *Clash of the Gods*, 68–72.

26 Mathews, *Clash of the Gods*, 91.

27 Mathews, *Clash of the Gods*, 62.

28 Quoted in Giorgio Agamben, *Pilate and Jesus*, trans. Adam Kotsko (Stanford: Stanford University Press, 2015), 10.

29 Mathews, *Clash of the Gods*, 63.

30 Lorrane Daston and Katherine Park provide an overview of this hermeneutic of anomalous bodies across the pre-Christian, patristic, and medieval West in *Wonders and the Order of Nature: 1150–1750* (New York: Zone Books, 1998), ch. 1.

31 Almut Caspary, "The Patristic Era: Early Christian Attitudes toward the Disfigured Outcast," in Brock and Swinton, *Disability in the Christian Tradition*, 24–64.

32 Bettany Hughes, *The Hemlock Cup: Socrates, Athens and the Search for the Good Life* (London: Vintage, 2011), 27–37.

33 That Christianity first spread among slaves was almost inevitable, given that a stable average of 30–35 percent of the populace of Greece and Italy were slaves from the fifth century BCE to the end of the Roman republic. M. I. Finley, *Ancient Slavery and Modern Ideology* (New York: Viking, 1980), 79–80, 126ff.; James Albert Harrill, *The Manumission of Slaves in Early Christianity* (Tübingen: Mohr, 1995), 11–76.

34 The history of early Christian persecution is sensitively surveyed in Bernard Green, *Christianity in Ancient Rome: The First Three Centuries* (London: T&T Clark, 2010), ch. 3.

35 "The world in which Christianity matured posed a choice between Truth and all that is worldly in a perspective that eliminated any possibility of mediation and compromise . . . The first acts of violence by the Empire aimed directly against the Christians were the events following the Great Fire of Rome in the year 64AD. . . . Paradoxically, in this way the law, which turned itself on the Church, brought out one of the deepest mysteries of Christianity. When he accepts the revealed Truth, the Christian transforms his life and he dies, 'to the whole order of things through which the order of death reveals itself here on earth: sin (Rom 6:11), the old self (Rom 6:6), the flesh with its passions and desires (Gal 5:24), the body (Rom 6:6, 8:10), the Law (Gal 2:9) and all the elemental powers of the world (Col 2:20).'" Karłowicz, *Archparadox of Death*, 139–40.

36 "The stage-set of Athens was littered with these perfect, permanently beautiful extras [perfectly lifelike statues], a reminder of what humans could and should be. And Athenian society also demanded a gold standard of physical perfection. The weak, the disabled were not welcome. We learn this from the bone graves, suggesting that a number were exiled (or abandoned), but also from a few throwaway words in the Platonic Dialogues, at the moment when, in 399 BCE, Socrates refuses to escape from his prison. His turn of phrase, his choice of analogy, highlights the difficulty of being 'imperfect' in the city: Socrates [Imagining the Laws of Athens speaking to him] 'But you preferred neither Lacedaemon nor Crete, which you are always saying are well-governed, nor any other of the Greek states or foreign ones, but you went away from this city less than the lame and the blind and the other cripples.'" Hughes, *Hemlock Cup*, 112, citing Plato, *Crito* 52e–53a, in *The Trials of Socrates: Six Classic Texts*, ed. C. D. C. Reeve (Indianapolis: Hackett, 2002). Martha L. Rose points out that grave excavations also indicate that deformities were nonetheless still visible in Greek societies, some 40 percent of individuals displaying some bone pathology. *The Staff of Oedipus: Transforming Disability in Ancient Greece* (Ann Arbor: University of Michigan Press, 2003), 38.

The Greek interlacing morality with the aesthetics of bodily comportment is explicitly stated in Plato: "The inexperienced in wisdom and virtue, ever occupied with feasting and such, are carried downward, and there, as is fitting, they wander their whole life long, neither ever looking upward to the truth above them nor rising toward it, nor tasting pure and lasting pleasures. Like cattle, always looking downward with their heads bent toward the ground and the banquet tables, they feed, fatten, and fornicate." Plato, *The Republic*, ed. and trans. Chris Emlyn-Jones and William Preddy (Cambridge, Mass.:

Harvard University Press, 2013), 586a. The theory was predictably mechanical in its root assumption. "As regards the most sovereign kind of soul in us, we must conceive of it in this way: god has given to each of us, as his daemon, that which we say resides in the summit of our body and which raises us from earth towards its kind in the heaven, since we are not an earthly but a heavenly plant, as they say most truly. For it is there, whence the soul first sprang into birth, that the divine <part of us> suspends our head or root and thus erects the whole body." Plato, *Timaeus* 90a2–b1, in *Timaeus and Critias*, trans. Desmond Lee (London: Penguin, 1977).

I have emphasized Plato's view in these paragraphs given his outsize influence on patristic theologians. Aristotle rejected many of Plato's physiological theories while agreeing with his conclusions on the topic at hand. Both agreed that humans are made to stand upright, infants proving the relation of posture to rational capacity. For Aristotle's view, see *Parts of Animals [De partibus animalium]: Movement of Animals. Progression of Animals*, trans. A. L. Peck and E. S. Forster (Cambridge, Mass.: Harvard University Press, 1937), 4.10. For an overview of the views of both thinkers on the moral and physiological implications of posture see Pavel Gregori , "Plato's and Aristotle's Explanation of Human Posture," *Rhizai: A Journal for Ancient Philosophy and Science* 2 (2005): 183–96.

These anthropological assumptions influenced many Christian thinkers and were only slowly critically engaged despite some of the evident deficiencies of this picture of the human. In the first work of Christian systematic theology see Lactantius' *The Divine Institutes*, in *Ante-Nicene Christian Library*, vol. 21: *The Works of Lactantius*, ed. Alexander Roberts and James Donaldson (Edinburgh: T&T Clark, 1881). This Greek anthropology and aesthetics of comportment is engaged in some detail (Plato's view is explicitly invoked at 3.20) but given a distinctly Christian spin.

> For that one and only Parent of ours, when He created man,—that is, an animal intelligent and capable of exercising reason,—raised him from the ground, and elevated him to the contemplation of his Creator. As an ingenious poet [Ovid] has well represented it: 'And when other animals bend forward and look to the earth, he gave to man an elevated countenance, and commanded him to look up to the heaven, and to raise his countenance erect to the stars. (2.1)

> Man does not immediately upon his birth walk upright, but at first on all fours, because the nature of his body and of this present life is common to us with the dumb animals; afterwards, when his strength is confirmed, he raises himself, and his tongue is loosened so that he speaks plainly, and he ceases to be a dumb animal. And this argument teaches that man is born mortal; but that he afterwards becomes immortal, when he begins to live in conformity with the will of God, that is, to follow justice, which is comprised in the worship of God, since God raised man to a view of the heaven and of Himself. And this takes place when man, purified in the heavenly laver, lays aside his infancy together with all the pollution of his past life, and having received an increase of divine vigor, becomes a perfect and complete man. (7.5)

> Those philosophers, therefore, who wish to free the mind from all fear, take away even religion [Lucretius, for example], and thus deprive man of his peculiar and surpassing good . . . What reason is there why they should also maintain that the mind is to be turned in the same direction to which the countenance is raised? For if we must look to heaven, it is undoubtedly for no other reason than on account of

> religion; if religion is taken away, we have nothing to do with heaven. Therefore we must either look in that direction or bend down to earth. We are not able to bend down to earth, even if we should wish, since our posture is upright . . . We must therefore devote ourselves to religion, and he who does not undertake this prostrates himself to the ground, and, imitating the life of the brutes, abdicates the office of man. (3.10)

37 Plato, *Republic* 407a–408b, 410a. See also Julia Annas, *An Introduction to Plato's Republic* (Oxford: Clarendon, 1981), 92–93.

38 Plato, *Republic* 406d–407a.

39 Anton J. L. van Hooff, "Ancient Euthanasia: 'Good Death' and the Doctor in the Graeco-Roman World," *Social Science & Medicine* 58, no. 5 (2004): 975–85, quotation from 980.

40 Van Hooff, "Ancient Euthanasia," 979. Though it would take us too far afield here, the contemporary philosophical and practical implications are obvious. Kateřina Kolářova succinctly states the philosophical problem: "What does it mean that, although the 'human right of the 21st century' is not articulated in terms of 'the right to health care' or 'the right of access, welfare, and solidary social provision,' 'the right to die' is regarded as such a momentous human right? And indeed, what are the ramifications of the discourse of the 'right to die' as a defining line of citizenship in times of biological precarity and under the neoliberal restructurings that, due to privatization, favor the upward redistribution of resources?" "Death by Choice, Life by Privilege: Biopolitical Circuits of Vitality and Debility in the Times of Empire," in *Foucault and the Government of Disability*, ed. Shelley Tremain (Ann Arbor: University of Michigan Press, 2015), 396–423, quotation from 401. The practical problems are no less stark. Irene Tuffrey-Wijne, Leopold Curfs, Ilora Finlay, and Sheila Hollins, "Euthanasia and Assisted Suicide for People with an Intellectual Disability and/or Autism Spectrum Disorder: An Examination of Nine Relevant Euthanasia Cases in the Netherlands (2012–2016)," *BMC Medical Ethics* 19, no. 17 (2018).

41 Van Hooff, "Ancient Euthanasia," 976.

42 L. Stephanie Cobb, *Divine Deliverance: Pain and Painlessness in Early Christian Martyr Texts* (Oakland: University of California Press, 2017).

43 Karłowicz, *Archparadox of Death*, 163–75. Augustine's treatment of these themes was highly influential on later Western views in so precisely delineating the difference between Christian and Greco-Roman accounts of the value of life and of the good death. See Augustine's *City of God*, 1.16–20. Jones explicates the anomaly of modern Christian defenses of euthanasia against the presentation of the tradition by theologians like Nigel Biggar. David Albert Jones, "Apostles of Suicide: Theological Precedent for Christian Support of 'Assisted Dying,'" *Studies in Christian Ethics* 29, no. 3 (2016): 331–38. Nigel Biggar, *Aiming to Kill: The Ethics of Suicide and Euthanasia* (Cleveland: Pilgrim, 2004).

44 Brown, *Body and Society*, 6–7.

45 Rose sounds an important note of caution: the textual evidence for widespread practices of exposure are limited, and there has been a strong tendency of nineteenth-century authors to spin that evidence to highlight the supposed humanity of modern culture.

> In our [modern] mythology, we describe the ancient Greek practice of infanticide in such extreme terms in order to justify our discomfort with disability and our culture's desire to rid the world of people with disabilities. In painting a society of Greeks who routinely disposed of their deformed infants, we are holding up

> our own, advanced society—in which there are two distinct groups, the able (us) and disabled (them)—up for comparison: We label them kindly, we treat them as "almost normal," and we do not stare. We treat disabled people better than the Greeks did because we treat them with compassion: we can cure them, rehabilitate them, make them "normal." If we determine that they do not have the potential to be a Helen Keller or a Stevie Wonder, we can ensure that they're not even born. (Rose, *Staff of Oedipus*, ch. 2, 29–49.)

To counter this modern interpretative bias, and in distinction from my argument, Rose is skeptical that the Greeks saw anomalous births as portents or signs of divine activity or that their lionization of physical beauty and utopian thought experiments ended in the practical devaluation of disabled lives.

46 O. M. Bakke, *When Children Became People: The Birth of Childhood in Early Christianity*, trans. Brian McNeil (Minneapolis: Augsburg Fortress, 2005), 110–51. Brown, *Body and Society*, 28. Henri-Jacques Stiker engages the practical realities and philosophical implications of Greek practices of exposure in some depth in *History of Disability*, ch. 3.

47 Plato, *Republic* 460c, 461c. "As for the exposure and nurture of infants, let there be a law against nourishing those that are deformed, but if exposing offspring because of the number of children one has is prohibited by a customary rule, then a numerical limit must be set upon procreation." Aristotle, *Politics Books VII and VIII*, trans. Richard Kraut (Oxford: Clarendon, 1997), 1335b19–20. My analysis parallels Kraut's in taking this espousal of infanticide as being related not only to economic questions but the premise of ancient virtue ethics: "Notice that [Aristotle's position] does not simply *allow* infanticide—it *requires* it. Those who have various physical defects cannot make the contributions to the community that are expected of all citizens. Here we have a striking illustration of Aristotle's conception of the relation between the individual and the political community. He does not conceive of individuals as possessors of a natural right not to be killed. Rather, human beings should be protected in various ways only on condition that they are able to make the same contribution to the good of others that is expected of all other full members of the community." Aristotle, *Politics*, p. 154 of the Kraut translation.

48 "The man who when he sees a quarrel on the streets coming to blows will try to quiet it or expresses his strong disproval, will in the stadium applaud fights far more dangerous; that he who shudders at the body of a man who died by nature's law the common death of all, will, in the amphitheater, gaze down with most tolerant eyes on the bodies of men mangled, torn in pieces, defiled with their own blood." Tertullian, *De spectaculis* 21, in *Tertullian: Apology, De spectaculis, Minucius Felix*, trans. T. R. Glover and Gerald Rendall, Loeb Classical Library 250 (Cambridge, Mass.: Harvard University Press, 1931); Novatian, *De spectaculis: A Translation with an Introduction and Notes*, trans. Jacoby Matthew Henry (Washington, D.C.: Catholic University of America Press, 1957).

49 "You will not murder offspring by means of abortion and you will not kill having been born." *Didache* (approx. 40–90 CE) 2.2, ed. Aaron Milavec, in *The Didache: Text, Translation, Analysis and Commentary* (Collegeville, Penn.: Liturgical, 2003).

50 "In our case, murder being once for all forbidden, we may not destroy even the fetus in the womb . . . To hinder a birth is merely a speedier man-killing; nor does it matter whether you take away a life that is born, or destroy one that is coming to the birth." Tertullian, *Apology* 9.25 (approx. 197 CE), in *Tertullian: Apologetical Works*, trans. R. Arbesmann, E. J. Daily, and E. A. Quain, Fathers of the Church 10 (Washington, D.C.: Catholic University of America Press, 1950). Tertullian's assumption is that Christians display a

harmony between word and deed. This essential premise of the apologetic literature of the first centuries is directly linked to their understanding of martyrdom. Karłowicz, *Archparadox of Death*, 131.

51 Brown, *Body and Society*, 101.

52 Betcher singles out Pseudo-Justin, Irenaeus, and Augustine for this criticism in "Disability and the Terror," 164–65.

53 Christians did not invent the idea of moral beauty trumping physical beauty, which was present in Stoic and Neoplatonic traditions. Their innovation was the weight it was given within their whole conceptual framework and the rich connections they drew from it for practical Christian life.

54 Augustine, *Expositions of the Psalms (Enarrationes in Psalmos) 51–72*, trans. Maria Boulding, Works of St. Augustine 3/17 (New York: New City Press, 2001), 275, emphasis added. It is worth noting how Augustine is modifying his sources. This passage likely draws from sentiments found in Cicero while jettisoning his presumption that it is normal and appropriate to be repulsed at human deformities. "[I]s there any evil greater than moral wrong? For if physical deformity excites a certain amount of aversion, how offensive ought the deformity and hideousness of a demoralized soul to seem!" Cicero, *De Officiis*, trans. G. P. Goold, Loeb Classical Library (Cambridge, Mass.: Harvard University Press, 1913), 3.29.

55 Commenting on the creation of humans in the book of Genesis, Augustine concluded that "it was in the very factor in which he surpasses nonrational animate beings that man was made to God's image." Because humans have been created rational, "the apostle too says: Be renewed in the spirit of your minds and put on the new man, who is being renewed for the recognition of God according to the image of him who created him [Rom 12:2; Eph 4:23-24; Col 3:10] . . . he makes it plain enough just in what part of man was created in God's image—that it was not in the features of the body but in a certain form of the illuminated mind." Augustine, *The Literal Interpretation of Genesis*, trans. Edmund Hill, Works of St. Augustine 1/3 (New York: New City Press, 2002), 3.20, 30. This definition of rationality as the meeting point of God's creative and redeeming works in the human breast hints that Augustine is not thinking of rationality in terms of modern understandings of rationality as a capacity of biological organisms.

56 An earlier and more comprehensive view of some arguments developed in this section can be found in Brian Brock, "Augustine's Hierarchies of Human Wholeness and Their Healing," in Brock and Swinton, *Disability in the Christian Tradition*, 65–100.

57 Augustine, *City of God* 11.7.

58 Augustine, *City of God* 11.7.

59 "For example, who could fail to see, on rational consideration, how marvelous it is that, despite the innumerable multitude of men, and despite the great similarity of their nature, each individual man has his own particular appearance?" Augustine, *City of God* 11.8.

60 Augustine, *City of God* 11.8.

61 "[J]ust as it was not impossible for God to create whatever natures he chose, so it is not impossible for Him to change those natures which He has created in whatever way he chooses." Augustine, *City of God* 11.8.

62 Augustine, *City of God*, 11.8, emphasis added.

63 Augustine, *City of God*, 16.8.

64 For a typical version of this warning see Augustine's *Confessions*, 10.35. Such warnings were doomed to centuries of repetition, as indicated for example, by Luther's exasperation with Melanchthon's belief in astrological signs. Luther, *Table Talk*, ed. Theodore G. Tappert, Luther's Works 54 (St. Louis: Concordia, 1967), 219–20. This combination of practical attraction and theological resistance to astrology continued right up to the modern period among Protestants, not least because until well into the seventeenth century it appeared a highly useful tool in the physician's armory. As many doctors were ordained ministers in late modern Christendom, only the rise of medical science as we know it finally ended the conflict. See Michael MacDonald, *Mystical Bedlam: Madness, Anxiety, and Healing in Seventeenth-Century England* (Cambridge: Cambridge University Press, 1981), ch. 2.

65 Romans 12:2; Augustine, *Literal Interpretation of Genesis* 3.20, 30.

66 See Augustine, *City of God* 1.20. The biblical sources Augustine has in view here are Gen 1:28, Rom 12:2; Eph 4:23-24; and Col 3:10.

67 Augustine, *City of God*, 12.19.

68 Augustine, *A Treatise on the Merits and Forgiveness of Sins, and on the Baptism of Infants* (412 CE) 1.32, in *Nicene and Post-Nicene Fathers* 1/5, ed. Philip Schaff (Grand Rapids: Eerdmans, 1978), citing 1 Cor 1:31.

69 John 9:3.

70 "Now a good deal may be said of men's strange vocations, —either such as we have read about, or have experienced ourselves. . . . If we follow those persons who suppose that souls are oppressed with earthly bodies in a greater or a less degree of grossness, according to the deserts of the life which had been passed in celestial bodies previous to the assumption of the present one, who would not affirm that those had sinned previous to this life with an especial amount of enormity, who deserve so to lose all mental light, that they are born with faculties akin to brute animals, —who are (I will not say most slow in intellect, for this is very commonly said of others also, but) so silly as to make a show of their fatuity for the amusement of clever people, even with idiotic gestures [*cerriti*], and whom the vulgar call, by a name, derived from the Greek, Moriones [that is, "fools" from the Greek μωρός]? And yet there was once a certain person of this class, who was so Christian, that although he was patient to the degree of strange folly with any amount of injury to himself, he was yet so impatient of any insult to the name of Christ, or, in his own person, to the religion with which he was imbued, that he could never refrain, whenever his gay and clever audience proceeded to blaspheme the sacred name, as they sometimes would in order to provoke his patience, from pelting them with stones; and on these occasions he would show no favour even to persons of rank." Augustine, *Treatise on the Merits and Forgiveness of Sins* 1.32.

71 Augustine's reading of monstrous births in the *City of God*, "sets the tone for the entire Middle Ages: God created prolifically and esthetically. In order to create a fine cloth, threads of different colors must be mixed, contrasts must be established. The cause and the role of monsters is the glorification of God." Stiker, *History of Disability*, 71.

72 Brown, *Body and Society*, 24–25.

73 Tim Stainton, "Reason, Grace and Charity: Augustine and the Impact of Church Doctrine on the Construction of Intellectual Disability," *Disability & Society* 23, no. 5 (2008): 485–96.

74 Augustine, *City of God*, 22.12–22.

75 Augustine, *City of God*, 22.19.

76 Gregory of Nazianzus, Oration 14 (CE 370), in *Gregory of Nazianzus*, ed. Brian E. Daley, The Early Church Fathers (London: Routledge, 2006).

77 Carol Harrison, *Augustine: Christian Truth and Fractured Humanity* (Oxford: Oxford University Press, 2000), 67.

78 Brian Daley, "Building the New City: The Cappadocian Fathers and the Rhetoric of Philanthropy," *Journal of Early Christian Studies* 7, no. 3 (1999): 431–61, quotation from 448.

79 C. Paul Schroeder provides an excellent overview of Basil's life and social work in his introduction to *On Social Justice: Basil the Great* (Crestwood, N.Y.: St. Vladimir's Seminary Press, 2009), 15–39.

80 Gregory of Nazianzus, Oration 14.8, emphasis added.

81 Gregory of Nazianzus, Oration 14.10, emphasis added.

82 Ola Sigurdson, *Heavenly Bodies: Incarnation, the Gaze and Embodiment in Christian Theology*, trans. Carl Olson (Grand Rapids: Eerdmans, 2016), 10–15.

83 Gregory and Basil both shared this interest in humanizing the faces of those in need, notes C. Paul Schroeder.

> In contrast with the "anonymous poor" found throughout much of the monastic literature, Basil's homilies are characterized by a deliberate attempt to humanize and personalize the plight of the poor. He wonders aloud more than once, "How can I bring the sufferings of the poor to your attention?" Basil brings his powerful gift of rhetoric to bear in order to reveal the face of the neighbour: the emaciated face of the starving person who has gone blind as a result of malnutrition, the agonized face of a parent forced to sell a child into slavery in order to save the rest of the family from starvation. He is determined that the faces of those who suffer should not remain hidden. (Schroeder, *On Social Justice*, 25.)

John Chrysostom draws attention to the voices of people with disabilities in the New Testament, taking an approach much like Nazianzus in highlighting the faith and fortitude of these biblical characters as exemplars for all Christians. John Chrysostom, "Homily on the Paralytic Let Down through the Roof: and Concerning the Equality of the Divine Father and Son," in *Nicene and Post-Nicene Fathers* 1/9, trans. W. R. W. Stephens, ed. Philip Schaff (Grand Rapids: Eerdmans, 1978), 209–32.

84 Gregory of Nazianzus, Oration 14.11, emphasis added.

85 Gregory of Nazianzus, Oration 14.12.

86 Gregory's account of the place of the leper in God's purposes was at the leading edge of a groundswell in early Christianity. At the dawn of the Christian era, Zotikos was martyred for having diverted money from Constantine's imperial treasury to found a leprosarium, an act which later led to the conversion of Constantine's son to the cause of funding institutions of care. Stiker, *History of Disability*, 73–75. The theme resurfaces even as a critique of these institutions at the late end of the medieval period. The author of the *Legend of the Three Companions* presents the conversion of St. Francis of Assisi as catalyzed by his admission of repulsion at lepers.

> One day he was riding his horse near Assisi, when he met a leper. And, even though he usually shuddered at lepers, he made himself dismount, and gave him a coin, kissing his hand as he did so. After he accepted a kiss of peace from him, Francis remounted and continued on his way. He then began to consider himself

less and less, until, by God's grace, he came to complete victory over himself. After a few days, he moved to a hospice of lepers, taking with him a large sum of money. Calling them all together, as he kissed the hand of each, he gave them alms. When he left there, what before had been bitter, that is to see and touch lepers, was turned into sweetness. . . . With the help of God's grace, he became such a servant and friend of the lepers, that, as he testified in his Testament, he stayed among them and served them with humility. (Quoted in Miguel J. Romero, "The Goodness and Beauty of Our Fragile Flesh: Moral Theologians and Our Engagement with 'Disability,'" *The Journal of Moral Theology* 6, Special Issue no. 2 [2017]: 250.)

87 Gary B. Ferngren, *Medicine and Religion: A Historical Introduction* (Baltimore: Johns Hopkins University Press, 2014), ch. 2.

88 Timothy S. Miller, *The Birth of the Hospital in the Byzantine Empire*, rev. ed. (Baltimore: Johns Hopkins University Press, 1985), 4; Gary B. Ferngren, *Medicine and Health Care in Early Christianity* (Baltimore: John Hopkins University Press, 2009); Andrew Crislip, *From Monastery to Hospital: Christian Monasticism and the Transformation of Healthcare in Late Antiquity* (Ann Arbor: University of Michigan Press, 2005), 125.

The tenor of the age is palpable in the apologetic tone of Basil's Letter 94, in which he defends the construction of the Basiliad as nonsubversive to Elias, the local governor.

> And whom do we wrong when we build hospices for strangers, for those who visit us while on a journey, for those who require some care because of sickness, and when we extend to the latter the necessary comforts, such as nurses, physicians, beasts for traveling and attendants? There must also be occupations to go with these men, both those that are necessary for gaining a livelihood, and also such as have been discovered for a decorous manner of living. And, again, they need still other buildings equipped for their pursuits, all of which are an ornament to the locality, and a source of pride to our governor, since their fame redounds to your credit. (Basil, *The Letters*, vol. 2, trans. Roy J. Deferrari, Loeb Classical Library 215 [London: William Heinemann, 1928], 151–53.)

89 Amanda Porterfield, *Healing in the History of Christianity* (Oxford: Oxford University Press, 2005); Miller, *Birth of the Hospital in the Byzantine Empire*, 66–67.

90 Charles Taylor, *Sources of the Self: The Making of the Modern Identity* (Cambridge, Mass.: Harvard University Press, 1989), ch. 2.

91 Originally the Greek term *ethos* designated the "stall" or "dwelling" of animals but came in classical Greek to designate a sense of place or habitable environment, the sociolinguistic clearing held open by relatively stable agreements about behavioral norms. Paul Lehman, *Ethics in a Christian Context* (New York: Harper & Row, 1963), 23–25; William Brown, *The Ethos of the Cosmos: The Genesis of Moral Imagination in the Bible* (Grand Rapids: Eerdmans, 1999), 11.

92 Important questions about the relation of thought to practice lie at this juncture. Modern Westerners are among the first generations who do not live in constant fear of starvation, deadly and widespread epidemics, and the depredations of war. The taken for granted in any ethos is directly linked with such material practices. Banner, *Ethics of Everyday Life*, 8–17. In a culture of survival, much in the traditional warnings against premarital sex (to take one example) made plain sense, both as human wisdom and rules promulgated by the Creator. But in the wake of modern contraception, abortion, and antibiotics, such

moral strictures can now appear not only antiquated but as arbitrary human constructions. These changes in material practices help make developments in the Western ethos visible at a point of particular relevance for disability discussions, the marked change in attitudes toward abortion and euthanasia over the last fifty years. Banner, *Ethics of Everyday Life*, chs. 2–3, 5–6.

Though the Western secular ethos contains obvious continuities with the ethos of Christendom, modern Westerners assume this is a historical accident rather than a heritage to be consciously preserved. Bonhoeffer, "Heritage and Decay," in *Ethics*, 103–33. Christians themselves contributed to this state of affairs by using Christian theology to legitimate imperial conquest and supporting rigid demarcations of "religion" from "public life" during the Enlightenment period. On the former, see Willie James Jennings, *The Christian Imagination: Theology and the Origins of Race* (New Haven, Conn.: Yale University Press, 2010); on the latter, see Timothy Fitzgerald, *Discourse on Civility and Barbarity: A Critical History of Religion and Related Categories* (Oxford: Oxford University Press, 2007). Whatever the processes involved, in important respects modern liberal societies are marked by a substantially different ethos which in important respects diametrically opposes the ethos that had earlier characterized Christendom. Christian theologians after Christendom increasingly encounter ethical debates that rule out any defense of the characteristic moral norms of previous Christian eras, whose intelligibility assumed the Christian ethos. With this comes a second more particularly modern dilemma, the secularization of primary theological terminology. This is the secularization internalized in Christians themselves.

These two thorny problems faced by Christians yield a third challenge: the need for the Christian church to face its own complicity in this state of affairs. Understandable psychological defenses protect Christians against admitting having been shaped by the ethos of modern secularity. The problem of disability demands facing this more difficult complicity. The rapidly shifting landscape of contemporary ethical discussions signals the maturation of a new Western ethos. The changes already well under way will not be adequately addressed by engaging the ethical arguments as currently configured within the modern ethos.

93 This point has been most influentially argued by Alasdair MacIntyre, *Three Rival Versions of Moral Inquiry: Encyclopedia, Genealogy, and Tradition* (London: Gerald Duckworth, 1990).

94 Hans Reinders, in *The Future of the Disabled in Liberal Society: An Ethical Analysis* (South Bend, Ind.: University of Notre Dame Press, 2000), arrived at this claim by way of internal critique of modern liberal political philosophy.

95 Miguel J. Romero states the problem more analytically: "Most contemporary theologians who intentionally engage or intentionally avoid 'disability' have, in some way, appropriated at least one of the following presumptions. *First* . . . that the ability-disability distinction is a self-evident and unproblematic natural division within humanity. *Second* . . . that the concept of 'disability' can function as an internally coherent, conceptually stable, ahistorical category for Christian theological discourse (i.e., that it can stand as a specialized field of inquiry). *Third* . . . that the Christian theological tradition holds human impairment, illness, and injury (i.e., 'disabilities') to be unequivocally bad, objectively ugly, and definitively tragic corporeal states . . . . none of [these three presumptions] comes even close, from the Christian perspective, to being historically demonstrable or theologically defensible in relation to Christian anthropology and the various ways that

human beings experience corporeal impairment, illness and injury. . . . the problem is a theologically unfounded confidence in the nature, meaning and valuation of the concept 'disability.'" "Goodness and Beauty of Our Fragile Flesh," 219–20 (emphasis in original).

96 Whatever the historical ambiguities surrounding the actual practices of infanticide in the ancient world, what is indisputable is that it was the Christian emperors who outlawed it (Constantine, in 318 CE), followed by the exposure of children (Valentinian, in 384 CE). Banner, *Ethics of Everyday Life*, 77.

97 The most influential instances of this gesture are found in Jean Vanier, *Made for Happiness: Discovering the Meaning of Life with Aristotle*, trans. Kathryn Spink (Toronto: Anasi, 2012), ch. 2; and Stanley Hauerwas and Charles Pinches, *Christians among the Virtues: Theological Conversations with Ancient and Modern Ethics* (South Bend, Ind.: University of Notre Dame Press, 1997), ch. 3.

98 Cicero, *De Officiis* 1.14.

99 Betcher accuses the theologians of the patristic era to have been the first to diverge from the biblical consensus by promulgating a thinly Christianized Platonic dream of resurrection to aesthetic perfection. Several church fathers are presented as precursors of the modern medicalized normalization project that is the main target of Betcher's critique. Pseudo-Justin, Irenaeus, and Augustine display admittedly problematic strands of patristic envisioning of the perfect symmetry and proportionality of the resurrected Christ. The laudably materialist disposition and social orientation of the earliest Christians is subverted by a high patristic Christology that reinjects ancient notions of beauty into Christian anthropology. A salutary attention to bodies, their brokenness, and their neediness among the earliest Christians thus ends up being consistently undermined: Betcher, "Disability and the Terror," 164–65. This extreme makeover of Christianity by Platonized notions of divine purity was a precursor to the modern medical normalizing project in effectively undermining the this-worldly hopes for healing and resurrection held by the earliest Christians.

While a deserved criticism of at least one strand of the patristic approach to disability, the problem is less that these early theologians fell prey to Platonic conceptualizations of the human and more the wide currency of those views today in developed societies and among the Christians in them. Airbrushed fantasies of human perfection every bit as idealized as the most extreme Greek views are projected on every available surface in the modern world, fantasies the medical establishment seems to hold out as achievable for the masses. To expose the violence of contemporary normalization regimes, Betcher has summoned the Christian artists of the first centuries as witnesses who repudiate such fantasies of perfection as un-Christian. But in doing so she has given short shrift to the complexity displayed in the works of patristic theologians.

Chapter 2: Wonders from Christendom to Modernity

1 Psalms 111:1-2, 4, NRSV translation modified. The word "wonders" here is not an adjective but a verb transliterated *pala*, and denotes a "dealing powerfully or extraordinarily." "God has established many commemorative commandments for His people to keep alive the memory of those miraculous events associated with the Exodus. These show Him not only as the Creator but also as the One Who cares for His creatures with compassion and mercy. Moreover, God performs miracles of compassionate deliverance in *every* generation; these are small-scale re-enactments of those ancient miracles." Hillel Danziger and Nosson Scherman, *The ArtScroll Tehillim* (Brooklyn: Mesora Publications, 2001), 244–45.

2 Refusing to push contagious people out of the city was part of a wider development in Christian culture that ultimately sprang from the Christian belief that Jesus had defeated death. Bernd Wannenwetsch, "From *Ars Moriendi* to Assisted Suicide: Bonhoefferian Explorations into Cultures of Death and Dying," *Studies in Christian Ethics* 24, no. 4 (2011): 428–40. In Christendom the dead were no longer to be buried outside the city walls but were brought inside, typically to be buried around the basilica. The veneration of the martyrs again played a pivotal role in this development. The condition of this development was that the dead body, like the body of the leper, had to cease to inspire fear. Philippe Ariès, *The Hour of Our Death* (London: Allen Lane, 1981), 30–36.

Irina Metzler surveys views of disability in medieval Christendom in *Disability in Medieval Europe: Thinking about Physical Impairment during the High Middle Ages, c.1100–1400* (Abingdon, U.K.: Routledge, 2006); and *Fools and Idiots? Intellectual Disability in the Middle Ages* (Manchester: Manchester University Press, 2016).

3 Stiker, *History of Disability*, 73–86, surveys the history of charity toward the disabled in the medieval period. Thomas E. Reynolds surveys the modern theological critique of the charity model of disability in *Vulnerable Communion: A Theology of Disability and Hospitality* (Grand Rapids: Brazos, 2008), 114–16. Nancy Eiesland's *Disabled God* (73–75) called the problem of charity one of the "cardinal sins" of traditional Christian theology.

4 Luke 6:36. The Latin term for "mercy," *misericordia*, combines the roots for "pity" and "heart." Mercy is born in a person's "heart going out" to another human being. Mercy can lead to "compassion"—again from the Latin *compassio*, literally "suffering with"—that derives in turn from the Greek for "sympathy." "Compassion" is one name for this moment of being made responsive, if we insist that it is no more than the moment of human recognition of the need for divine rescue for a specific creature here and now.

5 "The worst and true denial of the deity of Christ—every revolt in dogmatics rests on a revolt in ethics—is when we deny that Christ has come to seek and save the lost [cf. Luke 19:10], when we change the divine goodness that is at issue here into a human goodness, when we change the seeking and savings of the lost into the image of our own supposed improving, or arrogant and impotent desire to improve others, in which we do not affirm them but in the strongest and most refined and incorrigible manner affirm ourselves." Karl Barth, *Ethics*, trans. Geoffrey W. Bromiley, ed. Dietrich Braun (Edinburgh: T&T Clark, 1981), 341.

6 The messianic Adventus tradition so prominent among the earliest Christians not only remained alive among Christians through the centuries but continues to offer a potent theological emphasis for people thinking about disability today. Another order, another truth is revealed in the life, death, and resurrection of Jesus Christ. The plausibility of any deployments of this Adventus tradition today turns on how believable the descriptions are in such accounts of how the divine mercy that precedes and provokes human acts enters the life of individual subjects. A concrete account is needed that convincingly displays the disruption of the regimes of unmerciful habit and perception that characterize given generations in their resistance to God's merciful rule. Indicators will need to be set out about the clues to be watched for that indicate those unmerciful regimes are being eschatologically overturned. I take the rival order offered in Jesus Christ to be not only the hope of people labeled "disabled," but of all human beings. "Indeed, the bloody crucifixion of Jesus is such a revolutionary story precisely because it tells of his wounded flesh, his dead body, vis., that it was not left to rot on Easter Sunday, but immersed in a 'life' quite different from the life that comes and goes, the life analyzed by biochemists

and insurance companies' comments." Craig Keen, *After Crucifixion: The Promise of Theology* (Eugene: Cascade, 2013), 124.

Methodological implications follow. Whatever progress the church might make in enculturating the vision of Christ's peace in the world, it is not *itself* this redemption. This is no denigration of the presence of Christ animating the church, but an insistence that the animating Spirit be distinguished from the tangled incompleteness of the Body of Christ. Christ appears in the weakness of the church, and that appearance does reform the church in its practices and thinking, but not by drawing it upward in an unbroken ascent. That the life of a given culture is not transparently a downward descent is a sign of God's refusal to abandon the world. The technicalities of my tying these theological claims to specific contemporary cultural moments will in important respects resemble those deployed by Ted A. Smith in his *The New Measures: A Theological History of Democratic Practice* (Cambridge: Cambridge University Press, 2007), 30–39.

7 "Whatever else we might insist that the little three-letter word means, 'God' resounds particularly well when—from under the heel of the beast, pressed down as beasts always are by the weight of their provisions for a negotiable future—prayers for salvation tear out of the bellies and throats of 'expendables': 'God, Creator of Israel and of the world, rain fire down from heaven!' 'God, Creator of Israel and of the world, save your people!'" (cf. Rev 19:1; 20:9; Isa 43). Keen, *After Crucifixion*, 137.

8 The ancient categories of the marvelous or demonic give way to the language of deviance. "As modernity develops in Western culture freak discourse logs the change: the prodigious monster transforms into the pathological terata; what was once sought after as revelation becomes pursued as entertainment; what aroused awe now inspires horror; what was taken as a portent shifts to a site of progress. In short, wonder becomes error." Garland-Thomson, "Introduction: From Wonder to Error," 3.

9 "[A] pastor got a call that a young couple, after several years of hoping and nine months of embodied longing, had received their long awaited baby. But the grandparent calling the pastor wanted to make clear that the baby's mother did not want the pastor to visit them in the hospital. Understanding from the tone that more than mere modesty was involved in the request, the pastor gently asked if he could be of help in some way. Yes, through prayer, the caller responded, for the baby girl had been born with a cleft palate. Perhaps because he prayerfully respected the mother's wishes, the pastor was eventually invited to the hospital to pray with the couple and their baby. He told me later that he was able simply to say to the mother that the baby was beautiful. For she was, he explained to me, 'beautiful.' The young couple went on to struggle with their news, and the spreading of their news throughout the relatively small community. They did not bring the baby to church, so reluctant were they, perhaps, to deal with the awkward comments of others. And, somewhat to the pastor's confusion, they waited until the baby was well past the usual time to have her baptized. They waited until the series of reconstructive surgeries to erase the mark of disability was complete before they brought the child to be liturgically marked as God's own." Amy Laura Hall, *Conceiving Parenthood: American Protestantism and the Spirit of Reproduction* (Grand Rapids: Eerdmans, 2008), 6.

10 Brock, "Augustine's Hierarchies of Human Wholeness and Their Healing," 71–72; Martin Wendte, "On Hegel's View of People with Disabilities," in Brock and Swinton, *Disability in the Christian Tradition*, 251–85, reference to 257–59.

11 The medieval period continues in the patristic (Augustinian) view of wonder, setting the stage for its later rejection. Bynum, *Metamorphosis and Identity*, 48. While there was

no one medieval view of the wonder, there was a common core of beliefs. "Medieval theorists . . . understood wonder (*admiratio*) as cognitive, non-appropriative, perspectival, and particular. Not merely a physiological response, wonder was a recognition of the singularity and significance of the thing encountered. Only that which is really different from the knower can trigger wonder; yet wonder will always be in a context and from a particular point of view. To medieval thinkers, human beings cannot wonder at what is not there; but neither can we wonder at that which we fully understand." Bynum, *Metamorphosis and Identity*, 39.

12 Aristotle, *Metaphysics* 1.2, 982b10–18.

13 The details of this transition are surveyed in Daston and Park, *Wonders and the Order of Nature*, ch. 3. Thomas Aquinas' mature view of wonder is surveyed in *Summa contra Gentiles*, in *Basic Writings of Saint Thomas Aquinas*, vol. 2: *Man and the Conduct of Life*, ed. Anton C. Pegis (Indianapolis: Hackett, 1997), chs. 99–105.

Though deeply influenced by Augustine and embracing many of his views, including his insistence on the goodness of every human life created by God, Thomas Aquinas sought to reduce the role played by Augustine's inventive reading of the portent as a divine communication. Emphasizing the mighty works of God in this manner undermined serious investigations of natural causal mechanisms.

Both, for instance, believed in the influence of the stars on creaturely events (cf. *Confessions* 5.3; Thomas Aquinas, *Summa Theologica*, trans. Fathers of the English Dominican Province [London: Burns Oates & Washbourne, 1920], 1.96.3), but their reading of this domain in which the most obvious wonders and portents arise was strikingly different, as Daston and Park observe. Augustine worried that the astronomers' account of the heavens "prevented them from feeling appropriate wonder when faced with the marvels of creation, such as a solar eclipse—wonder that the laudably ignorant felt in full measure. On the other hand, it led them, and encouraged them to lead others, into error, usurping for themselves the wonder that ordinary Christians should direct not toward other humans, however learned, but rather should reserve for God. . . . Thus the Latin natural philosopher had an ambivalent relationship to the preternatural and to the passion of wonder that defined its boundaries. As a Christian—often a cleric—he was committed to a tradition that saw humble and accepting wonder as the proper passion with which to regard natural phenomena, particularly marvelous natural phenomena. Because wonder was associated with the ignorance of causes, however, it was a peculiarly unsuitable passion for one whose entire discipline was organized around the causal knowledge of nature . . . Aquinas and his contemporaries proved unable to resolve this dilemma in any satisfying way. Aquinas' solution . . . was to make a distinction between curiosity, which he retained as a vice, and acceptable forms of inquiry . . . for him, curiosity was aimless and half-hearted, while studiousness (*studiositas*), a virtue, was disciplined devotion to intellectual knowledge itself. On the basis of this distinction, he simply laid aside the heart of Augustine's argument, replacing it with another set of values, less sympathetic to wonder, and more sympathetic to curiosity." Daston and Park, *Wonders and the Order of Nature*, 124–25.

While Augustine had celebrated Jesus' emotions, such as his "wonder" at the faith of the centurion (Matt. 8:10), Thomas shifted the verbal emphasis to present Jesus' wonder as a "defect" (*defectum*) taken on for the edification of onlookers. Christ's wondering as a pedagogical act for the onlooking humans was an example of Christian *humility* and was not intended to encourage credulity. Aquinas, *Summa Theologica* 3.15.8.2.

Within the field of disability theology, Miguel J. Romero has vigorously contested this reading of Thomas Aquinas and the *defectum* in a manner with which I am highly sympathetic, explicitly reading Thomas within the lines of the theological tradition as I have presented it. "Goodness and Beauty of Our Fragile Flesh," 206–53. The issues at stake here cover a very wide territory, and in the end, I find myself in agreement with Louis Dupré's suggestion that Thomas wanted to limit the intrusions of grace into nature without severing the study of nature from grace. I take Romero to be true to Thomas in claiming that "in the light of Christ, what is fitting is revealed for its proper and dignified place in the order of creation" ("Goodness and Beauty of Our Fragile Flesh," 252). Though Romero also calls for the inversion of perception much as I have presented, the concept of human nature retains a basic solidity within his treatment. I think Dupré is right in suggesting that, to the extent that the Thomist concept of nature is theologically robust, it remains "overdetermined by the category of grace" so that "nature may be a formal and abstract object of investigation," but, despite the claims of subsequent Thomists, his account does not establish nature as "a concrete reality in its own right." Louis Dupré, *Passage to Modernity: An Essay on the Hermeneutics of Nature and Culture* (New Haven, Conn.: Yale University Press, 1993), 171.

Some interpreters present Luther and Aquinas on opposite sides of the question of wonder as presented in this chapter. Dennis Quinn, for instance, presents Aquinas as the pinnacle of the ancient (Aristotelian) wonder tradition, and fingers Luther as the beginning of the erasure of wonder in modernity. *Iris Exiled: A Synoptic History of Wonder* (Lanham, Md.: University Press of America, 2002). My account converges with Quinn's in the claim that the loss of wonder has theologically crucial import for Christians in modernity.

14 Dupré, *Passage to Modernity*, 70–79; Michael Allen Gillespie, *The Theological Origins of Modernity* (Chicago: University of Chicago Press, 2008), 204–6.

15 History suggests that this historical example is not unique. Stresses associated with social change tend to be discharged by a heightening of awareness of and debate about and sometimes exhibition of anomalous bodies. Garland-Thomson, "Introduction: From Wonder to Error," 11.

16 Martin Brecht, *Martin Luther: Shaping and Defining the Reformation, 1521–1532* (Minneapolis: Fortress, 1990), 98. If the explosion of public awareness of monstrous births was provoked by the social upheavals of the late medieval change, the Reformation's destabilization of fraying social orders seems to have contributed to the spread and extension of conflict about seemingly transnatural events like anomalous birth or mental illness. In England at least, the spread of reformed views both accelerated the conflict between religious elites who increasingly wanted to make wonders cease, and more populist strains of Protestantism that found supernatural readings of such phenomena religiously attractive (so repeating the early Christian attraction to Jesus as a threat to the regnant political power holders). MacDonald, *Mystical Bedlam*, ch. 5.

17 Daston and Park, *Wonders and the Order of Nature*, ch. 9; Foucault, *Abnormal*, 72–75; MacDonald, *Mystical Bedlam*, ch. 5.

18 Armand Maire Leroi, *Mutants: On the Form, Varieties and Errors of the Human Body* (London: Harper Perennial, 2005), offers an example of how the anomalous birth is today viewed entirely without wonder (so recalling Augustine's criticism of the misdirection of wonder among ancient astronomers). Contemporary thought continues to assume the separation of "scientific" from "fantasy" writing that demands people *either* see things as

"facts" or as miraculous and so "fiction." We live after the crystallization of a historically particular division of the "fact" from the miracle and wonder, which includes within it strict demarcations of serious intellectual investigation from the "imaginary" and "subjective" domain of wonder. See Mary Baine Campbell, *Wonder and Science: Imagining Worlds in Early Modern Europe* (Ithaca, N.Y.: Cornell University Press, 1999); and R. J. W. Evans and Alexander Marr, *Curiosity and Wonder from the Renaissance to the Enlightenment* (Aldershot: Ashgate, 2006).

19 "Even portents have been tamed: when hundreds of television viewers discerned the face of Jesus in a broadcast photograph of a nebula, no one anticipated riots." Daston and Park, *Wonders and the Order of Nature*, 365. A sociological analysis of the processes of this depoliticization is offered by Timothy Jenkins in, *Of Flying Saucers and Social Scientists: A Re-Reading of When Prophecy Fails and of Cognitive Dissonance* (New York: Palgrave Macmillan, 2013).

20 Stefan Heuser addresses the debates about these problematic passages in "The Human Condition as Seen from the Cross: Luther and Disability," in Brock and Swinton, *Disability in the Christian Tradition*, 185–89.

21 Luther, *Lectures on Genesis: Chapters 21–25*, ed. Jaroslav Pelikan, Walter A. Hansen, and George Schick, Luther's Works 4 (St. Louis: Concordia; Philadelphia: Fortress, 1964), 136–37. Luther keeps his options open as he enters the fray. Rejecting the belief in universals characteristic of scholasticism, he also rejected any idea that the being of God was continuous with the being of creation. God, being different in kind from the being of creation, remains free to work either directly or through secondary causes, through his *potestas ordinata* or his *potestas absoluta*. God has bridged the divide between Creator and creation in Jesus Christ in a manner that allows humans to leap from their side neither in practice nor theory. The being of God in his majesty is forever beyond humans because, as God explicitly states: "No one can see me and live" (Exod 33:20).

Asking about the role of contingent circumstances in guiding Christian discipleship by thinking about the provision of the ram for Jacob is not as far-fetched as it at first appears as a biblical locus. The pivotal moments in human lives often turn on how apparently happenstance occurrences are received. Theologically, the hermeneutics of contingent happenstance are thus directly connected to the hermeneutics of disabling conditions. Ross Hamilton, *Accident: A Philosophical and Literary History* (Chicago: University of Chicago Press, 2008), ch. 1.

22 Luther, *Lectures on Genesis*, 4:137.

23 Luther, *Lectures on Genesis*, 4:129–30.

24 "In keeping with his nominalist training, Luther was convinced that the reception of the word was a personal experience, but he insisted that it was not a private idiosyncratic revelation. Rather it was the result of an encounter with Scripture within an interpretative community of fellow worshippers. For Luther, Scripture is always powerfully present, a voice speaking to us here and now. This is the reason he emphasizes the spoken word as the most powerful manifestation of God—in fact, the word was one of Luther's most powerful metaphors for God himself." Gillespie, *Theological Origins of Modernity*, 117.

25 "Therefore the word of God must be given consideration first of all; and if someone were to perform all sorts of miracles, yes, even to raise the dead, and comes without the word he must be repudiated." Luther, *Lectures on Genesis*, 4:140.

26 Luther, "Psalm 2," in *Selected Psalms I*, ed. Jaroslav Pelikan, Luther's Works 12 (St. Louis: Concordia; Philadelphia: Fortress, 1968), 32. As counterintuitive as this passage sounds to

modern ears, Luther's position is a christological deepening of a position long present in Christian theology, as evident in passages like this one from Augustine:

> Moses was a holy servant of God. With him God spoke through a cloud, because, when God chose to communicate with any of his servants in time, he customarily did so through some created medium; that is to say, he did not speak through his own substance but by employing some material, created thing, through which his words might be transmitted and made audible to human, mortal ears. That was God's ordinary way of speaking to people; he did not speak to them as he speaks through his own substance. How does he speak in his own substance? The speaking of God is the Word of God, and Christ is the Word of God. That divine Word does not sound forth and then fade away. The Word through whom all things came into being [Jn. 1:3] abides immutably for ever. This Word is also the wisdom of God, and to the Word a psalm says concerning created things, *You will discard them, and so they will be changed, but you are the selfsame* (Ps. 102:26–27). . . . Wisdom stands firm—if we can properly say that she stands; the expression connotes immutability, not immobility—and stands in total self-consistency, varying in no place nor at any time. Nowhere is she other than she is here or there, never is she different from what she is now or was formerly. This is what God's utterance is. (Augustine, "Psalm 138," in Ramsey, *Expositions of the Psalms, 121–150*, 261.)

By insisting that the hypostatic union not be sidelined in a theology of revelation, Luther is forced to reject Augustine's Neoplatonic impulse to frame God's communicative works within changing/changeless and mutable/eternal binaries. Luther thus refuses Augustine's tendency to speak about God's revelatory work as circumventing and transcending mediation, as in this passage.

> When God speaks mysteriously before He acts, His speech is the unchanging cause of what He does. It has no noise of passing sound, and its force that works in time is eternally at rest. By such speech does He speak to the angels, but to us who are far from Him He speaks in another manner. When, however, we catch something of His words with our interior ears, we become like the angels. . . . Unchanging Truth either speaks to the minds of His rational creatures directly in a way that is indescribable, or He speaks by means of some changing creature, and, when He does so, He speaks to our spirit in spiritual images or to our senses by audible words. (Augustine, *City of God* 16.6.)

27 Here "no difference is perceptible between the word of Man and the word of God when uttered by a human being; for the voice is the same, the sound and the pronunciation are the same, whether you utter divine or human words." Luther, *Lectures on Genesis*, 4:140. Neoplatonic aspects of Augustine's thought persist in Luther's view to the extent that they are required to sustain this quasi-mystical theology. Martin Wendte, "Mystical Foundations of Politics? Luther on God's Presence and the Place of Human Beings," *Studies in Christian Ethics* 31, no. 4 (2018): 1–13. Attending to this mystical substrate of his account of mercy highlights the hermeneutical nature of Luther's account of mercy. By prioritizing divine mercy, a specific hermeneutic for understanding the world is set up that aims at genuine existential knowledge of the words "the mercy of God." These words cannot be understood without meditating on them and practicing them, which is why receiving Eucharist and practicing the hospitable embrace of other people is

indispensable for genuine understanding. Hans Burger, "God's Mercy and Practices of Mercy," in Schaeffer, den Hertog, and Paas, *Mercy*, 99–114.

28 Genesis 3:15. This promise of messianic salvation is the "source of all mercy and [the] fountainhead of all promises." Luther, *Lectures on Genesis: Chapters 1–5*, ed. George V. Schick, Luther's Works 1 (St. Louis: Concordia; Philadelphia: Fortress, 1958), 191.

29 Luther, *Lectures on Genesis*, 1:189.

30 "God is the God of the humble," Luther often repeats, "He gives grace to the humble and resists the proud (1 Pet. 5:5)." Luther, *Lectures on Genesis*, 1:244.

31 Luther, *Lectures on Genesis*, 1:245.

32 Luther, *Lectures on Genesis*, 1:249.

33 The constant need of the reestablishment of a true church is a theme that recurs in Luther's lectures. Luther, *Lectures on Genesis*, 1:327–28.

34 Luther, *Lectures on Genesis*, 1:250. This was an account of mercy as an outreaching hand of divine love that was to reenchant the world for many future generations of German theologians. It is clearly visible, for instance, in Dietrich Bonhoeffer's later use of the language of "orders of preservation" to emphasize the repentance-inducing aspects of the estates as manifest mercies. Bonhoeffer, "God's New Action," in *Creation and Fall: A Theological Exposition of Genesis 1–3*, ed. John De Gruchy, Dietrich Bonhoeffer Works, vol. 3 (Minneapolis: Fortress, 2004), 139–40.

35 Luther, *Lectures on Genesis*, 1:258–59, emphasis added.

36 Luther, *Lectures on Genesis*, 1:275.

37 Luther takes human rebellion to snowball (Gen 3:9-11) toward a crowning fatal blow: "to insult God and to charge Him with being the originator of sin. Unless hearts are given courage through trust in mercy, this nature cannot be urged on beyond this point if there are successive steps of sin." Luther, *Lectures on Genesis*, 1:179. At the same time, Luther also strongly affirms that even if the sinner has committed crimes as horrible as Manasseh (2 Chr 33:1-16), "when he recognizes his sin and is truly repentant, the Lord shows him mercy." Luther, *Lectures on Genesis*, 1:289. Even among those who have been born into deep rebellion, which rejects the divine word about all the institutions, can be plucked out of their disorientation by what Luther calls "pure mercy." Luther, *Lectures on Genesis*, 1:301.

38 "A human being, rather than his works, must be just, and that he is accepted by God without any works, solely through grace, which faith believes and apprehends. Nor does faith, as a work, make just, but it makes just because it apprehends the mercy which is offered in Christ. *The true church walks in this trust in God's mercy*, together with a humble confession of its sins and unworthiness, which hopes that God will grant His pardon through Christ. . . . *the works which follow are evidences, as it were, of this faith*; they please God, not simply on their own account but because of the believing person." Luther, *Lectures on Genesis*, 1:259, emphasis added.

39 Luther, *Lectures on Genesis*, 1:352.

40 Ephesians 2:10. Luther's account of the good work also grows from the seed of divine mercy. In neither the *politia*, *oeconomia*, nor the *ecclesia* are the admittedly good things that humans do constitutive of a good work—their goodness before God lies in their reality as acts of faith in the divine mercy and grace. "It is not the worth of the work itself that is of value in the sacrifice; it is the mercy and power of the divine promise." Luther, *Lectures on Genesis*, 1:250.

41 Karl Barth recovered and elaborated this theme in "The Perfections of Divine Love," in *Church Dogmatics* 2/1: *The Doctrine of God*, ed. G. W. Bromiley and T. F. Torrance (Edinburgh: T&T Clark, 1957), §30, 369–81.

42 Bonhoeffer, *Discipleship*, ed. John D. Godsey and Geffrey B. Kelly, Dietrich Bonhoeffer Works 4 (Minneapolis: Fortress, 2003), 107. Such an account of mercy wholly resituates how Christians understand their action in the world, Karl Barth pointed out. From the faith that seeks to follow the merciful working of the Trinitarian God flows "a political attitude, decisively determined by the fact that man is made responsible to all those who are poor and wretched in his eyes, that he is summoned on his part to espouse the cause of those who suffer wrong. Why? Because in them it is manifested to him what he himself is in the sight of God; because the living, gracious, merciful action of God towards him consists in the fact that God Himself in His own righteousness procures right for him, the poor and the wretched; because he and all men stand in the presence of God as those from whom right can be procured only by God Himself." Barth, *Church Dogmatics* 2/1: 387.

43 This phrasing is a gloss on Luther's more technical language of *promeity*. See Hans Joachim Iwand, "Wider den Mißbrauch des *pro me* as methodisches Princip in der Theologie," in *Briefe, Forträge, Predigtmeditationen*, ed. Peter-Paul Sänger (Berlin: Evangelische Verlagsanstalt, 1979), 225–30.

44 John 1:14. "In any other relation between God and creature except that attested in the Bible, the idea of personality in God is perhaps dispensable. But in the relation between the merciful God and the 'miserable' creature (i.e., in need of mercy) it emerges—and here at last it must emerge—that it is indispensable and expresses the truth." Barth, *Church Dogmatics* 2/1: 370.

45 Luther, *Lectures on Genesis*, 1:250.

46 Allowances for divine speaking are more common even in modernity than is often assumed. Leigh Eric Schmidt, *Hearing Things: Religion, Illusion, and the American Enlightenment* (Cambridge, Mass.: Harvard University Press, 2000).

47 The term "touch" gestures toward a range of bodily powers to become aware of what is happening outside the veil of our skin. "The organs of the external senses are open veils or envelopes. Through these doors we see, hear and experiences tastes and fragrances, through these walls, even when they are shut, we touch. The fabric of the pavilion, or the skin of the body, can either open or close, the external sense retaining its integrity. The internal sense is clothed in skin that is either impermeable or pierced with windows and forms its tent or pavilion, its habitat or tabernacle. Touch ensures that what is closed has an opening." Michel Serres, *The Five Senses: A Philosophy of Mingled Bodies (I)*, trans. Margaret Sankey and Peter Cowley (London: Continuum International, 2008), 55. See also David J. Linden, *Touch: The Science of Hand, Heart, and Mind* (London: Viking, 2015).

48 Maurice Merleau-Ponty once famously suggested that "what unites 'tactile sensations' in the hand and links them to visual perceptions of the same hand, and to perceptions of other bodily areas, is a certain style informing my manual gestures and implying in turn a certain style of finger movements, and contributing, in the last resort, to a certain bodily bearing. The body is to be compared, not to a physical object, but rather to a work of art." *The Phenomenology of Perception*, trans. Colin Smith (London: Routledge, 1962), 133. Bodies are like works of art for Merleau-Ponty because they can only be known firsthand, through direct contact, through some sort of touch. If this were not true, all

pictorial art, cinema, dance, novels, and even all figural forms of speech would be unintelligible, resting as they do on kinesthetic knowledge.

It would therefore be infinitely better, D. N. Rodowick suggests, if "the widely held default assumption that meaning, or sense, is *linguistically* constructed were renounced and the more expansive term 'expression' were substituted for 'language.' As even Wittgenstein well understood, human powers of expression are variegated and manifold, and every act of linguistic expression is not only embedded holistically in a variety of signifying actions (gestural, physiognomic, indicative, etc.), but also shot through with nonlinguistic elements that equally have the capacity to intend meaning and to demand interpretation." *Philosophy's Artful Conversation* (Cambridge, Mass.: Harvard University Press, 2015), 62 (the first sentence was a question in the original).

Theological hermeneutics of bodily gesture will have much more in common with modern literary views, with their much finer appreciation for the cultural embedding of the kinesic intelligence of human beings. Guillemette Bolens, *The Style of Gestures: Embodiment and Cognition in Literary Narrative*, foreword by Alain Berthoz (Baltimore: Johns Hopkins University Press, 2012), 1–49. A deep appreciation of the interweaving of gesture and gaze in communication lies at the heart of Kafka's work, and ties him to Benjamin and Foucault. Eleanor Kaufman, *The Delirium of Praise: Bataille, Blanchot, Deleuze, Foucault, Kosowski* (Baltimore: Johns Hopkins University Press, 2001), 73–77. My drawing these embodied and gestural themes into a christological account is a development of recent attempts to approach the theme of disability by way of a robustly theological epistemology of the body. See Creamer, *Disability and Christian Theology*, ch. 3, 53–73.

49 Cf. Mark 1:41; 8:2 and par; Matt 9:36; 18:27; 20:34; Luke 7:13; 10:33. English translations often obscure this Hebraism with the translation "pity."

50 Eiesland, *Disabled God*, 31. I would understand Eiesland's comment as follows (drawing on Bolens, *Style of Gestures*, 2–3, 10): The term "kinetic" refers to visible movements that can be measured by standard measurements, such as the laws of physics. "Kinesthesia" is the capacity to synchronize neurophysical sensations generated by proprioceptive nerves (mainly in the joints) to know the comportment of one's own body. "Kinesis" is the capacity to perceive movements performed by one's self or another person for their attributes—speed, the orientation and angling of limbs, changes in orientation of the head, etc. "Kinesic knowledge" arises as a learned recognition of characteristic body states. Kinesic sensations and knowledge are first-person knowledge, a "knowledge-how" which is only available to the agent, while kinesic information may be communicated in words or other media. Because kinesis is related to interpersonal relations, it can parse movements according to socially constructed conventions, even though gestures exceed culturally imbedded interpretations of them.

There is far more kinesic knowledge shaping all human action than is typically assumed. Taking the depth of this knowledge into account renders thought experiments that presume the "nonresponsive" person fatally implausible. John Swinton, "How Do We Know That Kelly Doesn't Know? Some Reflections on the Experiences of People with Profound Intellectual Disabilities," in *Knowing, Being Known, and the Mystery of God: Essays in Honor of Professor Hans Reinders, Teacher, Friend, and Disciple*, ed. Bill Gaventa and Erik de Jongh (Amsterdam: VU University Press, 2016), 175–82.

51 Descartes' pivotal moment of conceptual clarity about what it means to be a "self" came while dreaming in an overheated room. Bernard Williams, "Introductory Essay," in

René Descartes, *Meditations on First Philosophy with Selections from the Objections and Replies*, rev ed. (Cambridge: Cambridge University Press, 1996), xxii. Serres, in contrast, discovers the bodiliness of his "I" in the desperate straits of a fiery shipwreck. The individual "I" is, he concludes, "something everyone knows, unemotionally and as a matter of fact. You only have to pass through a small opening, a blocked corridor, to swing over a handrail or on a balcony high enough to provoke vertigo, for the body to become more alert. The body knows by itself how to say I. It knows to what extent I am on this side of the bar, and when I am outside. It judges deviations from normal balance, immediately regulates them and knows just how far to go, or not go. Coenesthesia says I by itself. . . . This internal sense proclaims, calls, announces, sometimes howls the I like a wounded animal. This common sense apportions the body better than anything else in the whole world." *Five Senses*, 19.

52 Serres, *Five Senses*, 20.

53 "A human being is created as a body; the Son of God appeared on earth in the body and was raised in the body. In the sacrament the believer receives the Lord Christ in the body, and in the resurrection of the dead will bring about the perfected community of God's spiritual-physical creatures. Therefore, the believer praises the Creator, the Reconciler and the Redeemer, God the Father, Son and Holy Spirit, for the bodily presence of the other Christian." Bonhoeffer, *Life Together and Prayerbook of the Bible*, ed. Geffrey B. Kelly, Dietrich Bonhoeffer Works 5 (Minneapolis: Fortress, 2004), 29.

54 "He who was God's eternal word, but was a fellowman and not an angel or a star, having assumed our *humanity*, our human *nature*, fundamentally reveals—whether we see and hear it or not is another question—each of our fellows to be a question, a promise, a supremely living reminder of *his* humanity. One cannot say that the revelation of Christ is the revelation of the fellowman in general. But one has to say that by this revelation the fellowman—not each person in general but the one that stands over against me—can and must and will become for me a witness, a messenger, a reminder and confirmation of revelation, of Christ himself. We cannot reinterpret God's incarnation in Christ as a general incarnation of God, but we have to take it seriously as an *illumination* by Christ's incarnation of those who confront us. As they confront me, so also the man Jesus Christ confronts me: in the same concealment in which at first and on its own the eye sees only sin, as in all others. . . . We do not exaggerate when we say with Isaiah 53:3 that 'he was the most despised and least esteemed of men.' The original light of God in Christ is not less but more hidden than the reflection of it in the life of the one who confronts me, so that if we neither can nor will see the latter, how can it be true that we have seen the former?" Barth, *Ethics*, 335–36, translation modified.

55 "The suffering and sin and abandonment and peril of these men not merely went to the heart of Jesus but right into His being, into Himself, so that their whole plight was now his own, and as such He saw and suffered it far more keenly than they did. It is not in vain, but with the immediate consequence of practical assistance, that Jesus undergoes this inner movement and makes the cause of this man His own. . . . The verb obviously refers to the action of Jesus, but it tells us that this has an inward source and is the movement of the whole man Jesus." Barth, *Church Dogmatics 3/2: The Doctrine of Creation*, ed. G. W. Bromiley and T. F. Torrance (Edinburgh: T&T Clark, 1960), 211.

56 Genesis 2:7; Bernd Wannenwetsch, "Loving the Limit: Dietrich Bonhoeffer's Hermeneutics of Human Creatureliness and Its Challenge for an Ethics of Medical Care," in *Bonhoeffer and the Biosciences: An Initial Exploration*, ed. Ralf K. Wüstenberg, Stefan

Heuser, and Esther Hornung (Frankfurt am Main: Peter Lang, 2010), 89–108, reference here to 101–4.

57 Ivan Illich, *Rivers North of the Future: The Testament of Ivan Illich as Told to David Cayley* (Toronto: Anansi, 2005), 222, 227; Serres, *Five Senses*, 279–81.

58 "I get upset when people tell me, 'You're doing a good job.' I'm not interested in doing a good job. I'm interested in an ecclesial vision for community and in living in a gospel-based community with people with disabilities. We are brothers and sisters together, and Jesus is calling us from a pyramidal society to become a body." Jean Vanier, in Stanley Hauerwas and Jean Vanier, *Living Gently in a Violent World: The Prophetic Witness of Weakness* (Downers Grove, Ill.: InterVarsity, 2008), 34–35.

59 "If we really see this *one* man Christ standing in our place, then over against *this* man we are really in need, and inevitably the concretion extends further and becomes even more serious. For inevitably we know that others are different, and our own relation to them is different, from what we first stated and believed to be true." Barth, *Ethics*, 334, translation modified.

60 Illich, *Rivers North of the Future*, 207.

61 I am pressing for an ever more fine-grained theological hermeneutics of the body. Jesus' story of the Good Samaritan is only intelligible in a community that has already developed a rich tradition of reading bodily gestures theologically, and which assumes every living person the capacity for gestural intelligence. Only such a view makes sense of observations like this, from Stanley Hauerwas: "Bonnie Rainey . . . was the social service staff on Protective Service. . . . One of our children was a young man named Boyce. Boyce may have been 12 or 13. He was profoundly mentally disabled. He spent most of his life laying in a beanbag. The presumption would be for most people seeing Boyce, they would think 'How sad, it would be better if he had never been born.' But Bonnie could walk in and greet Boyce and she would put her hand on his cheek and there would be the damndest smile you've ever seen in your life! You know, I thought, that's what it means to be human. But you need a Bonnie!'" Brian Brock and Stanley Hauerwas, *Beginnings: Interrogating Hauerwas* (London: Bloomsbury T&T Clark, 2017), 199–200.

The dominance of the post-Enlightenment distinction between fact and value that arose during the period, in which wonders were made to cease, is the main barrier to developing such a hermeneutic today. Charles Darwin assumed this post-Enlightenment bifurcation of fact and imagination when he read all bodily gestures through the lens of emotional projections grounded in neural reactions. Shared with animals, these neutrally programmed reactions are inherited from the long history of animal survival. Augustine's critique of the astronomer surely applies here too: this is a misdirection of the wonder at the complexity and depth of the human being created by God. Charles Darwin, *The Expression of the Emotions in Man and Animals*, 3rd ed., intro. and commentary by Paul Ekman (1889; London: HarperCollins, 1998).

62 "[W]hen we confess God to be merciful it is not even remotely possible to demonstrate this as a logically deducible truth. All that we can do is to acknowledge the actual reality of God. What else can we produce as a proof of this confession except the fact that God has given Himself to be known by us as merciful in the name of Jesus Christ?" Barth, *Church Dogmatics* 2/1: 373.

63 It bears reiteration at the close of this chapter that the grouping of humanity into the categories "able" and "disabled" accompanied the rise to dominance of modern medical and psychological sciences. The language of able and disabled, of deviance and abnormality,

were cultural constructions laboriously erected in the early modern period, most influentially described by Michel Foucault in *Madness and Civilization: A History of Insanity in the Age of Reason*, trans. Richard Howard (New York: Random House, 1965); Foucault, *Abnormal*; Foucault, *Society Must Be Defended: Lectures at the Collège de France, 1975–1976*, trans. David Macey (London: Penguin, 1997), 10–11. Throughout this book I will be in tacit and explicit dialogue with disability scholars drawing on Foucault's work, specifically the texts collected in Tremain, *Foucault and the Government of Disability*. Foucauldian genealogical analyses most often appear in disability theology teamed with liberation approaches. See Mary Jo Iozzio, "Solidarity: Restoring Communion with Those Who are Disabled," *Journal of Religion, Disability and Health* 25, no. 2 (2011): 139–52; Sharon V. Betcher, *Spirit and the Politics of Disablement* (Minneapolis: Fortress, 2007); and Carlson, *Faces of Intellectual Disability*, 17.

64 Pastorally speaking, it is completely understandable that Christians are drawn to this naturalist account of the genetically out-of-the-ordinary child. Aaron D. Cobb expresses this view in its most theologically supple form. "Neither [my wife nor I] believed that there were divine purposes in Sam's inheritance of an extra copy of the eighteenth chromosome. We were not worried about these questions. . . . We understood that God created a world with inherent limitations; we knew that fragility is an essential part of the world God has created. It is a good world, but its goodness is not predicated upon our immunity from difficulty." *Loving Samuel: Suffering, Dependence, and the Calling of Love* (Eugene, Ore.: Cascade, 2014), 31–32. Parts 4 and 5 will suggest that such a hermeneutic of the genetically anomalous new one is overdetermined by a doctrine of creation and its fallen conditions.

But as a parent in a not dissimilar position points out, the *pastoral* implications of this theology are disastrous.

> Essentially, our elders understood Christian faith to be a kind of blanket passive trust in divine goodness, whatever apparently terrible fate God, in His inscrutable sovereign will, has dished out for us. This did not strike us as a credible New Testament understanding of faith, of miracles, of petitionary prayer, or of God's character and sovereignty. But our church was not interested in crunching through these Scriptural and theological matters with us. Such matters were all a bit too threatening, all a bit too unhinging, and had the potential seriously to ruffle the existing status quo within our congregation. . . . In the ten years we were members of this congregation, by and large people whose wheels seriously fell off—marriage breakdown, mental illness, protracted unemployment, etc.—simply fell out of the church when this happened, and the church had no way of holding on to them or meeting their needs. Thinking of the many damaged and suffering people who had faded out of our congregational community in their extremity, we were now aware of a large body of evidence which demonstrated that the power of God was not present in our church to save people whose lives were crashing. And for the already crashed—the ruined people who floated around the edges of church life and whom the church tried to help in some manner—they simply remained ruined and did not find any transformative power of God in our midst. (Tyson, "Wounds of Faith and Medicine," 8–9.)

65 It should by now have become clear that I am intentionally highlighting the architectonic centrality of the doctrine of revelation for a Christian account of disability. A theologically nuanced account of the mediation of this revelation is important in order

that revelation not be misunderstood as radically otherworldly. Revelation is a divine self-presentation that enters and so remakes the creaturely realm. In part 1, I have foregrounded an older Christian usage of the language of "wonder" to draw attention to the breadth of the Christian tradition's thinking about the activity of God's self-revelation. See Colin E. Gunton, *A Brief Theology of Revelation* (Edinburgh: T&T Clark, 1995); and Jean-Luc Marion, *Givenness and Revelation*, trans. Stephen E. Lewis (Oxford: Oxford University Press, 2016).

66 Hans Reinders states this problem succinctly in his *Receiving the Gift of Friendship: Profound Disability, Theological Anthropology, and Ethics* (Grand Rapids: Eerdmans, 2008), 41–44.

67 Andrew Cameron, "A Care for the Aging," Social Issues Executive document (version 31 May 2011), Anglican Diocese of Sydney. In this situation, Christians in liberal societies can still affirm the compassionate acts of nonbelievers while preserving the uniqueness of the Christian understanding, see Ad de Bruijne, "Compassion as a Public Virtue," in Schaeffer, den Hertog, and Paas, *Mercy*, 73–86.

68 "The stammerings of the prophets were legitimated in the only way that, until the twentieth century, a pregnancy could be legitimated—postpartum—because the kid is there." Illich, *Rivers North of the Future*, 176.

69 To challenge the assumption that the Christian tradition is a barrier in the search for a humane modern Christianity, Christians will first need to admit their entanglement in the modern conceit that the task of the thinker is not to uphold and pass on a tradition, but to decontaminate and surpass it. Dupré, *Passage to Modernity*. The discipline of Christian ethics has been especially afflicted with this presumption due to the influence of Ernst Troeltsch in *The Social Teaching of the Christian Churches*, 2 vols., trans. Olive Wyon (Louisville: Westminster John Knox, 1992), which treated ethical claims as data to be analyzed and totally abandoned the task of teaching Christians how to theologically reason about their world *given their location in churches marked by sin*.

The term "tradition" itself is no less hotly contested than the term "disability." A relatively uncontentious definition designates the "Christian tradition" as the body of writings of a specific faith community oriented around authoritative Scriptures. An apparent anachronism lurks in even asking if premodern thinkers thought in terms of an idea (disability) invented in the modern era. One way to respond to this apparent anachronism is typical of methodologically disengaged modern scholarship, which holds that a tradition is intellectually interesting primarily as an artifact of archaic thought. More activist scholarship disputes the irrelevance of past scholarship and proceeds to rummage through the past to find ideas that can be coopted for contemporary moral crusades without allowing them to challenge the presuppositions of those who are appropriating them.

Christian disability theologians have often shied away from such genealogical investigations, given the ahistorical idioms dominant in modern Protestant theology, including American evangelicalism and the fundamentalism from which it sprang. George M. Marsden, *Reforming Fundamentalism: Fuller Seminary and the New Evangelicalism* (Grand Rapids: Eerdmans, 1987), 181–85. Such ahistorical approaches are no less prominent in the strains of liberal theology that were the seedbed of mainstream disability theology.

70 Walter Benjamin, "Excavation and Memory," in *Walter Benjamin: Selected Writings, Vol. 2, Part 2: 1931–1934*, trans. Rodney Livingstone, ed. Michael W. Jennings, Howard Eiland, and Gary Smith (Cambridge, Mass.: Belknap, 1999), 576.

71 Historically distant thinkers are often difficult to understand, morally alien, and regularly appear to hold untenable metaphysical beliefs. Yet confessing themselves members of a single tradition, Christians discipline themselves to gain access to and hand on the insights of previous generations, as the Latin root of the English word "tradition" emphasizes (*traditio*). It is important to recognize that this strife between rival visions of Christianity is constantly alive *within* the thought of individual Christians and is by no means absent from contemporary thinking about disability as well as Christian enactments of the human. The most eloquent voices raised in defense of a Christianity that valued fragile and marginal human life had to make themselves heard in the face of the fears and desire for power that were dominant in the *Christianity* of their times. No golden past beyond conflict exists, and agreement as well as disagreement are integral to the very idea of tradition. See Mark Edwards, *Catholicity and Heresy in the Early Church* (Farnham, U.K.: Ashgate, 2009).

To grapple seriously with the phenomenon of disability makes direct demands on the theological methods deployed. The first is that the theologian seriously entertain the idea that predecessors in the faith might have been more sensitive to "anomalous cases" than moderns typically assume. The work of making sense of the thought of believers of other ages develops transferrable empathetic skills. In becoming comfortable with the vast alienness of the lives of humans in ancient and distant cultures, the Christian is better prepared to attend to human lives in in the present that at first glance seem no less alien. The *moral* challenge levied by the lives of Christians in the patristic era is the almost unimaginable vigor with which they sought out countercultural ways to receive every human life as valuable.

72 Willie James Jennings, "Disfigurations of Christian Identity: Performing Identity as Theological Method," in *Lived Theology: New Perspectives in Method, Style and Pedagogy*, ed. Charles Marsh et al. (Oxford: Oxford University Press, 2017), 67–89, reference to 81.

Chapter 3: Practicing Welcoming in the New World of Genetic Testing

1 Tom Shakespeare, "'Losing the Plot'? Medical and Activist Discourses of Contemporary Genetics and Disability," *Sociology of Health and Illness* 21, no. 5 (1999): 669–88.

2 I have begun this chapter with a public ethical dispute because, as James Mumford points out, "ethics has a stake in description. Some of the most pivotal moral decisions we face, even decisions taken at moments of crisis, hinge upon competing descriptions. How we describe something—some phenomenon in the world, some situation in which we find ourselves involved—makes all the difference as to how we decide we are permitted to act." James Mumford, *Ethics at the Beginning of Life: A Phenomenological Critique* (Oxford: Oxford University Press, 2013), xi.

To elevate a divide over an ethical question (however deep) to a matter of rival ways of being human will seem perverse to some. I am assuming, however, that humanity is not a static form, but something that is enacted. I take this claim to be grounded in the New Testament's description of redemption as conformity to Christ. Every person is made to live in the form of Christ, but all are perfectly capable of performing their lives in ways that destroy their own created susceptibility to live as an image of Christ, and so destroy others. See Michael Banner, "A Doctrine of Human Being," in *The Doctrine of God and Theological Ethics*, ed. Alan Torrance and Michael Banner (London: T&T

Clark International, 2006), 146; and Tim Ingold, *The Life of Lines* (New York: Routledge, 2015), ch. 22, "To Human Is a Verb."

3 Bruno Latour, *Reassembling the Social: An Introduction to Actor, Network Theory* (Oxford: Oxford University Press, 2005); George Grant, *Technology and Empire* (Concord, Ontario: Anansi, 1969), 137.

4 Philip Bobbit, *Shield of Achilles: War, Peace, and the Course of History* (London: Penguin, 2003), 228–34.

5 Michel Foucault, *Discipline and Punish: The Birth of the Prison*, trans. Alan Sheridan (New York: Vintage Books, 1995).

6 Anne Waldschmidt, "Who Is Normal? Who Is Deviant? 'Normality' and 'Risk' in Genetic Diagnostics and Counselling," in Tremain, *Foucault and the Government of Disability*, 192.

7 "If the function of law in the nation-state is process-oriented, churning out impartial rules and regulations to promote desired behaviour, the market-state pursues its objectives by incentive structures and sometimes draconian penalties, not so much to assure that the right thing is done as to prevent the social instability that threatens material well-being." Bobbit, *Shield of Achilles*, 229. See also Anne Waldschmidt, "Who Is Normal? Who Is Deviant?" 191–207. Waldschmidt's account of normalistic norms is an elaboration of Jürgen Link's work in *Versuch über den Normalismus: Wie Normalität produciert wird* (Opladen, Germany: Westdeutscher Verlag, 1996). Ironically, the very business-people who invented the technologies on which biopolitical governance is based may be attempting to *increase* the activity in the long tail (the less numerous actions at both ends of a bell curve)—so disrupting the social cohesion the normalistic norm promised political leaders. Chris Anderson, *The Long Tail: Why the Future of Business is Selling Less of More* (New York: Hyperion, 2008).

8 Waldschmidt, "Who Is Normal? Who Is Deviant?" 195.

9 Mianna Meskus, "Personalized Ethics: The Emergence and the Effects in Prenatal Testing," *Biosciences* 7, no. 4 (2012): 373–92; Gareth M. Thomas and Barbara Katz Rothman, "Keeping the Backdoor to Eugenics Ajar? Disability and the Future of Prenatal Screening," *American Medical Association Journal of Ethics* 18, no. 4 (2016): 406–15.

10 Barbara Katz Rothman describes a mother coming to know her unborn child without prenatal testing as a work of family making even when the outcome is stillbirth or handicap. Inhabiting a pregnancy in this more traditional manner jars with commonly held understandings of pregnancy among hospital obstetricians, for whom the central concern is producing a live healthy child. "Spoiling the Pregnancy: Prenatal Diagnosis in the Netherlands," in *Birth by Design: Pregnancy, Maternity Care, and Midwifery in North America and Europe*, ed. Raymond De Vries, Cecilia Benoit, Edwin van Teijlingen, and Sirpa Wrede (New York: Routledge, 2001), 180–98.

11 In this case the doctor's nervousness sprang from the nonnegotiability of the legal limit for legal abortion in Germany that can only be breached in exceptional circumstances. Despite the much greater permissibility of later-term abortions in the U.K., Thomas documents the cultural processes in antenatal medical contexts which suggest this interchange is closer to the rule than an exception. Gareth M. Thomas, *Down Syndrome Screening and Reproductive Politics: Care, Choice, and Disability in the Prenatal Clinic* (Abingdon, U.K.: Routledge, 2017), 155.

12 Midwives are routinely sidelined in discussions of the ethics of prenatal testing, precisely because of their concern with fostering the integrity of the *woman's* experience of pregnancy. Rothman, "Spoiling the Pregnancy," 193–97.

13 Wondering at a child who is later discovered to face intellectual or physical challenges yields a markedly different experience from the "spoiling of a pregnancy" by prenatal testing. Once prenatal testing is introduced, a mother must first encounter a "defective" child who will only subsequently be discovered as a unique personality. Rothman highlights the importance of this attachment period in the formation of families using terms very like Rosenzweig's account of the role of the heart of wonder (the theme of ch. 7). Rothman, "Spoiling the Pregnancy," 189–91.

14 With great theological insight Søren Kierkegaard points out that this is an all too human thought, and just so, is sinful. Søren Kierkegaard, *Fear and Trembling, Repetition*, ed. and trans. Howard Hong and Edna Hong (Princeton: Princeton University Press, 1983), 74. Kierkegaard presses his reader squarely to face the fragility of supposedly disinterested parental love, which is prone, as is all human love, to falling under the "aesthetic illusion of magnanimity." Kierkegaard, *Fear and Trembling*, 93. See Amy Laura Hall, *Kierkegaard and the Treachery of Love* (Cambridge: Cambridge University Press, 2002), 71.

15 This interchange is by no means out of the ordinary in the U.K., as documented by Thomas, *Down Syndrome Screening and Reproductive Politics*, 83–86.

16 Those who have found themselves in the position of being advised to abort a genetically anomalous new one often narrate it in terms of a nearly crushing weight of grief accompanied by a drastic slowing of time. A painful sense of not having the time to become reconciled to what cannot be controlled grinds against the frustration of feeling pressured to make the time-sensitive decision to abort that rests on medical judgments that seem far beyond a parent's medical competence. Cobb, *Loving Samuel*, 14, 26–27.

17 Instinctive use of new technologies is an often-repeated pattern. The rise of ultrasound machines was associated with cutting-edge science, medical progress, and the culturally embedded assumption that newer and better technologies produced visual images. Such culturally embedded expectations drove the proliferation of ultrasound technology, even though doctors often knew that the information gleaned was not substantively different from what older manual examinations could supply. As one obstetrician observed during the period of transition to universal ultrasound screening, "there are few things my hands can't find that the ultrasound can. My hands are my eyes . . . but patients think it's more modern to use a machine. They themselves wouldn't trust just a manual exam. The doctor needs to show that he's modern too. That is, some will do an exam with a machine just because a woman will trust him more if he does." Mitchell and Georges, "Cross-Cultural Cyborgs," 386.

18 The doctor-patient power dynamics playing out in this clash are poignantly captured by Tyson.

> [The neonatologist] Dr. Brown was very concerned that we should not prolong Lucy's suffering, so she seemed to assume that a detached (clinical) and realistic (hopeless) outlook for Lucy was more humane and caring than our attached (nonmedical) and (hopeful) unrealistic outlook. . . . If we accepted her outlook, then we were all on the same page; Lucy would get the best palliative care, and we would be being both reasonable and "normal." I was genuinely respectful and appreciative of her medical expertise, but this reduction of Lucy's care to sit within medical determinism, and our sense that Dr. Brown was on a maternal

mission to help us get to where she was at, was received by us as deeply patronizing, profoundly ignorant of our beliefs and values, and—despite the smiles and kind tones—very forceful. In fact, we experienced her condescending assertiveness against our most basic belief commitments as a type of doctrinal violence, foisted onto us from a position of institutional and professional authority with the inbuilt assumed moral and intellectual superiority appropriate to her station. (Tyson, "Wounds of Faith and Medicine," 340.)

19 As far as scientists and paleontologists can tell, Down syndrome has always been part of human reproduction, a genetic translocation shared with some other mammals. CIBA Foundation Symposium 40, *Embryogenesis in Mammals* (Amsterdam: Elsevier, 1976).

20 The ethical implications of this standard feature of modern liberal democracies is insightfully examined by Simplican, *Capacity Contract*, ch. 3.

21 In the case of children, parents bear the burden of proving incapacity (Department for Work and Pensions, Disability and Carers Service, *Disability Living Allowance*). Our case was complicated by our citizenship status in Scotland. We were only eligible to receive some important disability benefits (including a social worker, the gatekeeper to most other benefits) once we were citizens and the extent of Adam's disabilities had been medically documented. This happened when he was eight years of age and in the middle of an entirely different medical crisis.

22 Michael Bérubé relates a similar experience in, *Life as We Know It: A Father, a Family, and an Exceptional Child* (New York: Pantheon Books, 1996), 5.

23 The Greek is *stoicheia*. See Col 2:8. Galatians 4 discusses the theme at some length, with *stoicheia* appearing in verse 3. These are the powers Christ has defeated, but not yet finally vanquished—and include alienated human powers of creativity and insight. Karl Barth, *Church Dogmatics* 4/4: *The Christian Life*, or *Lecture Fragments*, ed. and trans. Geoffrey W. Bromiley (Edinburgh: T&T Clark, 1981), 213–19.

24 "Because of the example of Christ, we also believe that love and fear are incompatible, and that love does not make decisions premised on a cost-to-benefit analysis that weights pleasure against suffering, or social acceptance against shame (1 John and Heb. 12:2). This is why, though Annette and I have a one in four probability of conceiving a child with [a terminal wasting disease], we did not stop having children after Daniel was born. This Christian logic of setting intrinsic values as primary in a decision-making process seems irrational, possibly indulgent, probably cruel, and certainly reckless and costly by the dominant naturalistic logic of our larger secular culture, where physical securities are considered primary and values and beliefs are considered secondary add-ons." Tyson, "Wounds of Faith and Medicine," 354n21.

25 "We would not have withheld our daughter from the great wonders of medical science, or from the genuine, deeply touching, often astonishingly beautiful practical care of medical professionals. But the cost for this care that we paid as Christians was the wound of medicine: our deepest hopes and convictions somewhat tolerated or politely overlooked, and our exteriority to the truths of modern scientific knowledge and sensible reality viewed with patronizing forbearance." Tyson, "Wounds of Faith and Medicine," 343.

26 Luther, "Exposition of Psalm 127, for the Christians at Riga in Livonia," *Christian in Society II*, ed. Walther Brandt, Luther's Works 45 (St. Louis: Concordia, 1968), 326. The insight is drawn from a wide range of biblical texts. Augustine makes the point by quoting 1 Cor 3:7 in *City of God* 22.24.

27 Luther makes the point elsewhere in a comment on the prayer of thankfulness for healing (through medical treatment) of Hezekiah in Isa 38:10-20: "For you heard in the song above that all things are kept and cared for by the Word. Then the ungodly cry: 'If the word does everything and provides nourishment for everything, we do not want to eat or take medicine.' For them he takes up this example. As for you, make use of means. Do not rely on them but use them, since God has created them. If they do not help, commit the matter to God. Do not say: 'Doctor, if this will not help this time, I refuse to take it anymore.' Yes, you want to have your own way! So we all go beyond the proper use of means by clinging to them. . . . Others despise works altogether, so does this song ascribe the power to the Word and not to the medicine. Yet it does not forbid that we use them, but the prophet's example supports their use, since he poultices the wound with a cake of figs." Luther, *Lectures on Isaiah: Chapters 1–39*, ed. Jaroslav Pelikan, Luther's Works 16 (St. Louis: Concordia, 1969), 344. On the contemporary implications of Luther's view of medicine see Wannenwetsch, "Loving the Limit."

28 "Clinical risk techniques . . . breach the distinction between disciplinary governance that acts on individual bodies and security governance that acts on populations." Lorna Weir, "Recent Developments in the Government of Pregnancy," *Economy and Society* 25 (1996): 372–92, quotation from 382. Cited in Waldschmidt, "Who Is Normal? Who Is Deviant?" 198.

29 Hannah Arendt, *The Human Condition* (Chicago: University of Chicago Press, 1958), ch. 6.

30 Theology and the empirical sciences will give different but mutually illuminating answers to the question of how appropriately to care for human bodies. For a more detailed discussion of the *theological* expectation that these different sorts of inquiry will meet, see Brian Brock, Walter Doerfler, and Hans Ulrich, "Genetics, Conversation and Conversion: A Discourse at the Interface of Molecular Biology and Christian Ethics," in Swinton and Brock, *Theology, Disability and the New Genetics*.

31 Mary Jo Iozzio, "Genetic Anomaly or Genetic Diversity: Thinking in the Key of Disability on the Human Genome," *Theological Studies* 66 (2005): 862–81.

32 Bonhoeffer, *Ethics*, 194.

33 Stanley Hauerwas, *Performing the Faith: Bonhoeffer and the Practice of Nonviolence* (Grand Rapids: Brazos, 2004), 230.

34 Barth, *Church Dogmatics* 3/1: *The Doctrine of Creation*, ed. G. W. Bromiley and T. F. Torrance (Edinburgh: T&T Clark, 1958), 423–24.

35 Chris Kaposy, *Choosing Down Syndrome: Ethics and New Prenatal Testing Technologies* (Cambridge, Mass.: MIT Press, 2018).

36 Bookstores are filled with stories in which "parents to be" conceive with the aim of producing a perfect child, and so narrate their story with their handicapped child in terms of how difficult it was to adjust to the letdown of a child with disabilities. Danny Mardell, *Danny's Challenge: The True Story of a Father Learning to Love His Son*, ed. Sally Weal (London: Short Books, 2005); and Mitchell Zuckoff, *Choosing Naia: A Family's Journey* (Boston: Beacon, 2002) are sobering examples of such a parental narrative which, at different levels of intellectualization, both portray the struggle to justify and respond to parenting a "different" child experienced in many ways as a burden. There are signs of an alternative and more positive cultural narrative emerging, such as the 2017 feature-length documentary directed by Rachel Dretzin, *Far from the Tree*.

Chapter 4: Prenatal Testing as Anti-Doxology

1 For an early but broad, sensitive, and prescient survey of modern screening modes and developmental trajectories focusing on the U.K. but with the developed world in view see Martin Richards, "Annotation: Genetic Research, Family Life, and Clinical Practice," *Journal of Child Psychology* 39, no. 3 (1998): 291–305. It is important to remember that "by and large, testing (or screening) is only available for the Mendelian single gene disorders or for chromosomal disorders. From the perspective of clinical psychology or psychiatry such disorders are the rarities and together only make up a very small proportion of the clinical burden. . . . For Mendelian disorders of all kinds genetic testing is likely to become more efficient and cheaper so that mutations at many loci may be looked for simultaneously. This means there is likely to be pressure to increase the extent of screening and testing" (294).

In practice, screening rates are rising across the developed world, though termination rates of conceptions found to be genetically anomalous have varied over the thirty years of widespread screening. A survey of these rates as of 2016 can be found in Thomas, *Down Syndrome Screening and Reproductive Politics*, 1–2. Iceland was an early adopter and universally administers a noninvasive genetic test. The result is a nearly 100 percent abortion rate for pregnancies found positive for Down syndrome. Denmark is right behind them at 98 percent, France at 77 percent, and the United States at 67 percent. Julian Quinones and Arijeta Lajka, "'What Kind of Society Do You Want to Live In?': Inside the Country Where Down syndrome Is Disappearing," *CBS News*, August 14, 2017. Even twenty years at the U.S. rate has some disturbing implications. In the United States alone, if we assume an average rate of 90 percent of children conceived with Down syndrome have been aborted, we are talking about one million missing people—leaving aside all those aborted after misdiagnosis. Simplican, *Capacity Contract*, 10. A 2016 BBC documentary hosted by Sally Phillips, *A World Without Down's Syndrome*, investigated the implications of universal screening for Down syndrome. The immediate backlash it ignited indicates the moral and political reasons why so many parties are keen that screening policy not be opened to public debate. Tracy McVeigh, "Sally Phillips's Film on Down's Is 'Unhelpful' for Families, Warns Antenatal Specialist," *The Guardian*, October 2, 2016.

2 Commenting on the situation in the UK, Gareth Thomas notes that

> similar to Down's syndrome screening at present—a practice which . . . has been entirely routinized in prenatal care—the controversies and complications of [noninvasive prenatal testing, a noninvasive blood test of a new one's genes] have also, mostly, been muffled . . . . we can draw a comparison with the public dialogues organised by the Human Fertilization and Embryology Authority on mitochondrial transfer. The public dialogues were arranged to assemble views on emerging techniques, specifically on their social and ethical dimensions, designed to prevent parents from passing on genetically inherited mitochondrial diseases to their children. Cutting edge reproductive technologies . . . are often extensively debated by the media yet no such debates were, or have since been organised regarding [noninvasive prenatal testing]. The speed with which a technique spreads does not necessarily reveal its social acceptability, thus masking possible controversial social values embedded within it. The routinization of Down's syndrome screening in many countries across the world, the UK included, has ensured that [noninvasive prenatal testing] (like its predecessor) has not been subjected to public scrutiny, other than within the

> campaigns of the disability rights groups . . . (Thomas, *Down Syndrome Screening and Reproductive Politics*, 184–85.)

3 Social research suggests that this is already well underway. See Thomas, *Down Syndrome Screening and Reproductive Politics*, 184–85.

4 Thomas, *Down Syndrome Screening and Reproductive Politics*, 29–33.

5 David Patterson and Alberto C. S. Costa, "History of Genetic Disease: Down Syndrome and Genetics—a Case of Linked Histories," *Nature Reviews Genetics* 6 (2005): 137–47.

6 Thomas, *Down Syndrome Screening and Reproductive Politics*, ch. 2.

7 Thomas, *Down Syndrome Screening and Reproductive Politics*, 162. Bruno Latour highlighted the political implications of the designation "incompatible with life." Recent French history presents cases in which disability groups mounted political pressure to force genetics researchers to investigate their condition. They resisted the assumption that their genetic condition should be taken as an unalterable fate.

> Thus, for [the French Association for the Fight against Muscular Dystrophy], gene action is a synonym for emancipation; the parents still remember the time when doctors, in the name of science, discouraged them from doing anything about their dreadful prognosis: "your child is condemned to certain death; there is nothing you can do; there is nothing we can do." Through the patients' action, doctors have been forced to learn a different science of handicap, and French molecular biologists, very reluctantly at first, have entered into an industrial-scale crash research program they would never have carried out without [the French Muscular Dystrophy Association] money and pressure.
>
> (Remember that, for the [the French Muscular Dystrophy Association], emancipation was gaining the right to identify genes and they managed to force surgeons, for instance, to learn how to practice tracheotomy, instead of letting their children die a 'natural' suffocating death.) . . . In this new fight . . . science is not innately always on the side of good; more specifically, each discipline, each scientist, each piece of science has to make a choice; to define which side of such body politics it is taking. (Bruno Latour, "Body, Cyborgs and the Politics of Incarnation," in *The Body*, ed. Sean T. Sweeney and Ian Hodder [Cambridge: Cambridge University Press, 2002], 127–41, quotations from 133 and 136, parenthetical sections original.)

8 Thomas, *Down Syndrome Screening and Reproductive Politics*, 118–21, 135.

9 Shakespeare, "'Losing the Plot'?" 669–88.

10 Dolmage, *Disability Rhetoric*, 39, 55.

11 Butler, *Precarious Life*, 26.

12 Mitchell and Georges, "Cross-Cultural Cyborgs," 383–84.

13 The most influential academic moral defense of abortion appeared at the watershed moment in the rise of prenatal testing regimes and depicted the question as a balancing of the rights of mother against the rights of the new one. Judith Jarvis Thomson, "A Defense of Abortion," *Philosophy and Public Affairs* 1, no. 1 (1971): 47–66.

14 Wolf Krötke, *Sin and Nothingness in the Theology of Karl Barth: With a New Foreword by the Author*, ed. and trans. Philip Ziegler and Christina-Maria Bammel, Studies in Reformed Theology and History (Princeton: Princeton Theological Seminary, 2005), x–xi.

15 Christian Führer, *Und wir sind dabei gewesen: Die Revolution, die aus der Kirche kam* (Berlin: Ullstein, 2009).

16 "Under 'singing,'" says Luther, "I include not only making melody or shouting but also every sermon or public confession by which God's work, counsel, grace, help, comfort, victory, and salvation are glorified before the world . . . . As [Ps 118:14] puts it: 'The Lord is my Strength and my Song; He has become my Salvation.'" Luther, "Psalm 118," in *Selected Psalms III*, ed. Jaroslav Pelikan, Luther's Works 14 (St. Louis: Concordia, 1968), 81.

17 Luther, "Treatise on Good Works," in *The Christian Society I*, ed. Helmut T. Lehmann and Lewis W. Spitz, Luther's Works 34 (St. Louis: Concordia, 1960), 40.

18 Luther, "Treatise on Good Works," 44, 46.

19 The language of "theology of testimony," "politics of praise," and "publicizing the miracle" are from Randi Rashkover, who uses it to describe the Jewish theology of Rosenzweig and the Christian theology of Barth on which my own work draws. "The God of revelation is the God whose being it is to act, and specifically to act lovingly toward humanity. Consequently, testimony to this reality must be practical in nature. . . . the key to Judaism's and Christianity's productive participation in the political arena rests in their ability to engage in a covenantal life of testimony or praise of God." Randi Rashkover, *Revelation and Theopolitics: Barth, Rosenzweig, and the Politics of Praise* (London: T&T Clark, 2005), 5–6.

20 Luther, "Treatise on Good Works," 61. I have developed this theme in more detail in my *Singing the Ethos of God: On the Place of Christian Ethics in Scripture* (Grand Rapids: Eerdmans, 2007), ch. 7.

21 Luther, "Admonition Concerning the Sacrament of the Body and Blood of our Lord," in *Word and Sacrament IV*, ed. Helmut T. Lehmann and Martin E. Lehmann, Luther's Works 38 (St. Louis: Concordia, 1976); "Treatise on Good Works," 108–9.

22 Luther, "Admonition Concerning the Sacrament of the Body and Blood of our Lord," 133.

23 Luther, "Admonition Concerning the Sacrament of the Body and Blood of our Lord," 133.

24 Judith Butler, *Frames of War: When Is Life Grievable?* (London: Verso, 2010), 20.

25 Reynolds, *Vulnerable Communion*, 58.

26 Butler, *Precarious Life*, 27, 43. In a North American context already prone to (over) emphasizing individual autonomy, the figuring of the new one in the womb as an autonomous agent has been accelerated by the public profile of abortion debates. Mitchell and Georges, "Cross-Cultural Cyborgs," 373–401.

27 "Although the term *human* is commonly used or understood as a straightforward descriptive term (that is, membership in the species human), *person* is a technical, philosophical, and normative term that refers to moral status and is not limited in its ascription to only one human, or even organic, life. It is a serious error . . . to assume that one's factual humanness will entail that one is recognized as normatively human—that is, as a person, with the entitlements and protections that the status 'person' confers. Yet . . . liberalist theorizing makes this error regularly, conflating fact with normative status and ignoring how 'socially recognized personhood' is ascribed independent of biological humanity." Ashley Taylor, "Expressions of 'Lives Worth Living' and Their Foreclosure through Philosophical Theorizing on Moral Status and Intellectual Disability," in Tremain, *Foucault and the Government of Disability*, 382. See

also John Swinton, "What's in a Name? Why People with Dementia Might Be Better Off without the Language of Personhood," *International Journal of Practical Theology* 18, no. 2 (2014): 1–14.

28 It should not be forgotten that only twenty-five years ago it was common practice in the Western world to bring about the death of infants with learning disabilities, particularly if the personal situations of the parents in question were "unfavorable." Janet Read and Luke Clements, "Demonstrably Awful: The Right to Life and the Selective Non-treatment of Disabled Babies and Young Children," in Clements and Read, *Disabled People and the Right to Life*, 148–75. Furthermore, in Western medical settings, disability itself has often been taken to be sufficient grounds to classify live-born infants as still-births or nonviable. Einarsdóttir, "Classification of Newborn Children," 253–61. To this day otherwise viable children with conditions such as Trisomy 18 are denied routine life-saving operations on the grounds that operating on children with such conditions is "not usual clinical practice." Joanne Warnock, "Fyvie Parents' Joy at Health Board's U-Turn on Willow's Life-Saving Operation," *Aberdeen Press and Journal*, May 8, 2018, 3.

29 Butler, *Precarious Life*, 22, 32.

30 Butler, *Precarious Life*, 34–35. Butler's own example is a rebuffed attempt to place an obituary in the *San Francisco Chronicle* for two Palestinian families killed by an Israeli military operation. If Socrates is granted the title of the founder of philosophy, then philosophy itself was born from the challenging of the boundaries of the publicly speakable.

31 Mumford, *Ethics at the Beginning of Life*, 193.

32 Ronald Dworkin, *Life's Dominion: An Argument about Abortion and Euthanasia* (London: HarperCollins, 1993), 15.

33 Thomas, *Down Syndrome Screening and Reproductive Politics*, 144.

34 Iozzio, "Genetic Anomaly or Genetic Diversity," 878.

35 Baroness Mary Warnock has been one of the most outspoken defenders of "medical advance" against disability activists and targets her response at social models of disability.

> For there is all the difference in the world between being profoundly deaf, say, and becoming part of the deaf world, and, in contrast, suffering from a devastating disease that entails a painful, miserable and short life. I cannot accept that there is at work here . . . a kind of latent discrimination against those who have been born with or have acquired a disability. If medicine, with the help of the new genetic understanding we are acquiring, can either prevent children from being born with genetic diseases or create genetically engineered drugs to treat those not at present capable of treatment, then I cannot see this as other than a benign advance in medicine, just as the discovery of insulin as a treatment for diabetes was. We should not allow ourselves to be browbeaten by the lobby of the existing disabled into either denying that they have disabilities or giving up the search for a remedy for future generations of children. (Mary Warnock, "The Bioethics of Reproduction: Have the Problems Changed?" in Sweeney and Hodder, *The Body*, 39–56, quotation from 49–50.)

36 See Reinders, *Future of the Disabled in Liberal Society*, ch. 4; and "Life's Goodness: On Disability, Genetics, and 'Choice,'" in Swinton and Brock, *Theology, Disability and the New Genetics*, 29–43.

37 Rayna Rapp, *Testing Women, Testing the Fetus: The Social Impact of Amniocentesis in America* (New York: Routledge, 2000), chs. 3, 6.

38 Ashley Taylor, "Expressions of 'Life Worth Living,'" 385.

39 Metasurveys of the limited empirical evidence suggests that, globally, people with disabilities experience 50–75 percent higher rates of domestic abuse (both physical and sexual) as well as disablist hate crime while having far lower access to social support networks. Christopher Mikton and Tom Shakespeare, "Introduction to Special Issue on Violence against People with Disability," *Journal of Interpersonal Violence* 29, no. 17 (2014): 3055–62; Karen Hughes, Mark A. Bellis, Lisa Jones, Sara Wood, Geoff Bates, Lindsay Eckley, Ellie McCoy, Christopher Mikton, Tom Shakespeare, and Alana Officer, "Prevalence and Risk of Violence against Adults with Disabilities: A Systematic Review and Meta-analysis of Observational Studies," *The Lancet* 379 (2012): 1621–29.

Journalists calculate that "people with disabilities are more than twice as likely to be the victims of violent crimes as those without disabilities, according to a [U.S.] Justice Department report based on Census Bureau surveys. And people with mental disabilities are the most likely to be victimized." Mitch Smith and Richard Pérez-Penajan, "Beating of a Disabled Teenager Highlights a Crime That's Often Unseen," *New York Times*, January 6, 2017, A8. This violence by individuals is often paralleled by disdainful treatment by service providers across the developed world. Angelique Chrisafis, "We're Fifty Years Behind on This: Anger Grows over Treatment of Autistic Children in France," *The Guardian*, February 8, 2018, 33.

40 Banner, *Ethics of Everyday Life*, 23–29.

41 These issues are sensitively discussed in Mitchell and Georges, "Cross-Cultural Cyborgs."

42 Mumford, *Ethics at the Beginning of Life*, 115.

43 Leisa Whitaker, quoted in Melinda Tankard Reist, *Defiant Birth: Women Who Resist Medical Eugenics* (North Melbourne: Spinifex, 2006), 214. This volume collects nineteen first-person narratives by women who experienced medicalized pre- and postnatal care as antagonistic to the continuation of their pregnancies. See also the narrative of Phillip Burcham, "War Against the Weak: Genetic Counselling and the New Eugenics," *ABC Religion and Ethics*, November 28, 2016.

44 There are two notable variations in practice and nomenclature for this practice. North Americans and Europeans typically label the technology ultrasound (the term "ultrasound" refers to the technology used to produce an image, the sonogram being the image produced). In Britain the more common nomenclature is sonography. In Britain this work is typically conceived as routine "hands-off work" and delegated to technicians (except in cases expected to be complicated), while in North America it is seen as the domain of the expert and is usually staffed by doctors trained in genetics. Thomas, *Down Syndrome Screening and Reproductive Politics*, ch. 3. Mara Buchbinder, "Down's Syndrome Screening and Reproductive Politics: Care, Choice, and Disability in the Prenatal Clinic," *New Genetics and Society* (2017): 47, DOI: 10.1080/14636778.2017.1368375.

45 The incompleteness of this knowledge has direct implications for how the mother perceives the shape and meaning of her pregnancy. Mumford, *Ethics at the Beginning of Life*, ch. 1.

46 "Visualizations are presented on a monitor quite similar to the ubiquitous television screen, and their impact is instantaneous. They hold a powerful place in women's narratives, and are recalled far more vividly than the 'caterpillar stick figures' of karyotype photographs. In the cases where spina bifida, anencephaly, or life-threatening heart, lung, and kidney problems were visualised, women from diverse sociocultural backgrounds . . . told virtually the same story: 'Pretty soon, it was a regular doctors'

convention in there. At some point, I must have had eight doctors muttering over that screen. I said to myself, my God, something is terribly wrong here, because they keep calling other people to come in and take a look. I know they wasted their opinions. But they wouldn't say anything to me.'" Rapp, *Testing Women, Testing the Fetus*, 221.

On cyborgs as a technically mediated human body see Latour, "Body, Cyborgs and the Politics of Incarnation," 127–41.

47 "Early ultrasounds had indicated serious concerns; we had come to learn how best to prepare for his arrival. Our slim hopes were assaulted by the silence that crept into the room as she [the sonographer] surveyed for signs of defects, for indicators of all the ways in which our son was already broken. Initially friendly and open, she stopped inviting questions about what she perceived; she did stop to point out his severely clubbed feet. And then she was done. With a sigh, she made her announcement. Trisomy 18. Lethal. Inevitable. Death. Would we terminate?" Cobb, *Loving Samuel*, 11.

48 Thomas, *Down Syndrome Screening and Reproductive Politics*, 98–100, 143.

49 For an anthropological account of the "cyborgification" of ultrasound and the "one-two punch" see Mitchell and Georges, "Cross-Cultural Cyborgs," 375–83.

50 Rapp, *Testing Women, Testing the Fetus*, 192.

51 Rapp, *Testing Women, Testing the Fetus*, 208; Shakespeare, "'Losing the Plot'?" 669–88.

52 Rapp, *Testing Women, Testing the Fetus*, 241.

53 This role is dominant in the American context but largely absent from British practice. Buchbinder, "Down's Syndrome Screening and Reproductive Politics."

54 As with sonographers, the vast majority of genetic counselors (95 percent) are female. Rapp, *Testing Women, Testing the Fetus*, 56–57; Sonja Eubanks Higgins, Patricia McCarthy Veach, Ian M. McFarlane, L. DiAnne Borders, Bonnie LeRoy, Nancy Callanan, "Genetic Counselling Supervisor Competencies: Results of a Delphi Study," *Journal of Genetic Counselling*, 22 (2013): 39–57. The skewing of this domain toward women undoubtedly reflects the cultural location of women in Western societies as the "genetic housekeepers of kinship." Richards, "Annotation," 296–97. This gender imbalance does have significant practical and moral implications, sensitively discussed by Carlson, *Faces of Intellectual Disability*, ch. 2 and p. 175.

55 Abby Lippman and Benjamin S. Wilfond, "Twice-Told Tales: Stories about Genetic Disorders," *American Journal of Human Genetics* 51 (1992): 936–37.

56 Rapp, *Testing Women, Testing the Fetus*, 56–57.

57 Waldschmidt, "Who Is Normal? Who Is Deviant?" 198.

58 Rapp, *Testing Women, Testing the Fetus*, 70.

59 Rapp, *Testing Women, Testing the Fetus*, 68.

60 The language of risk may well reveal the hidden engine of the modern problem of disability, tied up as that term has come to be with the need to correct supposedly anomalous human bodies. "The revolutionary idea that defines the boundary between modern times and the past is the mastery of risk: The notion that the future is more than a whim of the gods and that men and women are not passive before nature. Until human beings discovered a way across that boundary, the future was a mirror of the past or the murky domain of oracles and soothsayers who held a monopoly over knowledge of anticipated events." Peter L. Bernstein, *Against the Gods: The Remarkable Story of Risk* (New York: John Wiley & Sons, 1998), 1.

Perhaps this was inevitable, since, as Niklas Luhmann has pointed out, the rationalist presumption grounding this way of seeing the world is blind to its own blindness.

Such techniques are attempts to immunize decision making from failure. Early modern thinkers aspired to produce security as an objective state, displacing the medieval definition of security as the subject's sense of being at peace. "It is as if, in the face of an increasingly uncertain future, a secure basis for the making of decisions now had to be found. All this meant a vast expansion in the scope and pretentions of capability, and the old cosmological limitations. The constants of being and the secrets of Nature were replaced by distinctions falling within the domain of rational calculation. And this has determined the understanding of risk to this day." Niklas Luhmann, *Risk: A Sociological Theory*, trans. Rhodes Barrett (Berlin: Walter de Gruyter, 1993), 13.

The story of prenatal testing has highlighted that the belief in the power of rationality to control accidents springs directly from a psychology of fear, culturally elaborated. "This life of ours has proved to be different from the kind of life which the sages of the Enlightenment and their heirs and disciples envisaged and set out to design [in the hope] that the feat of taming fears and bridling the menaces that caused them would be a one-off affair. In [late modernity], however, the struggle against fears has turned out to be a lifelong task, while fear-triggering dangers, even when none of them is suspected to be *intractable*, have come to be believed to be permanent, *undetachable* companions of human life. . . . A *whole life* is now a long and probably unwinnable struggle against the potentially incapacitating impact of our fears, and against the genuine or putative dangers that make us fearful." Zygmunt Bauman, *Liquid Fear* (Cambridge: Polity, 2006), 7–8.

Sociologists have pointed out that this combination of blindness to the limits of human control and the globalization of fear-driven behaviors creates all sorts of paradoxical behaviors, such as fearing flying while undertaking the far more dangerous daily commute by car without thinking about it. Dan Gardiner, *Risk: The Science and Politics of Fear* (London: Virgin Books, 2008). As the quotation from Bernstein at the beginning of this note highlighted, the pitting of modernity and its techniques for attempting to control risk against religious beliefs presented as superstitious hocus pocus is typical modern antireligious polemic. But the use of this polemic in recent decades to justify and disseminate risk-laden market tools is an invitation to think again. In a society that lives with a pervasive fear of chance and the specter of loss, the practices of controlling chance have increasingly occupied the social function of ancient divination rituals. Joshua Ramey, *Politics of Divination: Neoliberal Endgame and the Religion of Contingency* (London: Rowan & Littlefield, 2016).

It is now clearer why theology must insist that the alternative to controlling risk can only be faith. "If the world is not believed in as that which is promised, then it will be experienced as a 'fearful natural realm,' as a relentlessly necessary, oppressive law, which says: you must squeeze some sense out of this chaos, this fearful natural realm in all its uncertainty; you have to be in charge of making sense in this and out of this chaotic world; you yourself have to establish its order!" Oswald Bayer, *Martin Luther's Theology: A Contemporary Interpretation*, trans. Thomas H. Trapp (Grand Rapids: Eerdmans, 2008), 102.

61 Thomas, *Down Syndrome Screening and Reproductive Politics*, 130.

62 Rapp, *Testing Women, Testing the Fetus*, 59. More recent empirical research does not encourage optimism that this training deficit has been rectified. Eubanks Higgins, et al., "Genetic Counselling Supervisor Competencies."

63 Barbara Katz Rothman, *The Tentative Pregnancy: Prenatal Diagnosis and the Future of Motherhood* (New York: Penguin Books, 1987), 256; Rapp, *Testing Women, Testing the Fetus*, 263.

64 Both modern notions of risk and normalcy rest on rationalist presumptions, cashed out through risk-controlling calculative methods based on faith in the powers of statistical accounting. In this context, however, the language of *risk* is designed to heighten awareness of features of historical occurrence that ought to be controlled, while the language of *normalcy* seeks to dampen this impulse by suggesting that a particular state is desirable. In modernity, the denotative translation of the term "risk" is "a state of affairs that *should be altered*," while those labeled normal, are "states of affairs that *are as they should be*." The term "normal" is thus seething with contradictions: does it tell us how things are, or how they should be? Does it indicate a given state of affairs or one that can and should be improved? "The normal stands indifferently for what is typical, the unenthusiastic objective average, but it also stands for what has been, good health, and for what shall be, our chosen destiny. That is why the benign and sterile-sounding word 'normal' has become one of the most powerful ideological tools of the twentieth century." Ian Hacking, *The Taming of Chance* (Cambridge: Cambridge University Press, 1990), 169.

65 Waldschmidt, "Who Is Normal? Who Is Deviant?" 197. The language of risk remains hegemonic despite the fact that the very economists from whom this language has been borrowed have pointed out there are deep conceptual problems with the use of the language of "rational expectations" as well as bell-curve-based accounts of risk modeling. Robert Skidelsky, *Keynes: The Return of the Master* (New York: Public Affairs, 2010), 31–36, 42–44. The reason is obvious: it remains a powerful and convincing way for a speaker to establish their expert status with its implied authority to announce what counts as rational behavior. This configuration of moral detachment and authoritative pronouncement is the most ethically problematic aspect of genetic counseling.

66 Rapp, *Testing Women, Testing the Fetus*, 312–13.

67 Iozzio, "Genetic Anomaly or Genetic Diversity," 874.

68 Thomas, *Down Syndrome Screening and Reproductive Politics*, 152–53.

69 Too little research has been done to determine whether widespread prenatal screening and abortion of new ones with Down syndrome is in fact cost efficient, especially if the costs of inadvertently propagating attitudes that restrict these people's independence and employment opportunities are taken into account. Unsurprisingly, surveys of people with Down syndrome reveal that they experience the culture of prenatal testing and the abortion of people with Down syndrome as deeply distressing. Priscilla Alderson, "Down's Syndrome: Cost, Quality, and Value of Life," *Social Science and Medicine* 53 (2001): 627–38.

70 Rapp, *Testing Women, Testing the Fetus*, 179.

71 Rapp, *Testing Women, Testing the Fetus*, 266–70.

72 Rapp, *Testing Women, Testing the Fetus*, 109.

73 Thomas, *Down's Syndrome Screening and Reproductive Politics*, 87–89.

74 Rapp, *Testing Women, Testing the Fetus*, 99–100.

75 Rothman, *Tentative Pregnancy*, 51, 83–85.

76 Rapp, *Testing Women, Testing the Fetus*, 225.

77 Thomas, *Down's Syndrome Screening and Reproductive Politics*, 154–60

78 Rapp, *Testing Women, Testing the Fetus*, 220.

79 Thomas, *Down Syndrome Screening and Reproductive Politics*, 182.

80 Rothman, *Tentative Pregnancy*, xiv.

81 Rapp, *Testing Women, Testing the Fetus*, 306–7.

82 Meskus, "Personalized Ethics," 373–92.

83 Rapp, *Testing Women, Testing the Fetus*, 247.

84 Rapp, *Testing Women, Testing the Fetus*, 308.

85 Thomas, *Down Syndrome Screening and Reproductive Politics*, 154.

86 "I know of no feminist who countenances abortion for sex-selection. An overwhelming number, along with at least 80 percent of the nation [United States] condone abortion for fetal 'deformities,' 'defects' or 'abnormalities.'" Adrienne Asch, "Can Aborting Imperfect Children Be Immoral?" in *Ethical Issues in Modern Medicine*, ed. John Arras and Bonnie Steinbock (Mountain View, Calif.: Mayfield, 1995), 237–40. Page 387 from another chapter in that volume, John Arras' "The Severely Demented," is quoted in Carlson, *Faces of Intellectual Disability*, 176. On the ways that genetic developments and new reproductive technologies are reshaping this discussion, see Clare Williams, "Framing the Fetus in Medical Work: Rituals and Practices," *Social Science & Medicine* 60 (2005): 2085–95.

87 Thomas, *Down Syndrome Screening and Reproductive Politics*, ch. 6; Rapp, *Testing Women, Testing the Fetus*, 248.

88 Rapp, *Testing Women, Testing the Fetus*, 264.

89 John Swinton, *Raging with Compassion: Pastoral Responses to the Problem of Evil* (Grand Rapids: Eerdmans, 2007), 200.

90 These criticisms are surveyed in Mumford, *Ethics at the Beginning of Life*, ch. 5.

91 Rapp, *Testing Women, Testing the Fetus*, 318.

92 Cobb, *Loving Samuel*, 9–11. Theologically speaking, a christological claim underlies such a reading of an anomalous birth, which "implicitly feeds on the resurrection of the one *angelos tou theou* who did not recoil from having his wings clipped (Phil. 2:5-8) or from sharing the human life of fear and anxiety, yet was triumphantly raised from the dead to offer transformation and new life to those who recognize him and their own existence as human beings in the faces of his most dependent brothers and sisters (Mt. 25:40)." Bernd Wannenwetsch, "Angels with Clipped Wings: The Disabled as Key to the Recognition of Personhood," in Swinton and Brock, *Theology, Disability and the New Genetics*, 182–200, quotation from 195.

93 Arendt, *Human Condition*, ch. 6.

94 "To ask for recognition, or to offer it, is precisely not to ask for recognition for what one already is. It is to solicit a becoming, to instigate a transformation, to petition the future always in relation to the Other. It is also to stake one's own being, and one's own persistence in one's own being, in the struggle for recognition." Butler, *Precarious Life*, 44.

95 Williams, "Framing the Fetus in Medical Work," 2085–95.

96 Cobb, *Loving Samuel*, 5–6.

97 "We had shared an ultrasound picture. We wanted our friends and family to see our son. I thought he had my profile. Craig saw in Samuel the image of God. This was a better image. And his was a good word. As our flesh and blood Samuel bore our humanity. In his humanity he was made to image God in a world where God often seems absent. . . . Jesus, the perfect image of God, humbled himself, subjected himself to the risks of conception and pregnancy, was born fully dependent upon a family, and was received with the love and welcome of a community who would nurture and care for him. His life was a gift and a sign of God's pursuing love. . . . in this way, Sam re-presented God to

me: Sam was the image of God even when God seemed most absent." Cobb, *Loving Samuel*, 36–37, cf. 15–16.

98 The social scientific literature is unambiguous on this point and reveals the typical types of stressors on parents across the developed Western world. Bengt Sivberg, "Coping Strategies and Parental Attitudes: A Comparison of Parents with Children with Autistic Spectrum Disorders and Parents with Non-autistic Children," *International Journal of Circumpolar Health* 61, no. 2 (2002): 36–50; J. M. Cramm and A.P. Nieboer, "Psychological Well-Being of Caregivers of Children with Intellectual Disabilities: Using Parental Stress as a Mediating Factor," *Journal of Intellectual Disabilities* 15, no. 2 (2011): 101–13; Benjamin Zablotsky, Catherine P. Bradshaw, Elizabeth A. Stuart, "The Association between Mental Health, Stress, and Coping Supports in Mothers of Children with Autistic Spectrum Disorders," *Journal of Autism and Developmental Disorders* 43 (2013): 1380–93; Sigan L. Hartley, Marsha Mailick Seltzer, Lara Head, and Leonard Abbeduto, "Psychological Well-Being in Fathers of Adolescents and Young Adults with Down Syndrome, Fragile X Syndrome, and Autism," *Family Relations* 61, no. 2 (2012): 327–42; R. Hassall, J. Rose, and J. McDonald, "Parenting Stress in Mothers of Children with an Intellectual Disability: the Effects of Parental Cognitions in Relation to Child Characteristics and Family Support," *Journal of Intellectual Disability Research* 49, no. 6 (2005): 405–18; Stephen Gallagher, Anna C. Phillips, Douglas Carroll, "Parental Stress Is Associated with Poor Sleep Quality in Parents Caring for Children with Developmental Disabilities," *Journal of Pediatric Psychology* 35, no. 7 (2010): 728–37; Cathy R. Cox, Sara Eaton, Naomi V. Ekas, and Erin A. Van Enkevort, "Death Concerns and Psychological Well-Being in Mothers of Children with Autism Spectrum Disorder," *Research in Developmental Disabilities* 45–46 (2015): 229–38.

It is remarkable how little support is needed to decrease these stresses significantly. Julie Barlow, Lesley Powell, Mollie Gilchrist, "The Influence of the Training and Support Programme on the Self-Efficacy and Psychological Well-Being of Parents of Children with Disabilities: A Controlled Trial," *Complementary Therapies in Clinical Practice* 12 (2006): 55–63.

99 Adrienne Asch, "Prenatal Diagnosis and Selective Abortion: A Challenge to Practice and Policy," *American Journal of Public Health* 89, no. 11 (1999): 1649–57.

100 Reinders, "Life's Goodness," 163–81. John Milbank, "Can a Gift Be Given? Prolegomena to a Future Trinitarian Metaphysic," *Modern Theology* 11, no. 1 (1995): 119–61.

101 Such attending, notes Anat Pick, cannot be a thin practice, and so brings with it important methodological implications. "Attention is antiphilosophical; it does not produce arguments or truth claims about its object. Vulnerability as an object of attention does not yield a moral 'reading.'" It thus forces us to consider "the ramifications (for thought and also for action) of being oriented toward vulnerability as a universal mode of exposure." Anat Pick, *Creaturely Poetics: Animality and Vulnerability in Literature and Film* (New York: Columbia University Press, 2011), 5.

102 Carlson, *Faces of Intellectual Disability*, 176–77.

Chapter 5: Orthodox Medical Ethics

1 Paul Ramsey's work, *The Patient as Person* (New Haven, Conn.: Yale University Press, 1970), is considered by many to be the formative text in the discipline. On the origins of the discipline and its secularization see John H. Evans, *Playing God: Human Genetic Engineering and the Rationalization of Public Bioethical Debate* (Chicago: University of

Chicago Press, 2002); Allen Verhey, *Reading the Bible in the Strange World of Medicine* (Grand Rapids: Eerdmans, 2003), 13–22; Stanley Hauerwas, "How Christian Ethics Became Medical Ethics: The Case of Paul Ramsey," in *Wilderness Wanderings: Probing Twentieth Century Theology and Philosophy* (Boulder: Westview, 1997), 124–40.

There are a few notable exceptions to this general rule. The earliest and most influential was Stanley Hauerwas' *Suffering Presence: Theological Reflections on Medicine, the Mentally Handicapped, and the Church* (Edinburgh: T&T Clark, 1986). Hauerwas discusses the origins of his thinking about disability as a challenge to the presumptions of mainstream medical ethics in Brock and Hauerwas, *Beginnings*, 195–214. For more recent engagements with disability in Christian medical ethics see Neil Messer, *Flourishing: Health, Disease, and Bioethics in Theological Perspective* (Grand Rapids: Eerdmans, 2013); Charles C. Camosy, *Too Expensive to Treat? Finitude, Tragedy, and the Neonatal ICU* (Grand Rapids: Eerdmans, 2010); John Wyatt, *Matters of Life and Death: Human Dilemmas in the Light of the Christian Faith*, rev. ed., foreword by John Stott (Nottingham: InterVarsity, 2009); James C. Peterson, *Genetic Turning Points: The Ethics of Human Genetic Intervention* (Grand Rapids: Eerdmans, 2001).

2 Alicia Ouellette has comprehensively surveyed the points of tension between disability activists and card-carrying members of the bioethics guild, concluding,

> Bioethicists tend to support individual choices to refuse medical care, family decision-making, and advanced directives. Members of the disability community are often sceptical of or oppose these practices. Some disability experts view medically assisted nutrition and hydration as a basic human right. Bioethicists tend to think of medically assisted nutrition and hydration as no different from other medical treatments. Bioethicists support efforts of doctors to fix physical impairments; disability scholars question the need to "fix" the bodies of individual [*sic*] with disability and look instead for societal solutions. Many bioethicists view persistent vegetative state as something entirely different from other disabling conditions; some disability activists deny those differences. Finally, many people in bioethics seek to resolve individual cases without taking into account social and community concerns, whereas social and community concerns are central to the disability community. (*Bioethics and Disability: Toward a Disability-Conscious Bioethics* [Cambridge: Cambridge University Press, 2011], 363–64.)

See also Tom Shakespeare, "Just What Is the Disability Perspective on Disability?" *Hastings Center Report* 46, no. 3 (2016): 31–32.

3 Ouellette, *Bioethics and Disability*, 12–46.

4 Douglas A. Mata, Marco A. Ramos, Narinder Bansal, Rida Khan, Constance Guille, Emanuele Di Angelantonio, and Srijan Sen, "Prevalence of Depression and Depressive Symptoms among Resident Physicians: A Systematic Review and Meta-analysis," *Journal of the American Medical Association* 314, no. 22 (2015): 2373–83; Lisa S. Rotenstein, Marco A. Ramos, Matthew Torre, J. Bradley Segal, Michael J. Peluso, Constance Guille, Srijan Sen, and Douglas A. Mata, "Prevalence of Depression, Depressive Symptoms, and Suicidal Ideation among Medical Students: A Systematic Review and Meta-analysis," *Journal of the American Medical Association* 316, no. 21 (2016): 2214–36; Stuart J. Slavin, "Medical Student Mental Health: Culture, Environment, and the Need for Change," *Journal of the American Medical Association* 316, no. 21 (2016): 2195–96; Alyssa F. Cook, Vineet M. Arora, Kenneth A. Rasinski, Farr A. Curlin, and John D. Yoon, "The Prevalence of Medical

Student Mistreatment and Its Association with Burnout," *Academy of Medicine* 89, no. 5 (2014): 749–54.

5 The book was first published in 1979 and is currently in its sixth edition. Tom L. Beauchamp and James F. Childress, *Principles of Biomedical Ethics*, 6th ed. (New York: Oxford University Press, 2008). Their four principles have become so universally absorbed in medical education in the U.S. that they are part of the MCAT, the standard admission test that every would-be doctor must take to be admitted to medical school. Renee C. Fox and Judith P. Swazey, *Observing Bioethics* (New York: Oxford University Press, 2008).

6 James Childress was a lifelong Quaker. Evans, *Playing God*, 87.

7 The page references to follow are to the fourth edition. Tom L. Beauchamp and James F. Childress, *Principles of Biomedical Ethics* (New York: Oxford University Press, 1994), 462.

8 Beauchamp and Childress, *Principles of Biomedical Ethics*, 464.

9 Beauchamp and Childress, *Principles of Biomedical Ethics*, 483.

10 The point of the concept of supererogation is to "Refrain from holding people to standards that are arduous, risky, and frightening." Beauchamp and Childress, *Principles of Biomedical Ethics*, 487.

11 Ironically, Immanuel Kant both recognized the Reformers' objections and bequeathed an account of moral duty that was taken up by twentieth-century neo-Kantians in a manner that once again collapsed the distinction between "optional" and "nonnegotiable" duties. Marcia Baron has argued that this distinction is in fact foreign to his thought, which assumed morality to be transtemporal and exceptionless in being based on universal reason. "Kantian Ethics and Supererogation," *The Journal of Philosophy* 84, no. 5 (1987): 237–62. Beauchamp and Childress draw on a neo-Kantian definition of supererogation.

12 See Aquinas, *Summa Theologica* 2-2.185.6.

13 Martin Luther, *95 Theses*, theses 44–45. The distinction had been propounded by Thomas Aquinas (and others), *Summa Theologica* 1-2.108.2–4.

14 Martin Luther, "The Freedom of a Christian," in *Career of the Reformer I*, ed. Harold J. Grimm and T. Lehmann, Luther's Works 31 (St. Louis: Concordia, 1957), 348; "Treatise on Good Works, 1520," in *The Christian in Society I*, ed. James Atkinson, Luther's Works 44 (St. Louis: Concordia; Philadelphia: Fortress, 1966), 33.

15 Resistance to this concept remained firm in Protestant theology right up to the modern era, as indicated, for instance by its anathematization in the Anglican Thirty-Nine Articles, finalized in 1571: "The works of supererogation cannot be taught without arrogancy and impiety" (Art. 14). Calvin summarized the protest of the magisterial Reformers against any bifurcation of moral claims in this manner: "Since we are unduly inclined to hypocrisy, this palliative ought by no means be added to soothe our sluggish consciences." John Calvin, *The Institutes of the Christian Religion*, 2 vols., trans. Ford Lewis Battles (Philadelphia: Westminster, 1960), 2.8.58.

16 The leveling and sacralization of all spheres of human activity was to have a deep and enduring effect on the ways moderns conceive their lives and work. It also explains why it is difficult today to sustain sharp distinctions between "personal" and "professional" ethics. Taylor, *Sources of the Self*, part 3, "The Affirmation of Ordinary Life."

17 See Reinhold Niebuhr, *Moral Man and Immoral Society: A Study in Ethics and Politics* (New York: Scribner's, 1932). Hans Ulrich presents the antidote to Niebuhr's view in *Wie Geschöpfe leben: Konturen evangelischer Ethik* (Münster: Lit Verlag, 2005), 109.

18 Benjamin S. Wall, *Welcome as a Way of Life: A Practical Theology of Jean Vanier*, foreword by John Swinton (Eugene, Ore.: Cascade, 2016).

19 Jean Vanier, *Community and Growth*, 2nd rev. ed. (London: Darton, Longman and Todd, 1989), ch. 3; Bernd Wannenwetsch, *Political Worship: Ethics for Christian Citizens*, trans. Margaret Kohl (Oxford: Oxford University Press, 2004), ch. 8. Wannenwetsch is commenting on the influential claim to this effect of Karl Barth in "The Christian Community and the Civil Community," in *Community, State, and Church: Three Essays*, intro. by David Haddorff (Eugene, Ore.: Wipf & Stock, 2004), section 14.

20 I present the case as faithfully to their framework as possible as a representation of one way their moral apparatus would be deployed in good faith in medical schools and many medical practices. It therefore represents the application of their ethical thought to an actual medical case in a way both typical of their casuistic case-study style that is extremely widespread in Anglophone medicine. An earlier version of this section originally appeared in Brian Brock and John Wyatt, "The Physician as Political Actor: Late Abortion and the Strictures of Liberal Moral Discourse," *Studies in Christian Ethics* 19, no. 2 (2006): 153–68. The case comes out of Wyatt's experiences as a consultant neonatal professor of medicine at a major British university research hospital. A comparable discussion of neonatal euthanasia derived from the four principles approach can be found in Mark Sklansky, "Neonatal Euthanasia: Moral Considerations and Criminal Liability," *Journal of Medical Ethics* 27 (2001): 5–11.

21 Burcham, "War Against the Weak," 4.

22 Beauchamp and Childress have constructed an ethical methodology that places a premium on the resolution of social disagreement and aims at political harmony. Their approach is a modification of the melding of Kant and Mill popularized by the political philosophy of John Rawls and described in ethical theory by William Frankena in his *Ethics*, 2nd ed. (Englewood Cliffs, N.J.: Prentice-Hall, 1973).

The common morality construct (derived from Rawls' conception of the "overlapping consensus") has been widely criticized: some have argued that it is unfair to call the four principles descriptive of any generic moral psychology (Markus Christen, Christian Ineichen, and Carmen Tanner, "How 'Moral' Are the Principles of Biomedical Ethics?—A Cross-Domain Evaluation of the Common Morality Hypothesis," *BMC Medical Ethics* 15 [2014]: 47); others, that the supposedly empirically derived four principles cannot possibly be held in the equipoise that Beauchamp and Childress propose, and in any case enact a moral imperialism (Angus Dawson and E. Garrard, "In Defence of Moral Imperialism: Four Equal and Universal Prima Facie Principles," *Journal of Medical Ethics* 32, no. 4 [April 2006]: 200–204). Some contest even the claim that these four principles cohere sufficiently to be called a single unified ethical approach (K. Danner Clouser and Bernard Gert, "A Critique of Principlism," *The Journal of Medicine and Philosophy: A Forum for Bioethics and Philosophy of Medicine* 152, no. 1 [April 1990]: 219–36).

23 Beauchamp and Childress, *Principles of Biomedical Ethics*, 109.

24 Beauchamp and Childress, *Principles of Biomedical Ethics*, 100–101, 107–9.

25 Sean Doherty, *Theology and Economic Ethics: Martin Luther and Arthur Rich in Dialogue* (Oxford: Oxford University Press, 2014), 163–74.

26 Beauchamp and Childress, *Principles of Biomedical Ethics*, 110.

27 Beauchamp and Childress, *Principles of Biomedical Ethics*, 104–5. Casuistry is understood as the process of refining the minimum moral grammar found in the overlapping consensus. The moral rules derived from this grammar are binding, yet negotiable. Beauchamp and Childress refuse to rank such moral rules in a hierarchy, suggesting that rules

must be continually balanced to achieve minimum infringement of the various rules in any given case.

28 Julian Savulescu and Udo Schuklenk, "Doctors Have No Right to Refuse Medical Assistance in Dying, Abortion or Contraception," *Bioethics* 31, no. 3 (2017): 162–70.

29 Carl Elliot, "The Drug Pushers," *Atlantic Monthly* 297, no. 3 (April 2006): 82–93.

30 Sara Lindforsa, Christina Eintreib, and Kristina Alexanderson, "Stress Factors Affecting Academic Physicians at a University Hospital" *Work* 34 (2009): 305–13.

31 Rebecca Jackson, Kimberly Gibson, Yvonne Wu, and Mary Croughan, "Perinatal Outcomes in Singletons Following In Vitro Fertilization: A Meta-analysis," *Obstetrics & Gynecology* 103 (2004): 551–63.

32 Howard Minkoff and Richard Berkowitz, "The Myth of the Precious Baby," *Obstetrics & Gynecology* 106 (2005): 607–9.

33 Rene Almeling, *Sex Cells: The Medical Market for Eggs and Sperm* (Berkeley: University of California Press, 2011); Debra Satz, *Why Some Things Should Not Be for Sale: The Moral Limits of Markets* (Oxford: Oxford University Press, 2010), ch. 5; Howard Minkoff, Kathleen Powderly, Frank Chervenak, and Lawrence McCullough, "Ethical Dimensions of Elective Primary Cesarean Delivery," *Obstetrics and Gynecology* 103 (2004): 387–92.

34 "Virtues in practice are habituated character traits that dispose persons to act in accordance with the worthy goals and role expectations of health care institutions." Beauchamp and Childress, *Principles of Biomedical Ethics*, 463.

35 Beauchamp and Childress, *Principles of Biomedical Ethics*, 474–83.

36 The reform of the deliberative principles themselves is possible, but only through "interpretation, specification and balancing" of moral principles accepted in the common realm. Beauchamp and Childress, *Principles of Biomedical Ethics*, 102.

37 The legal state of play is surveyed by Shawn H. E. Harmon, "Abortion and Conscientious Objection: Doogan—A Missed Opportunity for an Instructive Rights-Based Analysis," *Medical Law International* 16, nos. 3–4 (2016): 143–73. A survey of the arguments and counter arguments is provided by Christopher Kaczor, "Conscientious Objection and Health Care: A Reply to Bernard Dickens," *Christian Bioethics: Non-Ecumenical Studies in Medical Morality* 18, no. 1 (2012): 59–71.

38 As Alasdair MacIntyre has observed, the situation is ultimately grounded in the substitution of technical criterion for genuinely moral criterion in modern liberal societies. "For in the realm of professional practice matters which affect problems of immediate action cannot be allowed to go unsettled. One way or another, codes must be formulated, choices made, dilemmas resolved, with or without rational justification. Hence in this realm what is in fact inconclusive intellectual debate nonetheless issues in the practical resolution of problems, a resolution the arbitrariness of which is the function of both philosophical and professional rhetoric to conceal." *Three Rival Versions of Moral Enquiry*, 226–27.

39 Jacques Ellul, *The Technological Society*, trans. John Wilkinson (London: Jonathon Cape, 1964), 349–58.

40 "Dissent is built into the fabric of the modern system. We bureaucratize it as much as everything else." George Grant, *Lament for a Nation* (Ottawa: Carleton University Press, 1995), 91. See also Ellul, *Technological Society*, 356.

41 Trust is drastically eroded by those with a genetic condition when they sense complicity with "the practice of embryo destruction and the arbitrary bullying of victims of congenital disease by the culturally ascendant strong who consider themselves genetically

perfect, above criticism, and unaccountable. My fundamental contention is that *tolerance of this behaviour within the medical community—and its enabling by the modern state—is eroding the inner integrity of one of the greatest achievements of the modern world: a benevolent and egalitarian healthcare system*." Burcham, "War Against the Weak," 4, emphasis in original.

42 In fact, their anthropology rests entirely on the assertion of autonomy. Maureen Junker-Kenny, "Genes and the Self: Anthropological Questions to the Human Genome Project," in *Brave New World: Theology, Ethics and the Human Genome*, ed. Celia Deane-Drummond (London: T&T Clark, 2003), 124–25.

43 Beauchamp and Childress, *Principles of Biomedical Ethics*, 109. For their general ethical theory, see chs. 1–2. Their theory is thus susceptible to the whole range of limits that come with proceduralist utilitarian (more broadly, consequentialist) accounts of ethics. Michael Banner, *Christian Ethics: A Brief History* (Chichester: Wiley Blackwell, 2009), 118–24.

44 Beauchamp and Childress, *Principles of Biomedical Ethics*, 108.

45 Beauchamp and Childress, *Principles of Biomedical Ethics*, 124.

46 The phrase is Alasdair MacIntyre's *After Virtue*, 3rd ed. (London: Duckworth, 2007), 2.

47 In a first-century context, the Greek word *martus* is most often used in a juridical context to denote a person who relates an eyewitness account. The New Testament concentrates this meaning on the person and teaching of Jesus, who is presented as a (the) witness in the fullest sense of the word: trustworthy and faithful (Rev 1:5, 3:14), testifying to the truth (John 18:37), which he has seen and heard from the Father (John 3:11, 32). Human witnessing is to the life, death, and resurrection of Jesus Christ, and at the middle of the second century in the midst of fierce persecutions, the term begins to be applied to Christians who were not historical witnesses of the witness and resurrection of Christ, but who died speaking the truth of Christ. Karłowicz, *Archparadox of Death*, 88–89.

48 John 19:25-27 and par.; Matt 5:6; 5:10; Luke 6:22; 1 Pet 3:14; 4:14; Heb 11; Barth, *Church Dogmatics* 4/2: *The Doctrine of Reconciliation*, ed. G. W. Bromiley and T. F. Torrance (Edinburgh: T&T Clark, 1958), 190–91.

49 Michael Banner, *Christian Ethics and Contemporary Moral Problems* (Cambridge: Cambridge University Press, 1999), 68–83.

50 Stanley Hauerwas, *After Christendom: How the Church Is to Behave if Freedom, Justice, and a Christian Nation Are Bad Ideas* (Nashville: Abingdon, 1999), 38; Oliver O'Donovan, *The Desire of the Nations: Rediscovering the Roots of Political Theology* (Cambridge: Cambridge University Press, 1996), 109.

51 O'Donovan, *Desire of the Nations*, 215.

52 Søren Kierkegaard, *Practice in Christianity*, ed. and trans. Howard Hong and Edna Hong, Kierkegaard's Writings 20 (Princeton: Princeton University Press, 1991), 206–11, 227–28.

53 Beauchamp and Childress, *Principles of Biomedical Ethics*, 489.

54 "That is, if a Christian receiving medical care is committed to a belief and practice and outlook not defined by instrumental rationality, anti-metaphysical positivism, and modern naturalism, the hospital environment can powerfully assault central components of such a Christian understanding of healing, care, illness, and death." Tyson, "Wounds of Faith and Medicine," 331.

55 "Witnessing is not coercion, but a chance which can be rejected, while faith is not only a question of reason which judges the credibility of the witness, but above all, a grace. . . . The

witness of Christ is not in a situation entirely different from the situation of Christ himself. Through imitating the Savior, the witnesses of all epochs reproduce the mysterious presence of God in the world of the senses." Karłowicz, *Archparadox of Death*, 252.

56 This is a third era of martyrologic language. In the New Testament Jesus is presented as the *martus* (witness), while in the second century those who died witnessing to Christ were called *martures*. Now those who suffered for their profession of Christ, but without giving their lives, begin to be called *homologetai* (confessors). Augustine and Jerome called acts of patient perseverance in the face of adversity and resistance to Christian ways of life "white martyrdom." Karłowicz, *Archparadox of Death*, 88–89; Brad S. Gregory, *Salvation at Stake: Christian Martyrdom in Early Modern Europe* (Cambridge, Mass.: Harvard University Press, 1999), 50–62. The crucial conceptual point is that martyrdom is not the claim that "deeds speak louder than words" (the deed gives weight to words of confession) nor "I really believe in this" (a proof of subjective conviction) nor "virtue in suffering" (oriented to the perfection of the one undergoing martyrdom). Martyrdom is an intersubjective act whose intelligibility is tied to a real external truth. Christian martyrdom is therefore intrinsically related to a theology of the cross and so a vision and presence of Christ's righteousness. Karłowicz, *Archparadox of Death*, 95–99.

57 Michael Jensen, *Martyrdom and Identity: The Self on Trial* (London: Bloomsbury, 2013), 187.

58 Jensen, *Martyrdom and Identity*, 187.

59 Oliver O'Donovan, *Resurrection and Moral Order: An Outline for Evangelical Ethics*, 2nd ed. (Leicester: Apollos, 1994), 96.

60 O'Donovan, *Resurrection*, 97.

61 Bonhoeffer, *Ethics*, 286.

62 "The boundary of vocation has been broken open not only vertically, that is, through Christ, but horizontally, with regard to the extent of responsibility." Bonhoeffer, *Ethics*, 293. Bernd Wannenwetsch insightfully unpacks this Bonhoefferian view of vocation in the medical context in "Loving the Limit," 90–99.

63 "[T]he dignity of disabled life appears to be more than yet another 'topic' for Bonhoeffer. Rather, it represents a focal point in which numerous key insights developed in his theological work coincide." Bernd Wannenwetsch, "'My Strength Is Made Perfect in Weakness': Bonhoeffer and the War over Disabled Life," in Brock and Swinton, *Disability in the Christian Tradition*, 353–69, quotation from 353.

64 The specter of the Nazi euthanasia programs is too often and too quickly invoked in contemporary discussions of disability and eugenics. This ad hominem attack needlessly obscures the reality that the Nazi program was essentially indistinguishable from the core affirmations of modern liberal prenatal testing regimes: that testing makes good economic sense and that those who cannot be counted on to become economically productive members of society can legitimately be eliminated. Economics was the essential driver of the Third Reich euthanasia program. "Despite occasional posturing of humanitarianism, the essence of the Nazi argument for the destruction of the insane was economic. Euthanasia was defended as a means of cutting costs, or ridding society of 'useless eaters' . . . the purpose of the operation was not only to continue the 'struggle against genetic disease' but to free up hospital beds and personnel for the coming war. The philosophy behind this was simple: Patients were to be either cured or killed." Robert N. Proctor, "The Destruction of 'Lives Not Worth Living,'"

in *Deviant Bodies: Critical Perspectives on Difference in Science and Popular Culture*, ed. Jennifer Terry and Jacqueline Urla (Bloomington: Indiana University Press, 1995), 170–96, quotation from 171.

65 The head of Bethel, Friedrich Bodelschwingh the Younger, was later involved in a highly symbolic struggle for the head bishopric in the Lutheran church. "The nasty campaign against Bodelschwingh made plain that those who bought into the Nazis' ideologies understood perfectly well the symbolic significance of Bethel as a social embodiment of Christian anthropology." Wannenwetsch, "'My Strength Is Made Perfect in Weakness,'" 357.

66 "The strong booster injection of ecclesiological realism he received at Bethel allowed Bonhoeffer to denounce the Nazi elimination of disabled life not simply as wrong or morally corrupt, but more precisely as 'mad,' as completely out of touch with reality." Wannenwetsch, "'My Strength Is Made Perfect in Weakness,'" 355.

67 Bonhoeffer, "Sermon for Evening Worship Service on 2 Corinthians 12:9, London, 1934," in *London, 1933–35*, ed. Keith W. Clements, Dietrich Bonhoeffer's Works 13 (Minneapolis: Fortress, 2007), 402.

68 As Bonhoeffer notes, Bodelschwingh was protecting the patients in Bethel by refusing to fill out the questionnaires that were the basis of their selection for euthanasia. Wannenwetsch, "'My Strength Is Made Perfect in Weakness,'" 369. The contrast could not be more stark with the pastors of the Lutheran church as a whole, whose church records were the main documents establishing racial purity, and who by and large complied with requests to supply these documents to prove that specific Jews could not be Christians.

69 Bonhoeffer, *Ethics*, 287.

70 "The grammar of this political ethics is the witness to God's claim on the whole of reality by virtue of the togetherness of God and man in Christ. Institutional responsibilities are not exempt from this claim." Stefan Heuser, "The Cost of Citizenship: Disciple and Citizen in Bonhoeffer's Political Ethics," *Studies in Christian Ethics* 18, no. 3 (2005): 49–69.

71 Bonhoeffer, *Ethics*, 309–11.

72 See John Swinton and Brian Brock, eds., *A Graceful Embrace: Theological Reflections on Adopting Children* (Leiden: Brill, 2018). The essay by Sarah Shea is especially noteworthy in the context of the discussion in this chapter, "Theological Reflection on Intercountry Adoptions of Special Needs Children from Mainland China," 161–82.

Chapter 6: Quality of Life in an Industrialized Age

1 Alicia Ouellette surveys some of the reasons that disabled people find medical contexts threatening.

> From a disability perspective, the health care setting is a dangerous and difficult place. Babies are left to die because they are born with disabling or potentially disabling conditions. Healthy growth is stopped and functioning organs are removed from children with disabilities when such interventions would never be allowed for nondisabled children. Parents are charged with child neglect for failure to cede to social and medical pressure to use medical technologies to cure traits in their children deemed defects by medicine but a valuable human variant by their parents. Women with disabilities are denied their sexuality and gender identities by doctors who fail to ask about their

> sexual health or even equip their offices to provide basic screening services like pap smears and mammograms. Parents with disabilities are presumed to be incompetent strangers to their own sick and injured children. Fertility specialists deny services based on assumptions about the ability of persons with disabilities to parent. Doctors unquestionably accept as reasonable decisions by adults with disability to die regardless of the surmountable social problems faced by the patient. Finally, components of daily living for adults who live happily with disability—feeding tubes and ventilator support—are deemed artificial and optional by nondisabled surrogates. (*Bioethics and Disability*, 319.)

She also documents her claim that it is rare for bioethicists to grasp the threatening nature of health care for people with disabilities by citing a comment by Erik Parens that proves the rule.

> I am not proud to confess that when I first heard people with disabilities say [that disabling features are a central part of their identity], I practiced some armchair psychoanalysis: "yes, yes, that's very nice. You *say* that the problem is social responses to your disability, not your disability. But let's be honest; you're in denial." The more I heard about people [who] say that the most difficult thing about having a disability was the way temporarily able-bodied people like me treated them, however, the more I began to take them at their word. I became convinced that if, after a process of truly informed decision-making, someone with a disability refuses the use of medical means to improve her social experience, then there is no good alternative to respecting her decision, no matter how surprising I might find it. (Erik Parens, "Respecting Children with Disabilities—and Their Parents," *Hastings Center Report* 39, no. 1 [2009]: 22–23.)

Parens' admission only highlights the problem of the guild's paternalistic stance as he displays an inability to move beyond us-them language and does not challenge the expectations that render the self-descriptions of disabled people so surprising to him. The burden of proof is placed on disabled people to opt out of the treatments medical ethicists and doctors think appropriate. Parens does not even appear aware of the additional marginalization of those with intellectual disabilities, given their obvious incapacity to engage in a "process of truly informed decision-making" that is the central focus of mainline medical ethics. Ouellette, *Bioethics and Disability*, 318.

The portrayals of the theme of the hospital as purgatorial realm in literature and in cinema are almost too numerous to mention. See for instance the 2001 triumph of the human spirit film *Wit*, starring Emma Thompson, which is based on the play of the same title by Margaret Edson (which won a Pulitzer Prize in 1999). Other classics in the field that have shaped popular understandings of disability are the story told by Jean-Dominique Bauby's *Le scaphandre et le papillon* (1997), translated into English as *The Diving Bell and the Butterfly*, and made into a film.

Another book-to-film adaptation, the story of Joni Erickson Tada, *Joni: The Unforgettable Story of a Young Woman's Struggle against Quadriplegia and Depression* (1976), was widely distributed through churches in the United States in the 1980s, deeply shaping evangelical Protestant Christian sensibilities about disability and its proximity to hospitals, understood as fearful places of purgatorial suffering.

2 Kafka's stories "The Great Wall of China" and "The Trial" are paradigmatic instances of this type of inquiry. I am updating Walter Benjamin's pithy phrase "organization as

destiny." Walter Benjamin, "Franz Kafka, on the Tenth Anniversary of His Death," in Jennings, Eiland, and Smith, *Walter Benjamin*, 803–7.

3 Wendell Berry, *The Unsettling of America: Culture and Agriculture* (San Francisco: Sierra Club Books, 1977), 19.

4 Berry, *Unsettling of America*, 90.

5 Berry, *Unsettling of America*, 31–35, 177–78, 182–89.

6 Michel Foucault, *The Birth of the Clinic: An Archaeology of Medical Perception*, trans. A. M. Sheridan Smith (New York: Vintage Books, 1994), ch. 2, esp. 35.

7 Foucault, *Birth of the Clinic*, 29–30, 102.

8 Foucauldian disability theorists have explored this theme in some detail. See the chapters by Sullivan, Carlson, Snigurowicz, Waldschmidt, McGuire, and Kolářová in Tremain, *Foucault and the Government of Disability*.

9 The story was first broken by the BBC's *Panorama* television show on May 31, 2011. A timeline of the coverage and responses is collected at http://www.bbc.co.uk/news/uk-england-bristol-20078999. On March 28, 2013, the U.K. Department of Health released its report on the scandal in *Transforming Care: A National Response to Winterbourne View Hospital*, 2013, www.gov.uk. For more detailed narrative of some of the issues at stake see Sara Ryan's account of the death of eighteen-year-old Connor Sparrowhawk, found drowned in the bath in a specialist NHS unit in Oxford in 2014. Ryan offers an extremely instructive accounting of the mechanisms that protect poor care from being exposed. *Justice for Laughing Boy: A Death by Indifference* (London: Jessica Kingsley, 2018), esp. chs. 5–6 and 8. That the systemic problems remain troublingly ongoing is indicated by the story of Colette McCulloch, killed in her mid-twenties, hit by a truck after walking out of Pathway House, Bedford, in the early hours of July 28, 2016. Damien Gayle, "Family Seek to Replace 'Sarcastic' Coroner after Autistic Daughter Died," *The Guardian*, May 5, 2018, https://www.theguardian.com/society/2018/may/10/family-seek-to-replace-sarcastic-coroner-after-autistic-daughter-died. Such stories are distressingly easy to find and geographically widespread. Danny Hakimjune, "A Disabled Boy's Death, and a Troubled System," *New York Times*, June 6, 2011, A1.

10 Pauline Heslop, Peter Blair, Peter Fleming, Mat Hoghton, Anna Marriott, and Lesley Russ, *Confidential Inquiry into Premature Deaths of People with Learning Disabilities (CIPOLD)*, final report (Bristol, U.K.: Norah Fry Research Centre, 2013).

11 Heslop et al., *CIPOLD*, 12, 20. The survey reviewed all deaths in Bristol, Gloucestershire, North Somerset, South Gloucestershire, Bath, and northeast Somerset. The authors also noted that several large care institutions in the region had been closed in recent decades and their inhabitants settled in community settings, meaning that the proportion of learning-impaired people was statistically marginally higher in these counties than the national average.

12 The *CIPOLD* authors are keen to stress that the conclusions of this report are by no means new findings but are all the more disturbing in reiterating criticisms that appeared in earlier official government reports. Heslop et al. comment:

> *Valuing People* in 2001 committed the government to exploring the feasibility of establishing a Confidential Inquiry into mortality among people with a learning disability. *Treat Me Right* in 2004 concluded that a Confidential Inquiry into the deaths of people with learning disabilities would not only identify the causes of death, but would also be a powerful lever for improvement in the delivery of health services. A Disability Rights Commission report in 2006 considered it "alarming"

that little or nothing had been done to implement the recommendations of Mencap's *Treat Me Right* report by those with the power to do so. A Disability Rights Commission report in 2007 criticised the lack of strategic change and prioritisation that had taken place following its report the previous year, calling it "quite literally a matter of life and death." *Death by Indifference* described the circumstances surrounding the deaths of six people with learning disabilities while they were in the care of the NHS. It suggested that people with learning disabilities, their families, and carers were facing "institutional discrimination" in healthcare services. *Healthcare for All* is the report of the Michael Inquiry, which was established to learn lessons from the six cases highlighted in the Mencap report. It reported evidence of "a significant level of avoidable suffering and a high likelihood that there are deaths occurring which could be avoided." It recommended the establishment of a learning disabilities Public Health Observatory, and a time-limited Confidential Inquiry into premature deaths of people with learning disabilities "to provide evidence for clinical and professional staff on the extent of the problem and guidance on prevention."

13 Unexpected deaths were defined in the study as a "death which was not anticipated as a significant possibility 24 hours before the death or where there was a similarly unexpected collapse leading to or predicating events which led to death." Using this definition, the Overview Panel adjudged that over half, 57 percent, of deaths were expected, and 43 percent of deaths were unexpected. Heslop et al., *CIPOLD*, 34. The Panel also found that 42 percent of the unexpected deaths were preventable. Heslop et al., *CIPOLD*, 28.

14 As one mother whose son was diagnosed with autism in Oxford observed,

> I felt inordinately sad when I later found out [Connor] was never invited to the "First Fit" Clinic, an introductory clinic for newly diagnosed patients. The exclusionary roots run so blinking deep. . . . A general short-changing of life comes with the territory once you are diagnosed with a learning disability in the UK. Opportunities are closed off and mediocrity becomes the norm, or even considered as good. Families, particularly mothers, are expected to perform a range of tasks over and above typical parenting stuff with the spectre of the 'lack of resources' stick waiting in the wings to bat away the outrageous mother who dares to question the breadcrumbs thrown at her child or children. (Ryan, *Justice for Laughing Boy*, 46, 51.)

15 Heslop et al., *CIPOLD*, 2. Forty-two percent of those deemed to have died a premature death had at one time lived in a long-stay institution. "At the time of their deaths, 64% lived in residential care homes, most with 24-hour paid carer support. For 20% of the people with learning disabilities, safeguarding concerns had previously been raised; for a further 8% safeguarding concerns were raised to the CIPOLD review retrospectively—these had not been reported or investigated at any time previously." Heslop et al., *CIPOLD*, 4.

16 Heslop et al., *CIPOLD*, 56.

17 Heslop et al., *CIPOLD*, 57.

18 Heslop et al., *CIPOLD*, 58.

19 Heslop et al., *CIPOLD*, 58.

20 Heslop et al., *CIPOLD*, 63–66.

21 Heslop et al., *CIPOLD*, 65.
22 Heslop et al., *CIPOLD*, 102.
23 Heslop et al., *CIPOLD*, 66–67.
24 Heslop et al., *CIPOLD*, 83.
25 It is suggestive of appropriate responses to the dilemmas under discussion that simply by reflecting on the state of play during investigations, many healthcare professionals were already beginning to see reasons to adjust their attitudes and practices. Heslop et al., *CIPOLD*, ch. 12, 99ff.
26 The insights of Harvard Medical School doctors Leana Wen and Joshua Kosowsky are particularly relevant in this connection as both are emergency-room doctors concerned that the diagnosis of patients be quick, accurate, and responsive to changes in the development of a medical condition. *When Doctors Don't Listen: How to Avoid Misdiagnoses and Unnecessary Tests* (New York: St. Martin's, 2012), 7, 40.
27 Eric T. Juengst, "*What Does* Enhancement *Mean?*" in *Enhancing Human Traits: Ethical and Social Implications*, ed. Erik Parens (Washington, D.C.: Georgetown University Press, 1998), 29–47, esp. 35–37.
28 Wen and Kosowsky, *When Doctors Don't Listen*, 54–58, 106–9.
29 Wen and Kosowsky, *When Doctors Don't Listen*, 163–64.
30 Wen and Kosowsky, *When Doctors Don't Listen*, 200–224.
31 Abigail Zuger, "A Prescription for Frustration," *New York Times*, April 1, 2013, accessed online.
32 Wen and Kosowsky, *When Doctors Don't Listen*, 185, 189, 215.
33 For a theological critique of this concept of expertise, see Bernd Wannenwetsch, "Der Profi: Mensch ohne Eigenschaften: Warum die Kirche Amageure braucht," in *Alles ist Nichts: Evangelium Hören II*, ed. Arbeitskreis Kirche in der Marketgesellschaft (Nuremberg, Germany, 2001), 45–55.
34 Illich, *Rivers North of the Future*, 203.
35 Illich, *Rivers North of the Future*, 204.
36 Illich, *Rivers North of the Future*, 127, 162, 204.
37 By assembling an array of sources that have not previously appeared in disability theology, this section presents the critique of the medical model of disability in a slightly different key. As that critique is often condemnatory in tone, it is important to point out that the phenomenon of disability also presents an invitation to practitioners of modern medicine. Thinking hard about disability might help those living within the institutions of modern medicine think afresh about their practices and the premises on which they rest.

This invitation to a constructive imagination of medicine assumes that medicine itself is not a static entity. A significant number of philosophers of medicine, medical researchers, and doctors have recognized that, viewed in historical perspective, modern Western medicine takes a radically aggressive approach to treatment. The various thinkers drawn together in this section all agree that the virtues of multifaceted listening to the body and nonintervention have not been sufficiently appreciated in modern Western medicine. A greater degree of therapeutic and diagnostic humility would yield not only a more *humane*, but in fact a more *effective*, medicine.

The philosopher of science Jacob Stegenga has collated this work by physicians, epidemiologists, and science journalists to uncover the direct links between the aggressiveness of modern medicine, the dominance of test-based diagnostic practice, and modern medical research protocols. Focusing his analysis on modern pharmaceuticals, he displays the centrality of statistical models for analyzing therapeutic efficacy and the multiple ways in which these models can be, and are being, subverted in practice. The outcome is the marketing of a wide range of drugs and treatments whose positive effects cannot, in fact, be substantiated. Hence his call for a less aggressive, gentler medicine, which converges with the medicine recounted in this section that listens deeper and better to patients. Jacob Stegenga, *Medical Nihilism* (Oxford: Oxford University Press, 2018). See also Jonah Lehrer, "The Truth Wears Off," *New Yorker*, December 13, 2010, 52–57.

For a beautiful account of the gentling of one doctor, see Victoria Sweet, *God's Hotel: A Doctor, A Hospital, and a Pilgrimage to the Heart of Medicine* (New York: Riverhead Books, 2012).

38 The large number of instruments that have been developed for quality of life assessment are surveyed in Peter M. Fayers and David Machin, *Quality of Life: Assessment, Analysis, and Interpretation* (Chichester: Wiley and Sons, 2000), 3–42.

39 For a representative sample of how deeply this decision-making method has penetrated healthcare practice and thinking in the United States, see, R. Scott Braithwaite, David O. Meltzer, Joseph T. King Jr., Douglas Leslie, and Mark S. Roberts, "What Does the Value of Modern Medicine Say about the $50,000 per Quality-Adjusted Life-Year Decision Rule?" *Medical Care* 46, no. 4 (2008): 349–56. That the rise to prominence of this decision-making method is nearly as dominant in the United Kingdom can be seen in Katherine J. Stevens, "Working with Children to Develop Dimensions for a Preference-Based, Generic, Pediatric, Health-Related Quality-of-Life Measure," *Qualitative Health Research* 20, no. 3 (2010): 340–51. Looking wider afield into practice in other Anglo-Saxon countries would reveal that this approach to decision making about healthcare allocation has become the default decision-making framework against which all other approaches to healthcare allocation must defend their moral reasoning as rational.

40 Anne Soukhanov, ed., *The American Heritage Dictionary of the English Language*, 3rd ed. (Boston: Houghton Mifflin, 1992), 1479. Only in American dictionaries is the term presented as a separate item, and in most cases the middle-class resonances of the term are evident, as in this definition: "affecting the quality of urban life: *such quality-of-life crimes as farebeating and graffiti writing.* [1940–45]." Stuart Berg Flexner, ed., *The Random House Dictionary of the English Language*, 2nd ed. (New York: Random House, 1987), 1579. In British English the phrase has not become prominent enough to warrant its own entry, and in British dictionaries typically only appears as a specific case of the more general definition of comparison, "cases in which there is comparison (expressed or implied) with other things of the same kind; hence, the degree or grade of excellence possessed by a thing." J. A. Simpson and E. S. C. Weiner, eds., *The Oxford English Dictionary*, 2nd ed., vol. 12: *Poise–Quelt* (Oxford: Clarendon, 1989), 794.

41 Much is hidden in the growing gap between vernacular and technical uses of the language of "quality of life," with medical practitioners increasingly driven to use the term in a narrower technical sense, while vernacular usage continues to cover a much broader semantic range. The career of the phrase "quality of life" substantiates the linguist Uwe Poerksen's analysis of the social forces driving the translation of common language into quasiscientific terminology and indicate the effects of this translation on contemporary political culture. *Plastic Words: The Tyranny of a Modular Language*, trans. Jutta Mason and David Cayley (University Park: Pennsylvania State University Press, 1995).

42 David Wasserman, Jerome Bickenbach, and Robert Wachbroit, eds., *Quality of Life and Human Difference: Genetic Testing, Health Care, and Disability* (Cambridge: Cambridge University Press, 2005), 1–26.

43 Mary Jo Iozzio, "Radical Dependence and the *Imago Dei*: Bioethical Implications of Access to Healthcare for People with Disabilities," *Christian Bioethics* 23, no. 3 (2017): 234–60.

44 Banner, *Christian Ethics and Contemporary Moral Problems*, 139–40.

45 Banner, *Christian Ethics and Contemporary Moral Problems*, 161.

46 Banner, *Christian Ethics and Contemporary Moral Problems*, 143, 146–47.

47 Wannenwetsch, "Loving the Limit," 97.

48 Banner, *Christian Ethics and Contemporary Moral Problems*, 148, emphasis in original. For a more detailed discussion of the reasons for the continual expansion of this characteristic algorithmic reasoning across contemporary developed societies, see Brian Brock, *Christian Ethics in a Technological Age* (Grand Rapids: Eerdmans, 2010), 10–18.

49 With Charles C. Camosy, I will assume that this fundamental inability to resolve the very problem that was the reason for deploying the technique in the first place ultimately undermines all attempts to produce such models of healthcare allocation, seen in *Too Expensive to Treat?* David Wasserman, Adrienne Asch, and Jerome Bickenbach offer the strongest disability-aware defense of QUALY-style models, following Martha Nussbaum. "Mending, Not Ending: Cost-Effectiveness Analysis, Preferences and the Right to a Life with Disabilities," in Clements and Read, *Disabled People and the Right to Life*, 30–56.

50 Banner, *Christian Ethics and Contemporary Moral Problems*, 157. Another utilitarian, Peter Singer, who has famously advocated for the moral duty to legalize euthanasia, has recently been criticized for his decision to care lavishly for his mother, who is suffering from dementia. See Swinton's *Dementia*, 131–34.

51 Banner, *Christian Ethics and Contemporary Moral Problems*, 158.

52 Banner, *Christian Ethics and Contemporary Moral Problems*, 158–59.

53 Jacques Ellul, *Perspectives on our Age: Jacques Ellul Speaks on His Life and Work*, rev. ed., ed. Willem H. Vanderburg (Toronto: Anansi, 2004), 64. This claim has deeply theological roots and direct political implications.

> Those who receive the prophetic word of God breaking in and upheaving the realm of human control are typically 'those ill schooled in explanation and understandings. It comes to those who will settle for amazements they can neither explain nor understand.' Conversely, those who are deeply invested in the reality frame derived from the dominant human structures of power and control typically resist all divine in-breaking and all disruptive reality dissonance as vigorously as they can. Typically, the rich, the powerful, the knowledgeable, and the respected are invested heavily in the prevailing status quo. So it is largely with the outcasts that any distinctly prophetic and eschatological gospel of liberation finds reception. It is to those who yearn for a different reality and who are prepared to imagine radically alternative orders of power, knowledge, and wealth that the disruptive, the shockingly particular, and the incomprehensibly singular, in-breaking Word of God finds root. It is not surprising that . . . it is in the global underclass that the ancient spiritual dynamism and in-breaking power of the Holy Spirit is still vital in our times. (Tyson, "Wounds of Faith and Medicine,"

344–45, citing Walter Brueggemann, *The Prophetic Imagination* [Minneapolis: Fortress, 2001], 104.)

54 "Persons with disabilities [and those who love them] know too well how many hours and programs it takes to patch together subsistence livelihood, how hard it is to remain psychologically buoyant given culture's 'dis'/missal. A raised eyebrow, a simple offer of recognition among those on the . . . underside of humanism, registers appreciative awareness of the courage summoned and the indignities endured to get what one needs to make a life." Betcher, "Crippling Donald Trump's 'Crippled America,'" 145, quotation slightly altered.

55 Hauerwas, *Suffering Presence*, 200–201.

56 Hauerwas, *Suffering Presence*, 197.

57 The widespread overprescription of calming drugs (such as opioid analgesics) to people in institutions has been noted by many, including Heslop et al., *CIPOLD*, 46. Wen and Kosowsky even suggest personalized genetic medicine is a technique that attempts to formalize the replacement of listening to patent's accounts of their condition. *When Doctors Don't Listen*, 146–47.

58 Paul Shrier, "Messengers of Hope: A Boy with Autism, His Church, and the Special Olympics," *Journal of Disability & Religion* 21, no. 2 (2017): 230–44.

59 Creamer, *Disability and Christian Theology*, ch. 3.

60 More would need to be said about how theologically to understand the responsibilities of both parents *and* physicians to advocate for the best interests of the child, the parameters of which are well surveyed by Wannenwetsch, in "Loving the Limit," 96–99.

Chapter 7: Health in a Fallen World

1 Betcher, "Crippling Donald Trump's 'Crippled America,'" 143.

2 Dolmage, *Disability Rhetoric*, 31–61.

3 Hans G. Ulrich, "Bonhoeffer's Work—Challenging the Ethical Approach in the Field of Bioethics for a Critical Hermeneutics of Life: Shared Insights from a Multiple Dialogue," in Wüstenberg, Heuser, and Hornung, *Bonhoeffer and the Biosciences*, 169–74; see also Stefan Heuser, "Bonhoeffer and Bioscience: Dialogues on the Hermeneutics of Life," in that same volume, pp. 13–26.

4 Brendan Kelly, "Priesthood and Handicap—Some Personal Reflections," in *A Prophetic Cry: Stories of Spirituality and Healing Inspired by L'Arche*, ed. Tim Kearney (Dublin: Veritas, 2000), 86–96, quotation from 91–92.

5 Anne O'Sullivan, "The White Stone," in Kearney, *Prophetic Cry*, 98–104, quotation from 101–2.

6 The language is Debbie Creamer's, who describes the problem of sin as

> "Me versus Myself: Living a lie in relation to oneself." This lie recognizes that we tend to hold inaccurate self-representations, especially insofar as we deny or depreciate our own limits. This is closely related to traditional notions of sin . . . that sin is either thinking too highly of ourselves (pride, ignoring our own limits) or too lowly of ourselves (sensuality, defining ourselves solely based on our own limits). Lying about limits allows us to construct the categories of we and they, of able and disabled. This lie conditions us to believe that wearing glasses is normal but using a hearing aid is not (unless one is "old"), convinces us that it is a disability not to walk but normal not to fly, and highlights adaptive technology "for the disabled"

while blinding us (pun intended) to technological aids that are designed to adapt to other situations (e.g., a spacesuit, which may be the ultimate prosthesis). The lie that comes from a rejection of our own limits may at first be one of perception, but, just as . . . with the other lies, it eventually leads to the perpetration of injustices that cause harm to self and other beings and that impact the health and even survival of the body of God. (*Disability and Christian Theology*, 71.)

In a world where God is apparently silent or dead, many thinkers have been unsettled by the apparent paucity of conceptual materials available to stem the will to power that can no longer find grounds to preserve the givenness and proximity of the neighbor as a barrier or limit to human designs. The theologies of both Rosenzweig and Bonhoeffer are part of this movement. Benjamin Lazier, *God Interrupted: Heresy and the European Imagination between the World Wars* (Princeton: Princeton University Press, 2008), ch. 13.

7 Even amidst seemingly inexplicable events there is a "knowledge of God" in his living agency to be had and into which people can grow. "The leading question then becomes how God's Spirit may guide [creatures'] understanding toward what it will direct their eyes to see." Reinders, *Disability, Providence, and Ethics*, 160.

8 Judges 6:24; Eph 2:14. John Swinton, *From Bedlam to Shalom* (New York: Peter Lang, 2000), 53–63.

9 The Apostle Paul's approach is both informative and exemplary for the Christian theologian in that he does not set out definitions of these doctrinal themes in a discrete and sequential fashion but displays how the terms cohere as a pregnant linguistic constellation. The coherence on display in these words is also the template for the life of the apostle who writes them. In Paul, Christians are offered a worked exemplification of what is entailed in confessing one's self to be a Christian, an apostle, and a writer. His life displays why something crucial is lost if the hermeneutical and intertextual texture of theology is extracted from analysis of Christian moral existence. These claims are developed in more detail in Brian Brock and Bernd Wannenwetsch, *The Malady of the Christian Body: A Theological Exposition of Paul's First Letter to the Corinthians*, vol. 1 (Eugene, Ore.: Cascade Books, 2016), 53–62.

Medi Ann Volpe usefully surveys contemporary attempts to rethink the concept of *imago Dei* in light of the experience of disability without falling into the rationalist tenor of many traditional formulations. "Irresponsible Love: Rethinking Intellectual Disability, Humanity, and the Church," *Modern Theology* 25, no. 3 (2009): 491–501.

10 Bonhoeffer's *Creation and Fall* should be read as an extended exploration of the thematic unity of this very constellation of doctrinal themes as well as the theological method and style Paul exemplifies here. Only five months before he delivered the lectures published as *Creation and Fall*, Bonhoeffer took this complex of themes up in a two-part sermon preached on Col 3:1-4 in Berlin in 1932. Bonhoeffer, "Sermon Preached on Colossians 3:1-4 in Berlin in 1932," in *Ecumenical, Academic, and Pastoral Work: 1931–1932*, ed. Victoria J. Barnett, Mark Brocker, and Michael B. Lukens, Dietrich Bonhoeffer Works 11 (Minneapolis: Fortress, 2012), 450–65.

11 Bonhoeffer, "Sermon Preached on Colossians 3:1-4," 459, emphasis added.

12 It is often assumed in the theological and ethical discussions of health that the influential definition of the World Health Organization (WHO) is sufficient for the task. Not genuflecting to this, the WHO definition is to part ways with much of the discussion of disability and health. The reasons why simple agreement with the WHO definition is

theologically problematic are surveyed by Neil Messer, who also usefully outlines the problems that bedevil all such purportedly "value free" definitions of health. Messer, *Flourishing: Health, Disease, and Bioethics in Theological Perspective*, ch. 1.

13 Glatzer, *Franz Rosenzweig*, 138–42.

14 Glatzer, *Franz Rosenzweig*, 174–76.

15 "A thing receives a character of its own only within the flow of life. The question, 'what is this actually?' detached from time, deprived of it, quickly passes through the intermediate stage of the general term and comes into the pale region of the mere 'thing' [des Dinges überhaupt]. Thus emerges the concept of the one and only substance, the 'essential' nature of things. The singleness and particularity of the subject [Eigenheit des Gegenstandes] detached from time is transformed into a statement of its particular essence [Eigentlichkeit des Wesens]." Rosenzweig, quotation in Eric Santner, *On the Psychotheology of Everyday Life: Reflections of Freud and Rosenzweig* (Chicago: University of Chicago Press, 2001), 21.

16 Timothy Chappell, *Knowing What to Do: Imagination, Virtue and Platonism in Ethics* (Oxford: Oxford University Press, 2014), 282.

17 Chappell, *Knowing What to Do*, 160; Karłowicz, *Archparadox of Death*, 241.

18 Hilary Putnam, "Introduction" to Franz Rosenzweig's *Understanding the Sick and the Healthy: A View of World, Man, and God*, ed. and trans. Nahum Glatzer (Cambridge, Mass.: Harvard University Press, 1999), 9; Stanley Cavell, *The Claim of Reason: Wittgenstein, Relativism, Morality, and Tragedy* (New York: Oxford University Press, 1979), part 4.

19 As Rosenzweig put it in a letter to his mother, "The chief thing is not whether one 'believes' in the good Lord; what matters is that he opens all his five senses and sees the facts—at the risk that even the good Lord may be found among the facts." Cited in Putnam, "Introduction" to *Understanding the Sick and the Healthy*, 25. At this point Rosenzweig is also drawing on early modern German Romantics, such as Goethe's *Westlöstlicher Diwan*, which is appended as an epigraph in the English translation of *Understanding the Sick and the Healthy*.

> If we
> But perceived in proper time, how bland
> The truth would be, how fair to see!
> How near and ready to our hand!

20 Putnam, "Introduction" to *Understanding the Sick and the Healthy*, 31.

21 Glatzer, *Franz Rosenzweig*, 222.

22 "Things insist on their privilege of being named and going by a name." Rosenzweig, *Understanding the Sick and the Healthy*, 73.

23 Rosenzweig, *Understanding the Sick and the Healthy*, 72.

24 "There is no one for whom the Word of God is not meant, whose present is not implied by it; the word of humans implies the presence of the speaker and someone to whom the speech is addressed—and so also with the word of God." Rosenzweig, *Understanding the Sick and the Healthy*, 73.

25 "It is necessary for him to free himself from those stupid claims that would impose Juda-'ism' on him as a canon of definite, circumscribed 'Jewish duties' (vulgar orthodoxy), or 'Jewish tasks' (vulgar Zionism), or—God forbid—'Jewish ideas' (vulgar liberalism). If he has prepared himself quite simply to have everything that happens to him, inwardly and

outwardly, happen to him in a *Jewish way*—his vocation, his nationality, his marriage, and even, if that has to be, his Juda-'ism'—then he may be certain that with the simple assumption of that infinite pledge he will become in reality 'wholly Jewish.'" Glatzer, *Franz Rosenzweig*, 222–23. In one move Rosenzweig is simultaneously challenging *theistic dogmatisms* that attempt to circumvent human realities and material contexts, *humanisms* that assume they can sustain ethical lives without making universal truth claims or a final judge, and *materialist empiricisms* that presume that human life can happily proceed without seriously engaging moral and metaphysical claims.

26 "The historicity of the miracle of Revelation is not its content—this content is and remains its present actuality—but its ground and its guarantee." Franz Rosenzweig, *Star of Redemption*, trans. Barbara E. Galli (Madison: University of Wisconsin Press, 2005), 198. The fundamental difference between them is their different accounts of law.

27 Rosenzweig, *Understanding the Sick and the Healthy*, 82–83.

28 Santner, *On the Psychotheology of Everyday Life*, 119.

29 "He bears a name for our sake, so that we may call Him. It is for our sake that He permits Himself to be named and called by that name, since it is only by jointly calling upon Him that we become a 'We.'" Rosenzweig, *Understanding the Sick and the Healthy*, 91.

30 Rosenzweig, *Understanding the Sick and the Healthy*, 93, citing Deut 30:14.

31 Santner, *On the Psychotheology of Everyday Life*, 120.

32 "Moses and Aaron said to all the Israelites, 'In the evening you shall know that it was the Lord who brought you out of the land of Egypt, and in the morning you shall see the glory of the Lord, because he has heard your complaining against the Lord'" (Exod 16:6-7). The story foreshadows the more blatant rebellion of the Israelites at the very moment when God constitutes the people of Israel by giving the Ten Commandments on Sinai recounted in Exod 19.

33 Santner, *On the Psychotheology of Everyday Life*, 30–31. Santner labels this dynamic "Egyptomania," but in a treatment of disability it is important to be as precise as possible when specific diagnoses are introduced. I will therefore use the language of "Egypt obsession" which more precisely locates the problem of flight from reality not as an uncontrollable ecstasy but in a mental fixation on the past that, if exposed, can be rationally recognized as keeping them from recognizing what is most important in their present—and thus can be fought if the individual (or collective) so wills.

34 "Abraham had faith, and had faith for this life. In fact, if his faith had been only for a life to come, he certainly would have more readily discarded everything in order to rush out of a world to which he did not belong. But Abraham's faith was not of this sort, if there is such a faith at all, for actually it is not faith but the most remote possibility of faith that faintly sees its object on the most distant horizon but is separated from it by a chasmal abyss in which doubt plays its tricks." Kierkegaard, *Fear and Trembling*, 20. Kierkegaard's resistance to the sorts of faith that barricade believers against disappointment in this world is a common type of psychological defense mechanism that will be labeled in ch. 7 "Canaan obsession."

35 Santner, *On the Psychotheology of Everyday Life*, 44–45.

36 Rosenzweig believed that Franz Kafka had grasped with great profundity the predicament of fallen humans, especially in his novel *The Castle*. The tragedy of the human situation is to have eaten from the tree of knowledge and been cut adrift from life with God, while God from his side has separated himself from us by barring the way back to his tree of life. Rosenzweig sees in Kafka a worked-out awareness of the ocean of estrangement

that this unleashes into the human experience. "With the expulsion from Paradise man lost his name (Kafka's heroes go mainly by initials), lost his language (there is no real communication), lost his love (only sex remains); time which could now be man's is but confused, distorted, paralyzed eternity. Man (Kafka), World (village), and God (castle) exist, but their existences are not correlated." Putnam, "Introduction" to *Understanding the Sick and the Healthy*, 31–32.

37 Rosenzweig has Spinoza's God in mind here.

38 Rosenzweig, *Understanding the Sick and the Healthy*, 52–53.

39 Santner, *On the Psychotheology of Everyday Life*, 89.

40 Rosenzweig draws this claim from the Song of Songs 8:6: "Love is as strong as death." See discussion in Robert Gibbs, *Correlations in Rosenzweig and Levinas* (Princeton: Princeton University Press, 1992), ch. 4.

41 See Samuel Moyne, *Origins of the Other: Emmanuel Levinas between Revelation and Ethics* (Ithaca: Cornell University Press, 2005), 146–47.

42 By giving us reasons for this definition of estrangement, Rosenzweig helps us to make sense of Bonhoeffer's (nontraditional) insistence that "every one of us is also the 'first' sinner." Bonhoeffer, *Creation and Fall*, 115.

43 "And yet—love would not be the moving, the gripping, the searing experience that it is if the moved, gripped, seared soul were not conscious of the fact that up to this moment it had not been moved nor gripped. Thus, a shock was necessary before the self could become a beloved soul." Rosenzweig, quoted in Santner, *On the Psychotheology of Everyday Life*, 84.

44 "Not out of his own essence and out of the purity of his own heart does he discover the other, but out of the *happening* which happed to him and the deafness of his heart." Rosenzweig, quoted in Santner, *On the Psychotheology of Everyday Life*, 91

45 Richard A. Cohen, *Elevations: The Height of the Good in Rosenzweig and Levinas* (Chicago: University of Chicago Press, 1994), ch. 1.

46 Quoted in Santner, *On the Psychotheology of Everyday Life*, 112.

47 An emphasis on the Israel as simultaneously a historical and suprahistorical entity is a response to the dominant Hegelian accounts of history from Jewish-German philosophers between the two World Wars recounted by Susan Handelman in *Fragments of Redemption: Jewish Thought and Literary Theory in Benjamin, Scholem, and Levinas* (Bloomington: Indiana University Press, 1991).

48 Santner, *On the Psychotheology of Everyday Life*, 100–110; Moyne, *Origins of the Other*, 152.

49 "Thus at last we discover something which is the companion of everything, including every event which takes place in the world, and yet is external to them all: the Word. Language is not the world, nor does it make such claims. What actually is it? Unlike 'thought,' language cannot presume to be the 'essence' of the world. If the world is something which permits the existence of other things exterior to the world but not its essence, there is only one thing that language can be; it must be a bridge between the world and these other things." Rosenzweig, *Understanding the Sick and the Healthy*, 70–71.

50 It may come as a surprise to find that this Jewish thinker's ideas resonate strongly with those of the Christian theologian Dietrich Bonhoeffer. Lazier's *God Interrupted* explains why the second edition of Barth's *Römerbrief* proved a fertile meeting point for so many Jewish and Christian intellectuals in the interwar years and is more specifically related to Rosenzweig in Rashkover's *Revelation and Theopolitics*.

51 Bonhoeffer, *Creation and Fall*, 31–38.

52 Bonhoeffer, *Creation and Fall*, 57.
53 Bonhoeffer, *Creation and Fall*, 57.
54 Bonhoeffer, *Creation and Fall*, 63. "How can what is created be free? What is created is determined, bound by law, condition, not free. If the Creator wishes to create in the Creator's own image, then the Creator must create [the human] free. And only such an image, in its freedom, would fully praise God, would fully proclaim God's glory as Creator." Bonhoeffer, *Creation and Fall*, 61.
55 "In the free creature the Holy Spirit worships the Creator; uncreated freedom glorifies itself in view of created freedom." Bonhoeffer, *Creation and Fall*, 63–64.
56 Bonhoeffer, *Creation and Fall*, 85.
57 Bonhoeffer, "The Pious Question," in *Creation and Fall*, 103–14; *Ethics*, 381–87.
58 Bonhoeffer, *Creation and Fall*, 118.
59 Bonhoeffer, *Creation and Fall*, 87.
60 Bonhoeffer, *Creation and Fall*, 91.
61 Bonhoeffer, *Creation and Fall*, 116.
62 Bonhoeffer, *Creation and Fall*, 116–17.
63 Bonhoeffer, *Creation and Fall*, 98.
64 Wannenwetsch, "Loving the Limit," 102.
65 Bonhoeffer, *Creation and Fall*, 67.
66 Alasdair MacIntyre, *Dependent Rational Animals: Why Human Beings Need the Virtues* (Chicago: Open Court, 1999).
67 Bonhoeffer, *Creation and Fall*, 64.
68 Bonhoeffer, *Creation and Fall*, 79.
69 Bonhoeffer, *Creation and Fall*, 123.
70 "Self-centered, emotional love can never comprehend spiritual love, for spiritual love is from above." Bonhoeffer, *Life Together*, 43.
71 Bonhoeffer, *Life Together*, 43–47.
72 Bonhoeffer, *Life Together*, 44.
73 Hans Ulrich, "The Messianic Contours of Evangelical Ethics," in *The Freedom of a Christian Ethicist*, ed. Brian Brock and Mike Mawson (London: Continuum, 2015), 39–64.
74 Andrew Errington, "Every Good Path: Wisdom and Practical Reason in Christian Ethics and the Book of Proverbs" (PhD diss., University of Aberdeen, 2017).
75 Rowan Williams, "The Body's Grace," in *Theology and Sexuality: Classic and Contemporary Readings*, ed. Eugene F. Rogers Jr. (Oxford: Blackwell, 2002), 309–21.
76 Anne Gibson, "Entertaining Angels—A Faith and Light Experience," in Kearney, *Prophetic Cry*, 47–59, quotation from 54.
77 Tim Kearney, "The Upside-Down Kingdom," in Kearney, *Prophetic Cry*, 68–83, quotation from 71.
78 Interview with Vanier in Kearney, *Prophetic Cry*, 138.
79 John McCullagh, "The Prophetic Voice of the Poor," in Kearney, *Prophetic Cry*, 25–35, quotation from 29–30.
80 Stanley Hauerwas, "Why Jean Vanier Matters: An Exemplary Exploration," in *Knowing, Being Known, and the Mystery of God: Essays in Honor of Professor Hans Reinders: Teacher, Friend, and Disciple*, ed. Bill Gaventa and Erik de Jongh (Amsterdam: VU University Press, 2016), 229–39.
81 Tom Shakespeare, "Still a Health Issue," *Disability and Health Journal* 5 (2012): 129–31.
82 Elizabeth Barnes has labeled this "testimonial injustice." Barnes, *Minority Body*, ch. 4.

83 "Dogmatically speaking, we can say that Jesus as healer testifies to the incarnational dimension of Christian theology, underscoring the embodied and experiential character of Christian faith, as well as God's relation to, and taking part in all dimensions of human life with concern, care, mercy, and compassion." Henriksen and Sandnes, *Jesus as Healer*, 248.

84 "Modern western people . . . do not seem to live in a cosmos where we are able genuinely to believe that God *could* intervene in and override nature's laws. So, while modern Western Christians still readily pray for God to act providentially for the good of all and out of mercy, within what is possible in the natural order, so bizarre is the very notion of 'the miracle'—something that is naturally impossible—that we have no genuine expectation that we could even *ask* God to do a miracle. In reality, we only believe in God's activity where it is mediated to us through naturally understandable means. We cannot conceive of the actions of God outside of such mediation. A big part—actually, the very heart—of the world view of the New Testament (the miraculous) is lost to us, and we tend to read the Christian scriptures largely as a collection of exotic narratives and doctrinal propositions to be interpreted in discretely moral and theological terms. We no longer expect miracles to be part of the normal Christian life. It seems that David Hume's view of miracles has won in the west. We now tend to assume that any 'surprising' singular work of God—in time and space, yet beyond the bounds of natural law—is impossible, irrational, and embarrassingly naïve, or worse." Tyson, "Wounds of Faith and Medicine," 334–35.

85 Michael Nausner, "Participating in Christ: Therapeutic Dimensions in Christian Discipleship from a Wesleyan Perspective," in Wendte, *Jesus der Heiler*, 99–116.

86 Robert Vosloo, "Body and Health in the Light of the Theology of Dietrich Bonhoeffer," *Religion & Theology* 13, no. 1 (2006): 23–37, quotation from 36.

Chapter 8: Autism and Christian Hope

1 Young, *Face to Face*, 142. The divine claim that comes through other human beings is less visible in theologies that are oriented by a quest for "spiritual experience" or in Christian theologies that understand the realm of the "religious" as a numinous experience of the holy, as Rudolf Otto famously defended it in *The Concept of the Holy*. Traditional Christian theology strikes a very different stance to religious studies with its focus on describing "spiritual experience" as essentially related to special capacities of human agents. The Christian theology explored in this book assumes that God's self-revealing generates human insight framed by the thoughts, forms, and practices of a tradition that positions us in the world in a particular manner.

2 *Krisis* literally means "judgment" and is closely related to *apokalypsis*, meaning "manifesting or disclosing the truth." The Gospel of Matthew provides a sampling of the usage of *krisis* in the New Testament. See Matt 5:21-22; 10:15; 11:22, 24; 12:18, 20, 36, 41-42; 23:23, 33. *Apokalypsis* appears less frequently in the other Gospels (Luke 3:2) and is more regularly used by Paul. See Rom 2:5; 8:19; 16:25; 1 Cor 1:7; 14:6, 26.

The Greek term *krisis* is largely negative in valence (in that judgment is most often understood as a negative and exposing act) and is to be distinguished from *epiphany* meaning "manifestation" or "appearing." This positive vision of divine presence was christologically worked out in the New Testament, which the early Christians called in the Latin translation *adventus* (associating Christ with the pomp of an arriving political ruler) or associated with the *annunciation* of this rule (taken from the angelic annunciation of this coming ruler, Luke 1:26-38), which is as positive and particular as the incarnation that it heralds. Noticing the relative weighting of negative and positive valences in these two approaches is crucial.

3 If being trained into the language of the Christian tradition can foster *recognition* of this revelatory and redemptive work, this is not to suggest that new skills or capacities must be given in order to respond to it. Quite the opposite. God's capacity to communicate Godself *despite* human capacities and incapacities helpfully limits from the outset any claim that there might be some level of cognitive limitation below which people would be unable to respond to God. One secular thinker who has succinctly grasped this point is Alain Badiou in *Saint Paul: The Foundations of Universalism*, trans. Ray Brassier (Stanford: Stanford University Press, 2003). For a highly developed and influential Christian theological treatment of the theme see Karl Barth, *Church Dogmatics* 1/1, paragraph 4, and *Church Dogmatics*, 1/2, paragraphs 19–21.

4 Young, *Face to Face*, 62.

5 Young, *Face to Face*, 62, 63.

6 Framing autism within general conceptions like "religion" or "spirituality" abandons the claim that the language and conceptual structure of Christian belief purports to *reveal* the world. Terms like "spirituality" and "religion" are second order descriptions that do not necessarily emerge from any particular religions, and sometimes obscure the generative concepts of Christian theology. See John Swinton and Stephen Pattison, "Moving beyond Clarity: Towards a Thin, Vague, and Useful Understanding of Spirituality in Nursing Care," *Nursing Philosophy* 11 (2010): 226–37.

7 Steve Silberman's history of autism offers a perspicacious account of the rise of the diagnostic category of autism which is sensitively embedded in a string of more detailed accounts of the lives of people who lived before and after that diagnosis was invented. *Neurotribes: The Legacy of Autism and How to Think Smarter about People Who Think Differently* (London: Allen and Unwin, 2015).

8 "A wry saying popular in the autistic community, 'if you meet one person with autism, you've met one person with autism,' turns out to be true even for molecular biologists . . . . Most researchers now believe that autism is not a single unified entity but a cluster of underlying conditions. These conditions produce a distinctive constellation of behavior and needs that manifests in different ways at various stages of an individual's development. Adequately addressing these needs requires a lifetime of support from parents, educators, and the community, as Asperger predicted back in 1938." Silberman, *Neurotribes*, 14, 496. Olga Bogdashina, herself the parent of two autistic children, offers what is in my view the most persuasive accounting of the current state of scientific evidence. She holds that sensory impairments are the common denominator underlying these widely diverse autistic symptoms. Bogdashina, *Autism and the Edges of the Known World: Sensitivities, Language, and Constructed Reality* (London: Jessica Kingsley, 2010).

9 There is anxiety in some quarters at medicine's inability to prevent and cure autism. Some see this as deeply frustrating and threatening, even as a war-worthy threat, which is why the hawkish American Republican senator Ted Cruz proposed, and the hawkish American president George W. Bush officially signed into American law, funding for a medical assault on autism that was immediately dubbed the "war on autism." Anne McGuire, "'Life Worth Defending': Biopolitical Frames of Terror in the War on Autism," in Tremain, *Foucault and the Government of Disability*, 350–71. Sensing the problem here, some autism charities have intentionally distanced themselves of any talk

of "finding a cure for autism." Allison Fox, "Why Autism Speaks Dropped the Word 'Cure' From Its Mission Statement," *Huffington Post*, October 18, 2016.

10 See Thomas Sowell, "Autism Crusade Will Backfire on Children," *Redding.com*, November 14, 2007.

11 Luther gives us purchase on the soteriological implications of our conceptual beliefs and affective attachments with a pithy summary of the biblical witness: Your God is where you hang your heart. "A god is that to which we look for all good and in which we find refuge in every time of need . . . . The trust and faith of the heart alone make both God and an idol . . . . That to which your heart clings and entrusts itself is, I say, really your God." Martin Luther, "Large Catechism," in *The Book of Concord: The Confessions of the Evangelical Lutheran Church*, ed. T. G. Tappert (Philadelphia: Fortress, 1959), 365.

12 John Gillibrand, *Disabled Church, Disabled Society: The Implications of Autism for Philosophy, Theology and Politics* (London: Jessica Kingsley, 2010), 39, emphasis added. "As a bit of an aside, instead of tutting, staring or glaring at what you might think is the behavior of a naughty or spoiled child, it would ease the lives of families enormously if you could simply ignore the minor disruption to your life or just smile. . . . As the years passed, the responses of unknown others became less stinging and pretty much faded into irrelevance. Regular disruptions in public spaces become so commonplace that they evolved into a source of fascination and occasional amusement." Ryan, *Justice for Laughing Boy*, 43–44.

13 Reynolds, *Vulnerable Communion*, 113.

14 The novelist Kim Edwards captures the metamorphosis. Finding herself unexpectedly forced into raising a baby girl with Down syndrome, "set something into motion . . . For Caroline Gill was thirty-one, and she had been waiting a long time for her real life to begin." Kim Edwards, *The Memory Keeper's Daughter* (London: Penguin, 2005), 25.

15 Ryan, *Justice for Laughing Boy*, 31.

16 This complex of changes is nicely encapsulated in the rare Hollywood depiction of an autistic life, *Temple Grandin*, a 2010 biopic directed by Mick Jackson and starring Claire Danes.

17 "Going out in public with my [autistic] brother is risky. Inevitably, if I take him into a store, he manages to run out wildly, usually with stolen cans or bottles of caffeinated soda—a banned substance in his new institutional home. Humor and alliance are tools that we rely on to endure these risks. We look for alliances with strangers—cashiers, restaurant patrons, bystanders—who can respond with humor and not anxiety. We seek out alliances with his paid attendants; I know he has someone special if they laugh with us. When going public fails to go well, we recover by making the misadventure into a new yarn, laughing about the door he tore off the frame, the pants he took off in public, or the food he stole from the strangers at KFC." Simplican, *Capacity Contract*, 133.

18 Reynolds, *Vulnerable Communion*, 116.

19 John Swinton, *Becoming Friends of Time: Disability, Timefullness, and Gentle Discipleship* (Waco, Tex.: Baylor University Press, 2016).

20 Bynum, *Metamorphosis and Identity*, 19–21.

21 "Since the days of the pre-Socratics, change has been seen in the Western tradition as both horror and glory. If there is real replacement, we can after all both lose and transcend the self. And in the writers of the Western mainstream, there has been a tendency to fear these two—loss and transcendence—as the same thing." Bynum, *Metamorphosis and Identity*, 32.

22 Amos Yong is the most outspoken defender of this position and states it this way:

> Human bodies that are the temple of the Holy Spirit in this life (1 Cor 3:19, 6:19-20) anticipate being hosts of the resurrecting power of the same Spirit in the life to come. The resurrection body is hence both continuous with and yet transformed—sanctified and even beautified—by the life-giving Spirit of God . . . Precisely because the meanings of our lives are constituted by but irreducible to our bodies, so also will the resurrected body be the site through which the meaning of our narratives are transformed (and that eternally). . . . I further speculate that people with intellectual or developmental disabilities, such as those with Down Syndrome or triplicate chromosome 21—will retain their phenotypical features in their resurrection bodies. There will be sufficient continuity to ensure recognisability as well as self-identity. Thus, the redemption of those with Down Syndrome, for example, would consist not in some magical fix of the twenty-first chromosome but in the recognition of their central roles both in the communion of the saints and in the divine scheme of things. (Yong, *Theology and Down Syndrome*, 279, 282, 283.)

Though I will not pursue the argument here, it would also be possible to show that this modern anthropological appropriation of the patristic discussion of resurrection does not sufficiently engage the fact that these discussions were primarily focused less on recognition and more on the problem of changeable flesh being resurrected into eternal unchangeability. Caroline Walker Bynum, *The Resurrection of the Body in Western Christianity, 200–1336* (New York: Columbia University Press, 1995), 34–50.

23 Yong, *Theology and Down Syndrome*, 259–69.

24 The worry about the continuity of identity in the resurrection was more traditionally related to the problem of gathering scattered bodies and the desecration of improper burial: "the context of martyrdom, within which so much early theological writing emerged, made continuity of body important also. Irenaeus and Tertullian avoided any suggestion that the attainment of impassibility or glory entailed a loss of the particular self that offered up its own death for Christ. Identity was a crucial issue. As Tertullian said, all death (even the gentlest) is violent; all corpses (even the most respectfully buried) rot. Resurrection guarantees that it is *these very corpses* that achieve salvation. The promise that *we* will rise again makes it possible for heroes and ordinary Christians to face, for those they love and revere as well as for themselves, the humiliation of death and the horror of putrefaction. . . . Nothing can make the body unclean—neither nocturnal emissions of semen, nor menstruation and childbearing, nor even the putrefaction of the tomb. We Christians do not abominate a dead man because we know he will life again." Bynum, *The Resurrection of the Body*, 46–47, emphasis in original.

25 First John 3:2. Janet Martin Soskice, *The Kindness of God: Metaphor, Gender, and Religious Language* (Oxford: Oxford University Press, 2007), 76, 181–83.

26 Yong, *Theology and Down Syndrome*, 268–70.

27 Douglas Knight, *The Eschatological Economy: Time and the Hospitality of God* (Grand Rapids: Eerdmans, 2006), ch. 5.

28 Second Corinthians 6:16-18. Grant Macaskill, "Autism Spectrum Disorders and the New Testament: Preliminary Reflections," *Journal of Disability & Religion* 22, no. 1 (2018): 15–41, 28–30.

29 Jesus' presentation of his own works of healing makes this point unambiguously clearly, as in the paradigmatic healing of the paralyzed man lowered through the roof in Mark 2:1-12.

30 Though in sympathy with the range of considerations brought to bear in Yong's chapter on eschatology, I am inverting the order of his investigation in which discussion of the perfection of resurrected bodies precedes and situates discussion of reconciled human relationships. "If disability is never only a matter of individual embodiment but is always also an economic, political, and social experience, then the heavenly hope must redeem not only individual bodies *but also* heal and reconcile human relationships." Yong, *Theology and Down Syndrome*, 285, emphasis added.

31 Karłowicz, *Archparadox of Death*, 216–25; Bynum, *Resurrection of the Body*, 42–43.

32 One of the instabilities of Yong's argument is the extent to which he thinks of identity as what people generally recognize or whether he considers this identity in Christ determinative. Yong, *Theology and Down Syndrome*, 273–74.

33 See Matt 5:27-29. The phrase is Ola Sigurdson's (*Heavenly Bodies*, 190).

34 Paul Ramsey, *Basic Christian Ethics* (Louisville: Westminster John Knox, 1993), 94.

35 Here I wholeheartedly agree with Yong, *Theology and Down Syndrome*, 262.

36 The language is from Yong, *Theology and Down Syndrome*, 291.

37 Yong is well aware of the crucial importance of social reconciliation for a disability theology, but his account of it is fundamentally pneumatological. The upshot is that the central feature of eschatology is a shift in the Spirit's work, from reconciling relationships to also remaking bodies in heaven. Yong, *Theology and Down Syndrome*, 184–88, 278–81.

38 Silberman, *Neurotribes*, 17

39 Hauerwas, "Timeful Friends: Living with the Handicapped" and the response of Michael Bérubé, "Response: Making Yourself Useful," in *Critical Reflections on Stanley Hauerwas' Theology of Disability: Disabling Society, Enabling Theology*, ed. John Swinton, 11–26 and 31–36 (Binghamton, N.Y.: Hayworth Pastoral, 2004).

40 Yong's discussion of eschatology does end with a reminder that a "healed" future begins in the present; "the doctrine of the resurrection is not only a speculative idea concerning the life to come but also a concrete set of mandates regarding the Christian way of life in the here and now." Yong, *Theology and Down Syndrome*, 290. My proposal follows Francis Young's in working from the knowledge-how that is an essential part of Christian worship. Young dares not speculate what she and her son Arthur's resurrected bodies will be like, "but I do think that there will be a continuity between what we are now and what we will be then. . . . We will both be renewed. And we both have some inkling in the present of what that renewed life will be like, because we experience it in the fellowship and sacraments of the church." Young, *Face to Face*, 107.

41 "Emaciation displeases not us; for it is not by weight that God bestows flesh, any more than He does 'the Spirit by measure.' More easily, it may be, through the 'straight gate' of salvation will slenderer flesh enter; more speedily will lighter flesh rise; longer in the sepulcher will drier flesh retain its firmness." Tertullian, *On Fasting* 17, in *Ante-Nicene Fathers*, vol. 4: *Tertullian, Minucius Felix, Commodianus, Origen*, ed. Alexander Roberts and James Donaldson (Grand Rapids: Eerdmans, 1979). Elsewhere Tertullian carefully negotiates the concerns Yong has laid out (in common with much patristic thought). See his *On Resurrection*.

42 Augustine, *City of God* 22.13.

43 Augustine, *City of God* 22.14.

44 Augustine, *City of God* 22.15.
45 Augustine, *City of God* 22.17–18.
46 Augustine, *City of God* 22.19.
47 Augustine, *City of God* 22.20.
48 Augustine concludes as follows, differing only from Yong in suggesting that our infirmities will be immediately, rather than gradually healed. "So then: all are to rise with a body of the same size as they had, or would have had, in the prime of life. But it would in any case be no hardship even if the form of the body were to be that of a child or an old man, provided that no infirmity of mind or body remained. Thus, even if someone contends that everyone will rise with the same kind of body as he had when he died, we need not devote too much effort to the task of arguing the point with him." Augustine, *City of God* 22.16.
49 Even emphasizing the revelatory aspect of eschatology does not diffuse the problem of moral projection. It is almost impossible not to project culturally dominant images of health and happiness onto resurrection bodies. When, after the death of an infant that was by any account severely deformed, no less than three people independently came and told his parents that they had had visions of "a young boy with blondish hair and a striped shirt running while playing" (Cobb, *Loving Samuel*, 59–61) two questions should immediately be raised. Augustine asks: will this child have *no* signs of his vocation on earth in the resurrection? And Barth follows: would we be offended if he was resurrected bearing marks of that strange vocation? See discussion in Don Wood, "Barth on the Concrete Freedom of Human Life," in Brock and Swinton, *Disability in the Christian Tradition*, 392–93.
50 Hans G. Ulrich, *Eschatologie und Ethik: Die Theologische Theorie der Ethik in ihrer Beziehung auf die Rede von Gott siet Freidrich Schliermacher* (Munich: Chr. Kaier Verlag, 1988); Bernd Wannenwetsch, "Representing the Absent in the City: Prolegomena to a Negative Political Theology According to Revelation 21," in *God, Truth, and Witness: Engaging Stanley Hauerwas*, ed. L. G. Jones, R. Hütter, and C. R. Velloseo Ewell (Grand Rapids: Brazos, 2005), 167–92.
51 The Greek work translated "generous" here is *agathos*, the same goodness that Mark 10:18 and Luke 18:19 highlight is God's own work.
52 A theme also prominent in the character of the older brother in the parable of the prodigal son (Luke 15:25-30).
53 Cf. Ps 80:10-16; Isa 5:1-10; Matt 21:33-46; Mark 12:1-2; Luke 20:9-19.
54 The theme of the appearance of eschatological judgment as well as the problem of pious self-absorption is developed in more detail in Brock and Wannenwetsch, *Malady of the Christian Body*, 67–70.
55 See Hall, *Conceiving Parenthood*, chs. 1–2.
56 The phrase is from Wannenwetsch, *Political Worship*, 230.
57 The line comes from Rabbi Nahman of Bratzlav's *Tale of the Seven Beggars*, quoted in Yong, *Theology and Down Syndrome*, 289.
58 In an academic context such assertions are often accused of being "idealized" accounts of worship. Contemporary congregational studies suggest that such complaints are much more plausible to wealthy and comfortable Christians than those whose social location is much like the distinctly less well-heeled Christians of the first centuries. See Susan J. Dunlap, *Caring Cultures: How Congregations Relate to the Sick* (Waco, Tex.: Baylor University Press, 2009), ch. 1.

59 The idea is central to both Eastern and Western traditions. For the most influential Western assertion of this position see Augustine, *City of God* 19.24.

60 Thomas E. Reynolds, "Love without Boundaries: Theological Reflections on Parenting a Child with Disabilities," *Theology Today* 62 (2005): 193–209, quotation from 201, emphasis added.

61 M. A. Screech, *Laughter at the Foot of the Cross* (Boulder, Colo.: Westview, 1999), 37–39; Stanley Hauerwas, *The Work of Theology* (Grand Rapids: Eerdmans, 2015), ch. 12, "How to Be Theologically Funny," 229–49.

62 Luther, *Lectures on Genesis*, 3:156.

63 Bernd Wannenwetsch, "The Liturgical Origin of the Christian Politeia: Overcoming the 'Weberian' Temptation," in *Church as Politeia: The Political Self-Understanding of Christianity*, ed. Christoph Stumpf and Holger Zaborowski (Berlin: Walter de Gruyter, 2004), 322–40, reference to 333.

64 Bustion, "Autism and Christianity," 653–81.

65 A limited amount of good historical work has been done to uncover historical examples of the church functioning as a *community* that can carry and even value human difference, specifically autistic difference. See Christine Trevett, "Asperger's Syndrome and the Holy Fool: The Case of Brother Juniper," *Journal of Religion, Disability & Health* 13, no. 2 (2009): 129–50.

66 Reynolds, *Vulnerable Communion*, 53.

67 Thomas E. Reynolds, "Theology and Disability: Changing the Conversation," *Journal of Religion, Disability and Health* 16 (2012): 37. "A new conversation needs to begin that takes as it premise that disability is not a problem to be fixed or cured but an intrinsic feature of fragile and diverse human life that ought to be accommodated through concerted attention to removing barriers to a full social life and the resources necessary to engage in it. This is to highlight how language of disability covers a contested domain for problems of distributive justice that is acute in neoliberal societies, whose very definition of citizenship assumes that disability will be governed according to an ethics of normalization and minimization." Fiona Kumari Campbell, "Legislating Disability: Negative Ontologies and the Government of Legal Identities," in Tremain, *Foucault and the Government of Disability*, 108–30, quotation from 119.

68 Reynolds, "Theology and Disability," 33.

69 Reynolds' term.

70 Reynolds, "Theology and Disability," 39–40. Thanks to Martina Vuk for stimulating me to think much harder about the centrality of human vulnerability.

Chapter 9: Beyond Inclusion

1 "For people with disabilities, then, inclusion is often experienced via logic that is exclusionary at first (based on binary figuration), and subsequently assimilative (normalizing), all in the name of care and doing good." Reynolds, "Theology and Disability," 44–45. The problem is not that churches aim to widen their welcome, but "the mistaken assumption on which they are based: the need for an act of inclusion that, in turn, rests on an abstract and preconceived concept of personhood that is to be merely applied to disabled human life, instead of being won from a perceptive understanding of the phenomenon itself. . . . If we wish to transcend the ill-fated discourse of 'inclusion' and 'ascription,' we must be sensitized to the role that discovery or even revelation plays in this recognition process." Wannenwetsch, "Angels with Clipped Wings," 183–84.

2 Reynolds, "Theology and Disability," 45.

3 Jean-Francois Ravaud and Henri-Jacques Stiker, "Inclusion/Exclusion: An Analysis of Historical and Cultural Meanings," in *Handbook of Disability Studies*, ed. Gary L. Albrecht, Katherine D. Seelman, and Michael Bury (Thousand Oaks, Calif.: Sage, 2001), 490–515; Colin Barnes and Geoff Mercer, "Disability Culture: Assimilation or Inclusion," in Albrecht, Seelman, and Bury, *Handbook of Disability Studies*, 515–35. The internal conflicts and confusion of the various contemporary conceptualizations of inclusion are surveyed in Stacy Clifford Simplican, Geraldine Leader, John Kosciulek, and Michael Leahy, "Defining Social Inclusion of People with Intellectual and Developmental Disabilities: An Ecological Model of Social Networks and Community Participation," *Research in Developmental Disabilities* 38 (2015): 18–29.

Disability theology has had a largely reactive response to this, "the last civil rights movement," explicitly discussed in Nancy L. Eiesland, "Barriers and Bridges: Relating the Disability Rights Movement and Religious Organizations," in *Human Disability and the Service of God: Reassessing Religious Practice*, ed. Nancy L. Eiesland and Don E. Saliers (Nashville: Abingdon, 1998), 200–229; Jennie Weiss Block, *Copious Hosting: A Theology of Access for People with Disabilities* (New York: Continuum, 2002), 17–19; Eiesland, *Disabled God*, 19–20. For an account of the biographical complexities of this conceptual and existential synchronization of secular and theological uses of inclusion language see W. Graham Monteith, *Visibly Invisible: A Pilgrimage as a Disabled Minister* (Guildford, U.K.: Grovesnor House, 2010), chs. 2, 6.

4 Maarten Simons and Jan Masschelein, "Inclusive Education," in Tremain, *Foucault and the Government of Disability*, 208–28, quotation from 209.

5 Frances Young, for instance, finds in 1 Cor 12:21b-23a an intimation of the salutary shock that "unpresentable" members force on modern societies bent on performance and perfection, so representing Christ the outsider and challenger of convention. Frances M. Young, *Brokenness and Blessing: Towards a Biblical Spirituality* (London: Darton, Longman and Todd, 2007), 98–99.

6 Nancy Eiesland, for instance, reads 1 Cor 12:12-13, 27 as enjoining Christians to recognize the value of the created diversity of human life and so to commit to the struggle already under way for justice through full inclusion and accessibility. Eiesland, *Disabled God*, 108–9, 111. Jennie Weiss Block follows a similar procedure by elucidating the "gospel mandate" for churches to closely examine whom their practices and attitudes have excluded from full communion. Citing 1 Cor 12:20-22, she explains that this mandate destroys all forms of condescension and understands the gift of the Holy Spirit to be the comforting of those who have been thus excluded and looked down upon. Weiss Block, *Copious Hosting*, 120–22, 140–41.

7 Stewart D. Govig, *Strong at the Broken Places: Persons with Disabilities and the Church* (Louisville: Westminster John Knox, 1989), 118; Stephanie O. Hubach, *Same Lake, Different Boat: Coming alongside People Touched by Disability* (Philipsburg, N.J.: P&R Publishing, 2006), 175.

8 Arne Frison and Samuel Kabue, *Interpreting Disability: A Church of All and for All* (Geneva, Switzerland: World Council of Churches, 2004), 17; Michael S. Beates, *Disability and the Gospel: How God Uses Our Brokenness to Display His Grace* (Wheaton, Ill.: Crossway, 2012), 17–19, 63–64.

9 Taking 1 Cor 12:20-26 as his main text, Thomas Reynolds emphasizes Christ's teaching that all humans are vulnerable and needy to highlight the importance of weakness as a

central category for defining humans in general. This leads him to position disabilities as given realities that are themselves gifts to the church. Precisely because "disability is accorded less respect in the church, it should be privileged and accorded special respect and honor." Reynolds, *Vulnerable Communion*, 231–38. In an earlier essay he developed an idea that comes close to my own, the idea that Paul's image of the body depicts a politics emerging from a heightened empathy and connectivity among Christians. Empathy augmentation retrains Christian sympathies in the body of Christ much like neuromuscular reflex therapy. Repatterning physical behaviors remake people's neural (empathetic) connections. Brent Webb-Mitchell, "Crafting Christians into the Gestures of the Body of Christ," in Eiesland and Saliers, *Human Disability and the Service of God*, 267–80.

10 Like Vanier and several of the other authors just mentioned, in *Beyond Accessibility* Brent Webb-Mitchell also places his emphasis on disabled people being more than *welcome* in the church—rather, as *integral* to it. He ties this point much more explicitly both to the secular discourse of inclusion, and to details of the text of 1 Cor. 12. However, his call to empathy and care in the ecclesia makes Paul's theme of weakness much less central by laying greater weight on Paul's injunction to all believers to take on the "mind of Christ." He concludes that before Christ no one is disabled. Brent Webb-Mitchell, *Beyond Accessibility: Toward Full Inclusion of People with Disabilities in Faith Communities* (New York: Church Publishing, 2010), cf. chs. 2–4, esp. 61–65.

11 Two recent books dwell at some length on the theology of Paul with the aim of setting out a fully rounded theological account of inclusive community. Amos Yong's *The Bible, Disability, and the Church* comments directly on the biblical text in the course of developing a full biblical theology of disability. Within the context of the biblical canon as a whole, 1 Cor 12 is taken to be the biblical *locus classicus* and paradigm account of the politics of ecclesial inclusion. Amos Yong, *The Bible, Disability, and the Church: A New Vision of the People of God* (Grand Rapids: Eerdmans, 2011), esp. 90–95. Earlier versions of Yong's position can be found in "Disability and the Gifts of the Spirit: Pentecost and the Renewal of the Church," *Journal of Pentecostal Theology* 19, no. 1 (2010): 76–93; and *Theology and Down Syndrome*, 204–5, 218–19. In *Epistles of Inclusion*, W. Graham Monteith focuses more narrowly on the Pauline biblical canon while going into more detail than Yong on many of the interpretative questions. Monteith maps the conceptual convergences between Paul's argument and the modern concept of inclusion. Monteith, however, is more critical of previous interpretations of Christian accounts of inclusion, and specifically of the deployment of Pauline language of "the weaker member," which he feels have unnecessarily limited the contributions expected from parishioners with disabilities to the life of the church. He criticizes the approach of Stanley Hauerwas for instrumentalizing disabled people for the spiritual advancement of others as well as representatives of the L'Arche movement who, while treating people with disabilities as genuine participants in the ecclesial community, still too directly equate Paul's "weaker members" with disabled persons. W. Graham Monteith, *Epistles of Inclusion: St. Paul's Inspired Attitudes* (Guildford: Grovesnor House, 2010), esp. chs. 3–4. Statements like this one from Alasdair MacIntyre draw his most heated censure. "A great many people initially write off the disabled, not recognizing how much there is to be learnt not only from them and with them. Only by learning from such others can we rid ourselves of illusions of self-sufficiency, illusions that stand in the way of our recognizing our need for some of the virtues that we need to flourish." Alisdair MacIntyre, from Alex Voorhoeve, *Conversations on Ethics* (Oxford: Oxford University Press, 2009), 130. Hauerwas

often echoes this formulation of MacIntyre. See Hauerwas' *Suffering Presence*, 175–77; and *Dispatches from the Front: Theological Engagements with the Secular* (Durham: Duke University Press, 1994), 177–78. Hans Reinders can also fall into a similar narrowing in comments such as, "*The* mission of people with disabilities . . . consists in what being with them can teach *us*." Reinders, *Receiving the Gift of Friendship*, 310, emphasis added.

12 "Another fundamental text for L'Arche is 1 Cor. 12, which remains an enigma for me." Jean Vanier, in Stanley Hauerwas and Jean Vanier, *Living Gently in a Violent World*, 36. Vanier later comments, less modestly, that the chapter "is the heart of faith, what it means to be the church . . . In other words, people who are the weakest and least presentable are indispensable to the body" (74). This sentiment was already evident in the 1989 first edition of Vanier's foundational *Community and Growth*, in which the dominant imagery is arguably that of the community conceived as a body exchanging spiritual gifts and anchored in its vulnerable members (as seen especially 1 Cor 12:22, 24-26). Vanier, *Community and Growth*, 49.

Vanier's seminal work on friendship is surveyed in Jason Reimer Greig, *Reconsidering Intellectual Disability: L'Arche, Medical Ethics, and Christian Friendship* (Washington, D.C.: Georgetown University Press, 2015), ch. 6. Vanier's account of friendship provides the theological core of Hans Reinders' *Receiving the Gift of Friendship*. These appropriations develop a more explicit ontological grounding for Vanier's account of friendship based on the perichoretic divine self-giving. The redemption of human relationships is positioned as flowing out of this intertrinitarian love, via the work of the Holy Spirit, to create a community of friendship.

13 Both Yong and Monteith explicitly discuss these three questions at a sophisticated level (theologically and in terms of the experience of disability, if not exegetically), though Monteith does so at more length.

14 I cannot here set out in detail my exegetical reasoning for this reading of the opening of the chapter. Interested readers may consult Brian Brock and Bernd Wannenwetsch, *The Therapy of the Christian Body: A Theological Exposition of Paul's First Letter to the Corinthians, Volume 2* (Eugene, Ore.: Cascade Books, 2018), 73–76.

15 Ralph Martin, "Gifts, Spiritual," in *The Anchor Bible Dictionary*, vol. 2, ed. David Freedman (New York: Doubleday, 1992), 1015–18; James D. G. Dunn, *Jesus and the Spirit: A Study of the Religious and Charismatic Experience of Jesus and the First Christians as Reflected in the New Testament* (London: SCM Press, 1975), ch. 8.

16 The Greek term is *charizesthai*. James D. G. Dunn, *The Theology of Paul the Apostle* (Grand Rapids: Eerdmans, 1998), 553.

17 Paul is not offering a typology of three sorts of distinct entities. Spiritual gifts are not like trophies to be collected, but something that are *already* present in the congregation, as he emphasized at the outset of the letter. "I give thanks to my God always for you because of the grace of God that *has been given* you in Christ Jesus." 1 Cor 1:4. The NRSV translation of *eisin* as "there are" obscures this point. If translated instead, "There *is* different *apportioning* of gifts" it becomes clear that Paul is extending his previously elaborated resistance to the Corinthian desire to accumulate more prestigious spiritual gifts, in 1 Cor 1:11-15.

18 Gerhard Kittel, ed., *Theological Dictionary of the New Testament*, vol. 2, trans. and ed. Geoffrey W. Bromiley (Grand Rapids: Eerdmans, 1964), 652–54.

19 They are gifts because God *has* given them and refer neither to God's unseen desires to bestow these at some future date nor to latent capacities in the individual that must be brought to life by training or development.

20 Anthony Thiselton, *The First Epistle to the Corinthians: A Commentary on the Greek Text* (Grand Rapids: Eerdmans, 2000), 936.

21 Gerhard Friedrich, ed., *Theological Dictionary of the New Testament*, vol. 9, trans. and ed. Geoffrey W. Bromiley (Grand Rapids: Eerdmans, 1974), 6.

22 Having emphasized the *moment* of discovery as a marker of spiritual gifts and the concurrent need to affect a principled dissociation of the *charisma* from social role and status, it should be noted that this is not an absolute, but a relative independence. The *independence* of the Spirit's gifts from individual capacities needs to be underlined to mark out the appropriate space for the Holy Spirit's operation to actively donate instead of merely provide. But it is a *relative* independence because room for discovery may well entail discovery of natural talents that might have been suppressed or hidden from the person herself as well as others, but which might only now become the occasion for God to give to the body through this person what it needs.

It would be foolish to stress the principled independence of professional roles from spiritual gifts. To do so would produce a dogmatic insistence on nonconvergence that would disallow, for example, an accountant being the church treasurer when someone who was available was clearly unable to count. Any decision made in principle and in advance about whether someone's spiritual gifts will line up or not with their worldly roles ignores the decisive factor: whether the communicative sensitivity a member has to the body and to other members is either hampered or nourished by the arrangement of which they are made part. To take a different example: while the spirit of pragmatic arrangement that ties together natural talent or social role with *charisma* would intuitively suggest the busy teacher of the local kindergarten as the ideal leader of the church's crèche, the grumpy old lady who has been there every Sunday for ages and without fail, due to her "nervous connection" to the church and the children in their midst, might be offering precisely the gift that really matters for this peculiar ministry.

23 The explosive rise of monasticism in early Christianity can be read as a recognition of the inextricable reliance of *koinonia* on *energema*:

> "It is impossible, indeed," adds Basil [in his monastic rule], "to rejoice with him who receives an honor or to sympathize with him who suffers when, by reason of their being separated from one another, each person cannot, in all likelihood, be kept informed about the affairs of his neighbor." In the community of life (*en tēi tēs zōēs koinoniai*), by contrast, the gift of each becomes common to those who live together with him (*sympoliteuomenōn*) and the activity (*energeia*) of the Holy Spirit in each is communicated to all others. On the contrary, "he who lives alone . . . and has, perhaps, one gift renders it ineffectual through inoperativity (*dia tēs argias*) since it lies buried within him (*katoryxas en eautōi*)." (Giorgio Agamben, *The Highest Poverty: Monastic Rules and Form-of-Life*, trans. Adam Kotsko [Stanford: Stanford University Press, 2013], 9.)

My reading of 1 Cor 12 diverges from Basil's account of the problem of believers having no contact with each other. I contend that the problem of lack of physical presence is not a problem because they keep the gifts of the Holy Spirit "buried within them," but that they are not in the position to enact gifts of service that the Spirit must give to others through them, and to them through others in turn. In other words, they do not discover who they are meant to be because they are not in community. The most fundamental isolation of the believer is the refusal to enter that "in-between" space that is the operating theater of the Holy Spirit.

24 Friedrich, *Theological Dictionary of the New Testament*, 405.

25 Dunn, *Theology of Paul the Apostle*, 559–60. "According to the New Testament, the church is to exemplify—to some extent—a collective way of life that is enabled by the miraculous *dynamis* of the very Spirit of the living God. This *dynamis* is active in this world, as a foretaste of the eschatological world to come. The church is thus a very human and this-world-concerned community, but it is not *just* a human community (2 Corinthians 4:7), and its engagement with the world is always eschatologically and miraculously framed." Tyson, "Wounds of Faith and Medicine," 330–31.

26 Yung Suk Kim, *Christ's Body in Corinth: The Politics of a Metaphor* (Minneapolis: Fortress, 2008); Ernst Käsemann, "The Theological Problem Presented by the Motif of the Body of Christ," in *Perspectives on Paul*, trans. Margaret Kohl (London: SCM Press, 1971), 102–21.

27 Andreas Lindemann, "Die Kirche als Leib: Beobachtungen zur 'demokratischen' Ekklesiologie bei Paulus," *Zeitschrift für Theologie und Kirche* 92 (1995): 143–46. Lindemann identifies four principal ways the metaphor was applied, referring to passages in the works of Plato, Aristotle, Cicero, Livy (who cites Menenius Agrippa), Seneca, Epictetus, and others. See also M. Eugene Boring, Klaus Berger, and Carsten Colpe, *Hellenistic Commentary to the New Testament* (Nashville: Abingdon, 1995), 694–96. Victor Paul Furnish, *The Theology of the First Letter to the Corinthians* (Cambridge: Cambridge University Press, 1999), 89n17.

28 Livy, *Historia*, 2.32.9–12, translated in Dunn, *Theology of Paul the Apostle*, 550n103.

29 The NRSV translation overreaches at this point. *Hutous kai ho christos* has no verb, and if literally rendered would read, "for just as the body is one and has many members . . . so too the Christ."

30 Gerhard Kittel, ed., *Theological Dictionary of the New Testament*, vol. 4, trans. and ed. Geoffrey W. Bromiley (Grand Rapids: Eerdmans, 1967), 561–65.

31 Paul is taking account of the related New Testament language of Christ as the "head" of the church in this depiction.

32 Mark 2:2-12 and par. The story, it should be emphasized, highlights the important fact that Jesus does not pursue the blind, the lame, the cripple, or the leper to heal them. They come to him with the request for healing, and Jesus sees this as legitimate faith. But had they simply asked for forgiveness of sins, we have no indication he would have imposed healing on them against their will (as is rightly protested when it occurs in modern healing institutions).

33 Amy Julia Becker, "The Ministry of the Disabled," *Christianity Today* 62, no. 4 (May 2018): 34ff.

34 Wannenwetsch, *Political Worship*, 305.

35 Such an ecclesial recognition of the gift of healing would need to be oriented by a theological account of healing along the lines of the one offered at the end of chapter 7.

36 "The deepest truth behind anything, whether it be a body in nature or an event in history, is the relationship with God that it mediates; this relational truth can never be known except by the '*Affekt* of friendship,' the relational form of knowing exhibited in friendship. . . . our own selves and psyches, no less than nature and history, are relational

media; *loci* in which God can consolidate his relationship with us . . . empirical, experiential knowing is the true essential medium of knowledge, yet the end of knowledge is not material; or at least, no more material than human love." Gwen Griffith Dickson, *Johann Georg Hamann's Relational Metacriticism* (Berlin: Walter de Gruyter, 1995), 67–68.

37 Raymond F. Collins, *First Corinthians* (Collegeville, Penn.: Liturgical, 1999), 460.

38 The human body has a communicative surface by which individuals are present to one another. This claim is more explicitly developed by Paul's reasoning as he criticizes some of the Corinthian Christians who are visiting brothels and others who are ostentatiously eating meat offered to idols in chs. 6, 7, and 11.

39 John Chrysostom, *Homily* 29, cited in Judith Kovacs, trans. and ed., *1 Corinthians: Interpreted by Early Christian Commentators* (Grand Rapids: Eerdmans, 2005), 201.

40 Bernd Wannenwetsch, "'Members of One Another': *Charis*, Ministry and Representation: A Politico-Ecclesial Reading of Romans 12," in *A Royal Priesthood? The Use of the Bible Ethically and Politically: A Dialogue with Oliver O'Donovan*, ed. Craig Bartholomew, Jonathan Chaplin, Robert Song, and Al Wolters (Carlisle, U.K.: Paternoster, 2002), 196–220.

41 Reynolds, *Vulnerable Communion*, 237–38; Webb-Mitchell, *Beyond Accessibility*, 64–65; Yong, *Bible, Disability, and the Church*, 92–93; Yong, *Theology and Down Syndrome*, 222; Monteith, *Epistles of Inclusion*, 73, 77–78, 84. My reading comes closest to that of Young, *Brokenness and Blessing*, 98–100; and Vanier, *Community and Growth*, 47–49.

42 Cf. Brian Dillon, *Tormented Hope: Nine Hypochondriac Lives* (London: Penguin, 2010).

43 The full quote reads: "Adam and Eve not only were ashamed because of their nakedness, which previously was most honorable and the unique adornment of man, but they also made girdles for themselves, as though it were something most shameful, that part of the body which by its nature was most honorable and noble. What in all nature is nobler than the work of procreation?" Luther, *Lectures on Genesis*, 1:167, comment on Gen 3:7.

44 Giorgio Agamben, *The Church and the Kingdom*, trans. Leland de la Durantaye (London: Seagull Books, 2012); Giorgio Agamben, *The Use of Bodies*, trans. Adam Kotsko (Stanford: Stanford University Press, 2016), 273–74.

45 See discussion in Kelly S. Johnson, *The Fear of Beggars: Stewardship and Poverty in Christian Ethics* (Grand Rapids: Eerdmans, 2007), ch. 1.

46 Chrysostom, *Homily* 29, quoted in Kovacs, *1 Corinthians*, 208.

47 Chrysostom, *Homily* 29, quoted in Kovacs, *1 Corinthians*, 208.

48 This formulation draws on the work of Peter Capretto, who discerns this pattern in contemporary disability theology, specifically the work of Nancy Eiesland, Amos Yong, and John Swinton. Capretto, "On Not Operationalizing Disability in Theology," 902–7.

49 My account is very close to Reynolds at this point, though he does not explicitly tie *energema* and *diakonia* as I have argued Paul does in this chapter, deploying instead the more diffused language of "Spirit infused relationship." *Vulnerable Communion*, 235–40.

50 Kelly S. Johnson, "Interceding: Poverty and Prayer," in *The Blackwell Companion to Christian Ethics*, 2nd ed., ed. Stanley Hauerwas and Sam Wells (Oxford: Blackwell 2011), 246–48.

51 Again, my account comes close to that of Reynolds in intentionally drawing on the language of the "in between" originating in the ethics of Paul Ricoeur. Affirming the importance of those insights, the burden of my treatment here is to show how, at least in this chapter of the New Testament, these insights are set within a much more robustly Trinitarian, pneumatological, and so ecclesial frame of reference than is found in the philosophical literature. Reynolds, "Love without Boundaries," 193–209.

52 In this my experience parallels that described by Thomas Reynolds.

> Chris's genuine otherness continually breaks through my self-pity and astonishes me as something surprisingly precious in its own right. His is a young life seeking to affirm itself, thwarted by conditions that he did not ask for and for which he is not responsible. This vulnerability and beauty rouse me to attend to him in ways that lure me outward beyond self-preoccupation. The first taste of this conjures something akin to repentance. Confronted by Chris's vulnerability, I am humbled and brought to recognize how my own needs, expectations, and ideals have closed me in on myself and set up boundaries that condition and thereby limit my capacity to be open toward him, to be there with and for him in *his* struggle. On occasions too numerous to mention, parenting has highlighted my own shortcomings, my own poverty and brokenness as a human being. ("Love without Boundaries," 200.)

53 Consider also Sarah Williams, *The Shaming of the Strong: The Challenge of an Unborn Life* (Lottbridge Drove, U.K.: Life Journey/Kingsway Communications, 2005).

54 The challenge to the church in suggesting that if it is to rejoice and suffer with the most disabled, is that new forms of bodily communication will need to be explored that allow us to respond in ecclesial life as well to the divine invitation that they hold out into a genuine pneumatic giving and receiving. There is work going on in churches that is exemplary in this regard, as well as research that attempts to highlight the issues of communication that I have raises as they shape care in long term care homes. For the former see Björn Nalle Öhman, *Kropp, handling och ritual: hur förstå religion och personer med grava funktionshinder?* [trans. "Body, Action, and Ritual: How to Understand the Relation between Religion, and People with Severe Disabilities?"] (Åbo, Finland: Åbo Akademis förlag, 2008). For the latter, see Hans S. Reinders and Lydia Helwig Nazarowa, *Looking for Quality: Assessing Quality of Care in Long Term Services, toward a Narrative Approach* (unpublished conference paper).

55 Stanley Hauerwas, personal communication, July 30, 2018.

Chapter 10: A Remarkable Stroke in a Strange and Remarkable War

1 Michelle Gray, Haley Cripps and Avneet Johal, *British Social Attitudes Survey: Attitudes Toward the Rights of Disabled People*, Research Report 588 (Norwich, U.K.: Department of Work and Pensions, 2009).

2 Susan Schweik, *The Ugly Laws: Disability in Public* (New York: New York University Press, 2009).

3 Bernd Wannenwetsch, "But to *Do* Right . . . Why the Language of 'Rights' Does Not Do Justice to Justice," *Studies in Christian Ethics* 23, no. 2 (2010): 138–46.

4 David Brooks, "The Organization Kid," *Atlantic Monthly* 287, no. 4 (2001): 40–54.

5 "Harlan Hahn, a leader in the disability rights movement and disability studies, once joked that people with disabilities were a cultural minority because they, like other minorities, shared a cultural diet: fast-food drive-throughs. Drive-throughs side stepped the difficulties of physical and social barriers. Eating and living in private—due to physical and stigmatizing barriers—has defined what it has meant to be disabled. Being disabled *and* public can change what it means to be disabled and, at the same time, change the dynamics of the public—as a physical and political space." Simplican, *Capacity Contract*, 119.

6 Reinders, *Future of the Disabled in Liberal Society*, 14.
7 Wannenwetsch, *Political Worship*, 305–6.
8 I here recounted our experience at Blacknall Presbyterian Church in Durham, North Carolina.
9 This depiction of the communion of saints has been schooled by Orthodox Christians. Traditional Orthodox cathedrals are circular at their base and topped by a dome open to sunlight and are covered in gold leaf. The circularity represents eternity, as does the gold leaf, and at the top of the dome the sun's light represents the throne of God. Circling the walls and surrounding the communion table are icons of the saints, whose eyes and hands are artistically emphasized. The intentional effect of the whole is to present the church's worship as the vestibule of heaven and to remind living worshipers that they are vastly outnumbered by those who have preceded them. Victoria Hammond, *The Dome in European Architecture* (Princeton: Princeton Architectural Press, 2005), 164–69; Mathews, *Clash of the Gods*, ch. 6.
10 Jeffrey Stout, *Democracy and Tradition* (Princeton: Princeton University Press, 2004).
11 Wannenwetsch, *Political Worship*, 229–30.
12 "Monstrosity" has given way to "moron," then "retarded," then "handicapped," "disabled," and now "having special needs" or "a learning disability." Reinders, *Receiving the Gift of Friendship*, 45–46.
13 Tom Greggs, *Theology against Religion: Constructive Dialogues with Bonhoeffer and Barth* (New York: T&T Clark, 2011).
14 Reinders, *Receiving the Gift of Friendship*, 335n26.
15 Evin Winkelman Richardson and Zolinda Stoneman, "The Road to Membership: The Role of Resilience in Seeking and Maintaining Membership in a Faith Community for Families of Children with Disabilities," *Journal of Disability and Religion* 19, no. 4 (2015): 312–39. Bob Smietana summarizes the obvious first steps for churches who wish to understand and rectify this situation in, "Few Churches Are Autism Friendly," *Facts & Trends.net*, July 30, 2018.
16 Katie Bahr, "Real Presence: What Catholics with Developmental Disabilities Bring to the Table," *U.S. Catholic* 78, no. 12 (2013): 12–17.
17 Simplican, *Capacity Contract*.
18 Many of the stories in this chapter originate in the American South. I have made the perhaps indefensible decision not to highlight the significant threads of race that weave through all these stories, in part to protect some of the characters, and in part to keep the stories focused. To be a white disabled child in Durham, North Carolina, for instance, is to be forced across the race line. Adam was picked up by a black taxi driver for his trip to school, driven over to the black side of town, where he was one of a tiny minority of white children in a sea of black faces. As white Americans, Adam forced us to learn what it means for a black child to be classed as disabled. One school meeting to consider Adam's disability classification was particularly memorable in being attended by no less than a dozen white professionals. Only later did we learn that this overwhelming show of expertise had been arranged because African American parents often resist the labeling of their child as multiply handicapped. There is good reason for this resistance, as such a label virtually guarantees a child will never escape the backwaters of social-service provision. The most heartwarming event of that year was the spontaneous volunteering of a few of Adam's African American elementary school classmates to go through school dining hall trash cans in an attempt to find a missing hearing aid. That is gratuity.

I would love to have done more justice to the racialized aspects of this story. But the subject of disability and race in America deserves its own book. It is a history full of horrors very much ongoing. As J. Kameron Carter once observed to me, the root of these trajectories was the premise of the founding fathers that black people were too intellectually feeble to govern themselves. Dea H. Boster, *African American Slavery and Disability: Bodies, Property, and Power in the Antebellum South, 1800–1860* (New York: Routledge, 2013); Larry M. Logue, *Race, Ethnicity, and Disability: Veterans and Benefits in Post-Civil War America* (Cambridge: Cambridge University Press, 2013); Beth Harry and Janette K. Klingner, *Why Are So Many Minority Students in Special Education? Understanding Race and Disability in Schools* (New York: Teacher's College Press, 2006).

19 Ulrich, *Wie Geschöpfe leben*, ch. A6.

20 Philip Ziegler, *Militant Grace: The Apocalyptic Turn and the Future of Christian Theology* (Grand Rapids: Baker Academic, 2018), ch. 13.

21 See Williams, *Shaming of the Strong*, ch. 25.

22 J. M. Coetzee, *Life and Times of Michael K* (London: Secker & Warburg, 1983).

23 Karłowicz, *Archparadox of Death*, part 2.

24 "It is He first who with a pity which is not idle but active, angry, militant, aggressive and therefore genuine, takes pity on [human kind's] aberration and confusion, its infirmity and misery." Barth, *Church Dogmatics* 4/3.1: *The Doctrine of Reconciliation*, ed. G. W. Bromiley and T. F. Torrance (Edinburgh: T&T Clark, 1961), 328.

25 Barth, *Church Dogmatics* 4/3.1: 240. Translation altered for gender inclusivity.

26 "We humans and even we Christians usually talk past one another except when a miracle occurs. We do this even when we are talking to ourselves. We cannot, then, derive certainty, the certainty of victory, from any genuine superiority in us. But Jesus Christ in His word can and does. He is the Neighbor who can and does really speak to the other as Neighbor to neighbor, and therefore in this sense too, He is superior and radiates certainty." Barth, *Church Dogmatics* 4/3.1: 271–72.

27 "This total inversion is the content of His prophetic Word." Barth, *Church Dogmatics* 4/3.1: 241.

28 Modern developed societies are saturated with discourses of risk and terror which, Anne McGuire observes, "shape the biopolitical enemy as invisible, encroaching, life-threatening, and amoral . . . also work to delimit the terms of responses . . . as both necessary and moral. Vis-à-vis a death-driven enemy, a life loving and life-saving allied warrior is born confronted with an enemy that hides in plain sight [whether an affected conception, an incipient debilitating disease or injury, or a malignant terrorist]. The 'ally' must increase its surveillance techniques, fortify its borders, and hone its techniques of war." McGuire, "'Life Worth Defending,'" 367.

29 Maureen Swinger, "The Teacher Who Never Spoke: How My Brother Who Could Never Walk or Talk Coached Dozens of His Peers into Manhood," *Plough Quarterly* 12 (2017): 18–27, quotation from 26.

30 Thanks to Angelika Bocchetti for this story. On the theology of such peacemaking gestures see Brian Brock and Stephanie Brock, "Disability and Reconciliation: The Old Woman's Model," in *Joining Lives: A Primer on the Ministry of Reconciliation*, ed. Andy Odle (Eugene: Cascade, 2017), 78–88.

31 "Socrates' profession of ignorance was therefore a recognition of reality; not a philosophical doctrine, a methodological doubt, an unassailable position of skepticism—and there is a world of difference between the two. One is a live animal, the other a skeleton. . . .

Socrates' ignorance was the perfect prescription for the faults and follies of his contemporaries; we can fill in for ourselves that Jesus too was sent to the people of his time with the proper antidote to their hypocrisies and errors . . . Socrates no less than Jesus, St. Paul or the Hebrew prophets was sent by God as a witness to the truth." Dickson, *Hamann's Relational Metacriticism*, 48, 54.

32 Plato, *Apology* 30d–31a, in *The Trials of Socrates: Six Classic Texts*, trans. and ed. C. D. C. Reeve (Indianapolis: Hackett, 2002). Cf. 29c–31c.

33 "In short, Socrates lured his fellow citizens from the labyrinths of their learned sophists to a *truth which lay concealed*, to a *secret wisdom* and from the idols' alters of their pious and politically shrewd priests to the service of an unknown God." J. G. Hamann, "Socratic Memorabilia," NII 77, translated in Dickson, *Hamann's Relational Metacriticism*, 395, emphasis in original. Citing Ps 51:6; 1 Cor 2:7; Acts 17:23.

34 Karłowicz, *Archparadox of Death*, 143.

Bibliography

Agamben, Giorgio. *The Church and the Kingdom*. Translated by Leland de la Durantaye. London: Seagull Books, 2012.

———. *The Highest Poverty: Monastic Rules and Form-of-Life*. Translated by Adam Kotsko. Stanford: Stanford University Press, 2013.

———. *Pilate and Jesus*. Translated by Adam Kotsko. Stanford: Stanford University Press, 2015.

———. *The Use of Bodies*. Translated by Adam Kotsko. Stanford: Stanford University Press, 2016.

Albrecht, G. L., Katherine D. Seelman, and Michael Bury, eds. *Handbook of Disability Studies*. Thousand Oaks, Calif.: Sage, 2001.

Alderson, Priscilla. "Down's Syndrome: Cost, Quality, and Value of Life." *Social Science and Medicine* 53 (2001): 627–38.

Almeling, Rene. *Sex Cells: The Medical Market for Eggs and Sperm*. Berkeley: University of California Press, 2011.

Anderson, Chris. *The Long Tail: Why the Future of Business Is Selling Less of More*. New York: Hyperion, 2008.

Annas, Julia. *An Introduction to Plato's Republic*. Oxford: Clarendon, 1981.

Aquinas, Thomas. *Summa Contra Gentiles*. In *Basic Writings of Saint Thomas Aquinas*, vol. 2: *Man and the Conduct of Life*. Edited by Anton C. Pegis. Indianapolis: Hackett, 1997.

———. *Summa Theologica*. 2nd rev. ed. 22 vols. Translated by Fathers of the English Dominican Province. London: Burns, Oates & Washbourne, 1912–1936.

Arendt, Hannah. *The Human Condition*. Chicago: University of Chicago Press, 1958.

Ariès, Philippe. *The Hour of Our Death*. London: Allen Lane, 1981.

Aristotle. *Parts of Animals [De Partibus Animalium]: Movement of Animals. Progression of Animals*. Translated by A. L. Peck and E. S. Forster, 52–435. Cambridge, Mass.: Harvard University Press, 1937.

———. *Politics, Books VII and VIII*. Translated by Richard Kraut. Oxford: Clarendon, 1997.

Arras, John. "The Severely Demented." In Arras and Steinbock, *Ethical Issues in Modern Medicine*, 383–90.

Arras, John, and Bonnie Steinbock, eds. *Ethical Issues in Modern Medicine*. Mountain View, Calif.: Mayfield, 1995.

Asch, Adrienne. "Can Aborting Imperfect Children Be Immoral?" In Arras and Steinbock, *Ethical Issues in Modern Medicine*, 237–40.

———. "Prenatal Diagnosis and Selective Abortion: A Challenge to Practice and Policy." *American Journal of Public Health* 89, no. 11 (1999): 1649–57.

Augustine. *Augustine: Political Writings*. Edited by E. M. Atkins and R. J. Dodaro. Cambridge: Cambridge University Press, 2001.

———. *The City of God against the Pagans*. Edited and translated by R. W. Dyson. Cambridge: Cambridge University Press, 1998.

———. *The City of God, Books VIII–XVI*. Translated by Gerald G. Walsh and Grace Monahan. Washington, D.C.: Catholic University of America Press, 1952.

———. *Confessions*. Translated by Henry Chadwick. Oxford: Oxford University Press, 1991.

———. *Expositions of the Psalms (Enarrationes in Psalmos) 51–72*. Translated by Maria Boulding. Works of St. Augustine 3/17. New York: New City Press, 2001.

———. *Expositions of the Psalms (Enarrationes in Psalmos) 121–150*. Translated by Maria Boulding. Works of St. Augustine 3/20. New York: New City Press, 2004.

———. *The Literal Interpretation of Genesis*. Translated by Edmund Hill. Works of St. Augustine 1/3. New York: New City Press, 2002.

———. *A Treatise on the Merits and Forgiveness of Sins, and on the Baptism of Infants*. In *Nicene and Post-Nicene Fathers* 1/5. Edited by Philip Schaff. Grand Rapids: Eerdmans, 1978.

Badiou, Alain. *Saint Paul: The Foundations of Universalism*. Translated by Ray Brassier. Stanford: Stanford University Press, 2003.

Bahr, Katie. "Real Presence: What Catholics with Developmental Disabilities Bring to the Table." *U.S. Catholic* 78, no. 12 (2013): 12–17.

Bakke, O. M. *When Children Became People: The Birth of Childhood in Early Christianity*. Translated by Brian McNeil. Minneapolis: Augsburg Fortress, 2005.

Banner, Michael. "Children and Commodities: A Commentary on Mantegna's *Adoration of the Magi*." Paper presented at the Research Seminar in Theological Ethics, University of Aberdeen, March 17, 2018.

———. *Christian Ethics: A Brief History*. Chichester, U.K.: Wiley Blackwell, 2009.

———. *Christian Ethics and Contemporary Moral Problems*. Cambridge: Cambridge University Press, 1999.

———. "A Doctrine of Human Being." In *The Doctrine of God and Theological Ethics*, edited by Alan Torrance and Michael Banner, 139–46. London: T&T Clark International, 2006.

———. *The Ethics of Everyday Life: Moral Theology, Social Anthropology, and the Imagination of the Human*. Oxford: Oxford University Press, 2014.

Barlow, Julie, Lesley Powell, and Mollie Gilchrist. "The Influence of the Training and Support Programme on the Self-Efficacy and Psychological Well-Being of Parents of Children with Disabilities: A Controlled Trial." *Complementary Therapies in Clinical Practice* 12 (2006): 55–63.

Barnes, Colin, and Geoff Mercer. "Disability Culture: Assimilation or Inclusion." In Albrecht, Seelman, and Bury, *Handbook of Disability Studies*, 515–35.

Barnes, Elizabeth. *The Minority Body: A Theory of Disability*. Oxford: Oxford University Press, 2016.

Baron, Marcia. "Kantian Ethics and Supererogation." *The Journal of Philosophy* 84, no. 5 (1987): 237–62.

Barth, Karl. "The Christian Community and the Civil Community." In *Community, State, and Church: Three Essays*. Introduced by David Haddorff. Eugene, Ore.: Wipf & Stock, 2004, 149–90.

———. *Church Dogmatics*. 14 vols. Edited by G. W. Bromiley and T. F. Torrance. Edinburgh: T&T Clark, 1936–1977.

———. *Ethics*. Edited by Dietrich Braun. Translated by Geoffrey W. Bromiley. Edinburgh: T&T Clark, 1981.

Basil. *The Letters*. Vol. 2. Edited by Roy J. Deferrari. Loeb Classical Library 215. London: William Heinemann, 1928.

Basselin, Timothy J. *Flannery O'Connor: Writing a Theology of Disabled Humanity*. Waco, Tex.: Baylor University Press, 2013.

Bauman, Zygmunt. *Liquid Fear*. Cambridge: Polity, 2006.

Bayer, Oswald. *Martin Luther's Theology: A Contemporary Interpretation*. Translated by Thomas H. Trapp. Grand Rapids: Eerdmans, 2008.

Beates, Michael S. *Disability and the Gospel: How God Uses Our Brokenness to Display His Grace*. Wheaton, Ill.: Crossway, 2012.

Beauchamp, Tom L., and James F. Childress. *Principles of Biomedical Ethics*. 4th and 6th eds. New York: Oxford University Press, 1994, 2008.

Becker, Amy Julia. "The Ministry of the Disabled." *Christianity Today* 62, no. 4 (2018): 34ff.

Benjamin, Walter. "Excavation and Memory." In Jennings, Eiland, and Smith, *Walter Benjamin*, 576.

———. "Franz Kafka, on the Tenth Anniversary of His Death." In Jennings, Eiland, and Smith, *Walter Benjamin*, 803–7.

Bernstein, Peter L. *Against the Gods: The Remarkable Story of Risk*. New York: John Wiley & Sons, 1998.

Berry, Wendell. *The Unsettling of America: Culture and Agriculture*. San Francisco: Sierra Club Books, 1977.

Bérubé, Michael. "Family Values." In *Mental Retardation in America: A Historical Reader*, edited by Steven Noll and James W. Trent Jr., 494–500. New York: New York University Press, 2004.

———. *Life as We Know It: A Father, a Family, and an Exceptional Child*. New York: Pantheon Books, 1996.

———. "Response: Making Yourself Useful." In Swinton, *Critical Reflections on Stanley Hauerwas' Theology of Disability*, 31–36.

———. *The Secret Life of Stories: From Don Quixote to Harry Potter, How Understanding Intellectual Disability Transforms the Way We Read*. New York: New York University Press, 2016.

Betcher, Sharon V. "Crippling Donald Trump's 'Crippled America.'" In *Faith and Resistance in the Age of Trump*, edited by Miguel A. De La Torre, 137–45. Maryknoll: Orbis, 2017.

———. "Disability and the Terror of the Miracle Tradition." In *Miracles Revisited: New Testament Miracle Stories and their Concepts of Reality*, edited by Stefan Alkier and Annette Weissenrieder, 161–82. Berlin: Walter de Gruyter, 2013.

———. *Spirit and the Politics of Disablement*. Minneapolis: Fortress, 2007.

Biggar, Nigel. *Aiming to Kill: The Ethics of Suicide and Euthanasia*. Cleveland: Pilgrim, 2004.

Bloch, Ernst. *The Principle of Hope*. 3 vols. Translated by Neville Plaice, Stephen Plaice, and Paul Knight. Cambridge, Mass.: MIT Press, 1986.

Block, Jennie Weiss. *Copious Hosting: A Theology of Access for People with Disabilities*. New York: Continuum, 2002.

Bobbit, Philip. *Shield of Achilles: War, Peace, and the Course of History*. London: Penguin, 2003.

Bogdashina, Olga. *Autism and the Edges of the Known World: Sensitivities, Language, and Constructed Reality*. London: Jessica Kingsley, 2010.

Bolens, Guillemette. *The Style of Gestures: Embodiment and Cognition in Literary Narrative*. Foreword by Alain Berthoz. Baltimore: Johns Hopkins University Press, 2012.

Bonhoeffer, Dietrich. *Dietrich Bonhoeffer Works*. 17 vols. Edited by Wayne Whitson Floyd Jr. Minneapolis: Fortress, 1996–2014.

Boring, M. Eugene, Klaus Berger, and Carsten Colpe. *Hellenistic Commentary to the New Testament*. Nashville: Abingdon, 1995.

Boster, Dea H. *African American Slavery and Disability: Bodies, Property, and Power in the Antebellum South, 1800–1860*. New York: Routledge, 2013.

Braithwaite, R. Scott, David O. Meltzer, Joseph T. King Jr., Douglas Leslie, and Mark S. Roberts. "What Does the Value of Modern Medicine Say about the $50,000 per Quality-Adjusted Life-Year Decision Rule? *Medical Care* 46, no. 4 (2008): 349–56.

Brecht, Martin. *Martin Luther: Shaping and Defining the Reformation, 1521–1532*. Minneapolis: Fortress, 1990.

Brock, Brian. "Augustine's Hierarchies of Human Wholeness and Their Healing." In Brock and Swinton, *Disability in the Christian Tradition*, 65–78.

———. "Autism, Care, and Christian Hope." *The Journal of Religion, Disability and Health* 13, no. 1 (2009): 7–28.

———. *Christian Ethics in a Technological Age*. Grand Rapids: Eerdmans, 2010.

———. "Health in a Fallen World: Meditations on the Healthiest Guy I Know." In Wendte, *Jesus der Heiler*, 117–44.

———. "Introduction: Disability and the Quest for the Human." In Brock and Swinton, *Disability in the Christian Tradition*, 1–23.

———. "Looking at 'Us,' Attending to 'Them,' Seeking the Divine: Revisiting *Disability in the Christian Tradition*," *Journal of Religion, Disability and Health*, Special Issue on *Disability in the Christian Tradition* 17, no. 3 (2013): 327–37.

———. "Menschliche Freiheit in der Medizinethik." In *Gezwungene Freiheit? Personale Freiheit in pluralistichen Gesellschaften*, 1st and 2nd eds., edited by Markus Mühling, 222–43. Göttingen, Germany: Vandenhoeck & Ruprecht, 2009.

———. "Mercy, Compassion and the Flesh: On the Inbreaking of Divine Mercy." In Schaeffer, den Hertog, and Paas, *Mercy*, 31–49.

———. "Praise: The Prophetic Public Presence of the Mentally Disabled." In Hauerwas and Wells, *Blackwell Companion to Christian Ethics*, 139–51.

———. "Quality of Life and the Statistical Outlier: On Caring in an Industrialized Age." *The Journal of Disability & Religion* 18, no. 4 (2014): 318–39.

———. *Singing the Ethos of God: On the Place of Christian Ethics in Scripture*. Grand Rapids: Eerdmans, 2007.

———. "Supererogation and the Riskyness of Human Vulnerability." In *The Paradox of Disability: Responses to Jean Vanier and L'Arche Communities from Theology and the Sciences*, edited by Hans Reinders, 127–39. Grand Rapids: Eerdmans, 2010.

———. "Theologizing Inclusion: 1 Corinthians 12 and the Politics of the Body of Christ." *The Journal of Religion, Disability and Health* 15, no. 4 (2011): 351–76.

Brock, Brian, and Stephanie Brock. "Disability and Reconciliation: The Old Woman's Model." In *Joining Lives: A Primer on the Ministry of Reconciliation*, edited by Andy Odle, 78–88. Eugene: Cascade, 2017.

———. "The Disabled in the New World of Genetic Testing: A Snapshot of Shifting Landscapes." In Swinton and Brock, *Theology, Disability and the New Genetics*, 29–43.

Brock, Brian, and Stanley Hauerwas. *Beginnings: Interrogating Hauerwas*. London: Bloomsbury T&T Clark, 2017.

Brock, Brian, and John Swinton, eds. *Disability in the Christian Tradition: A Reader*. Grand Rapids: Eerdmans, 2012.

Brock, Brian, and Bernd Wannenwetsch. *The Malady of the Christian Body: A Theological Exposition of Paul's First Letter to the Corinthians*. Vol. 1. Eugene, Ore.: Cascade Books, 2016.

———. *The Therapy of the Christian Body: A Theological Exposition of Paul's First Letter to the Corinthians*. Volume 2. Eugene, Ore.: Cascade, 2018.

Brock, Brian, and John Wyatt. "The Physician as Political Actor: Late Abortion and the Strictures of Liberal Moral Discourse." *Studies in Christian Ethics* 19, no. 2 (2006): 153–68.

Brock, Brian, Walter Doerfler, and Hans Ulrich. "Genetics, Conversation and Conversion: A Discourse at the Interface of Molecular Biology and Christian Ethics." In Swinton and Brock, *Theology, Disability and the New Genetics*.

Brooks, David. "The Organization Kid." *Atlantic Monthly* 287, no. 4 (2001): 40–54.

Brown, Peter. *The Body and Society: Men, Women, and Sexual Renunciation in Early Christianity*. London: Faber and Faber, 1990.

Brown, William. *The Ethos of the Cosmos: The Genesis of Moral Imagination in the Bible*. Grand Rapids: Eerdmans, 1999.

Brueggemann, Walter. *The Prophetic Imagination*. Minneapolis: Fortress, 2001.

Buchbinder, Mara. "Down's Syndrome Screening and Reproductive Politics: Care, Choice, and Disability in the Prenatal Clinic." *New Genetics and Society* (2017). DOI: 10.1080/14636778.2017.1368375.

Burcham, Phillip. "War Against the Weak: Genetic Counselling and the New Eugenics." *ABC Religion and Ethics*, November 28, 2016.

Burger, Hans. "God's Mercy and Practices of Mercy." In Schaeffer, den Hertog, and Paas, *Mercy*, 99–114.

Bustion, Olivia. "Autism and Christianity: An Ethnographic Intervention." *Journal of the American Academy of Religion* 85, no. 3 (2017): 653–81.

Butler, Judith. *Frames of War: When Is Life Grievable?* London: Verso, 2010.

———. *Precarious Life: The Powers of Mourning and Violence*. London: Verso, 2006.

Bynum, Caroline Walker. *Metamorphosis and Identity*. New York: Zone Books, 2001.

———. *The Resurrection of the Body in Western Christianity, 200–1336*. New York: Columbia University Press, 1995.

Calvin, John. *The Institutes of the Christian Religion*. 2 vols. Translated by Ford Lewis Battles. Philadelphia: Westminster, 1960.

Cameron, Andrew. "A Care for the Aging." Social Issues Executive document. Version 31, May 2011. Anglican Diocese of Sydney.

Camosy, Charles C. *Too Expensive to Treat? Finitude, Tragedy, and the Neonatal ICU*. Grand Rapids: Eerdmans, 2010.

Campbell, Fiona Kumari. "Legislating Disability: Negative Ontologies and the Government of Legal Identities." In Tremain, *Foucault and the Government of Disability*, 108–30.

Campbell, Mary Baine. *Wonder and Science: Imagining Worlds in Early Modern Europe*. Ithaca, N.Y.: Cornell University Press, 1999.

Capretto, Peter. "On Not Operationalizing Disability in Theology." *Journal of the American Academy of Religion* 85, no. 4 (2017): 889–919.

Carlson, Licia. *The Faces of Intellectual Disability: Philosophical Reflections*. Bloomington: Indiana University Press, 2010.

Caspary, Almut. "The Patristic Era: Early Christian Attitudes toward the Disfigured Outcast." In Brock and Swinton, *Disability in the Christian Tradition*, 24–39.

Cavell, Stanley. *The Claim of Reason: Wittgenstein, Relativism, Morality, and Tragedy*. New York: Oxford University Press, 1979.

Chappell, Timothy. *Knowing What to Do: Imagination, Virtue and Platonism in Ethics*. Oxford: Oxford University Press, 2014.

Chrisafis, Angelique. "We're Fifty Years Behind on This: Anger Grows over Treatment of Autistic Children in France." *The Guardian*, February 8, 2018, 33.

Christen, Markus, Christian Ineichen, and Carmen Tanner. "How 'Moral' Are the Principles of Biomedical Ethics?—A Cross-Domain Evaluation of the Common Morality Hypothesis." *BMC Medical Ethics* 15 (2014): 47. DOI: 10.1189/1472-6939-15-47.

Chrysostom, John. "Homily on the Paralytic Let Down Through the Roof: And Concerning the Equality of the Divine Father and Son." *Nicene and Post-Nicene Fathers* 1/9. Edited by Philip Schaff, translated by W. R. W. Stephens. Buffalo, N.Y.: Christian Literature Publishing Co., 1889.

CIBA Foundation Symposium 40. *Embryogenesis in Mammals*. Amsterdam: Elsevier, 1976.

Cicero. *De Officiis*. Edited by G. P. Goold. Loeb Classical Library. Cambridge, Mass.: Harvard University Press, 1913.

Clark, David L., and Catherine Myser. "Being Humaned: Medical Documentaries and the Hyperrealization of Conjoined Twins." In Garland-Thomson, *Freakery*, 338–55.

Clements, Luke, and Janet Read, eds. *Disabled People and the Right to Life: The Protection and Violation of Disabled People's Most Basic Human Rights*. London: Routledge, 2008.

Clifton, Shane. *Crippled Grace: Disability, Virtue Ethics, and the Good Life*. Waco, Tex.: Baylor University Press, 2018.

Clouser, K. Danner, and Bernard Gert. "A Critique of Principlism." *The Journal of Medicine and Philosophy: A Forum for Bioethics and Philosophy of Medicine* 152, no. 1 (1990): 219–36.

Cobb, Aaron D. *Loving Samuel: Suffering, Dependence, and the Calling of Love*. Eugene, Ore.: Cascade, 2014.

Cobb, L. Stephanie. *Divine Deliverance: Pain and Painlessness in Early Christian Martyr Texts*. Oakland: University of California Press, 2017.

Coetzee, J. M. "Confession and Double Thoughts: Tolstoy, Rousseau, Dostoyevsky (1985)." In *Doubling the Point: Essays and Interviews*, edited by David Atwell, 251–93. Cambridge, Mass.: Harvard University Press, 1992.

———. *Life and Times of Michael K*. London: Secker & Warburg, 1983.

Cohen, Richard A. *Elevations: The Height of the Good in Rosenzweig and Levinas*. Chicago: University of Chicago Press, 1994.

Collins, Raymond F. *First Corinthians*. Collegeville, Penn.: Liturgical, 1999.

Connolly, William E. *Capitalism and Christianity, American Style*. Durham, N.C.: Duke University Press, 2008.

Cook, Alyssa F., Vineet M. Arora, Kenneth A. Rasinski, Farr A. Curlin, and John D. Yoon. "The Prevalence of Medical Student Mistreatment and Its Association with Burnout." *Academy of Medicine* 89, no. 5 (2014): 749–54.

Cox, Cathy R., Sara Eaton, Naomi V. Ekas, and Erin A. Van Enkevort. "Death Concerns and Psychological Well-Being in Mothers of Children with Autism Spectrum Disorder." *Research in Developmental Disabilities* 45–46 (2015): 229–38.

Cramm, J. M., and A. P. Nieboer. "Psychological Well-Being of Caregivers of Children with Intellectual Disabilities: Using Parental Stress as a Mediating Factor." *Journal of Intellectual Disabilities* 15, no. 2 (2011): 101–13.

Creamer, Deborah Beth. *Disability and Christian Theology: Embodied Limits and Constructive Possibilities*. New York: Oxford University Press, 2009.

Crislip, Andrew. *From Monastery to Hospital: Christian Monasticism and the Transformation of Healthcare in Late Antiquity*. Ann Arbor: University of Michigan Press, 2005.

Daley, Brian E. "Building the New City: The Cappadocian Fathers and the Rhetoric of Philanthropy." *Journal of Early Christian Studies* 7, no. 3 (1999): 431–61.

———, ed. *Gregory of Nazianzus*. The Early Church Fathers. London: Routledge, 2006.

Danziger, Hillel, and Nosson Scherman. *The ArtScroll Tehillim*. Brooklyn: Mesora Publications, 2001.

Darwin, Charles. *The Expression of the Emotions in Man and Animals*. 3rd ed. Introduction and commentary by Paul Ekman. 1889. London: HarperCollins, 1998.

Daston, Lorrane, and Katherine Park. *Wonders and the Order of Nature: 1150–1750*. New York: Zone Books, 1998.

Dawson, Angus., and E. Garrard. "In Defence of Moral Imperialism: Four Equal and Universal Prima Facie Principles." *Journal of Medical Ethics* 32, no. 4 (2006): 200–204.

de Bruijne, Ad. "Compassion as a Public Virtue." In Schaeffer, den Hertog, and Paas, *Mercy*, 73–86.

de Mooij, Marjolein. "People Are Born from People: Van den Bergh on Mentally Disabled People." In Brock and Swinton, *Disability in the Christian Tradition*, 152–64.

Dickson, Gwen Griffith. *Johann Georg Hamann's Relational Metacriticism*. Berlin: Walter de Gruyter, 1995.

Dillon, Brian. *Tormented Hope: Nine Hypochondriac Lives*. London: Penguin, 2010.

Doherty, Sean. *Theology and Economic Ethics: Martin Luther and Arthur Rich in Dialogue*. Oxford: Oxford University Press, 2014.

Dolmage, Jay Timothy. *Disability Rhetoric*. Syracuse: Syracuse University Press, 2014.

Douglas, Mary. *Purity and Danger: An Analysis of Pollution and Taboo*. London: Routledge Classics, 2002.

Dunlap, Susan J. *Caring Cultures: How Congregations Relate to the Sick*. Waco, Tex.: Baylor University Press, 2009.

Dunn, James D. G. *Jesus and the Spirit: A Study of the Religious and Charismatic Experience of Jesus and the First Christians as Reflected in the New Testament*. London: SCM Press, 1975.

———. *The Theology of Paul the Apostle*. Grand Rapids: Eerdmans, 1998.

Dupré, Louis. *Passage to Modernity: An Essay on the Hermeneutics of Nature and Culture*. New Haven, Conn.: Yale University Press, 1993.

Dworkin, Ronald. *Life's Dominion: An Argument about Abortion and Euthanasia*. London: HarperCollins, 1993.

Edwards, Kim. *The Memory Keeper's Daughter*. London: Penguin, 2005.

Edwards, Mark. *Catholicity and Heresy in the Early Church*. Farnham, U.K.: Ashgate, 2009.

Eiesland, Nancy L. "Barriers and Bridges: Relating the Disability Rights Movement and Religious Organizations." In Eiesland and Saliers, *Human Disability and the Service of God*, 200–229.

———. *The Disabled God: Toward a Liberatory Theology of Disability*. Nashville: Abingdon, 1994.

Eiesland, Nancy L., and Don E. Saliers, eds. *Human Disability and the Service of God: Reassessing Religious Practice*. Nashville: Abingdon Press, 1998.

Einarsdóttir, Jónína. "The Classification of Newborn Children: Consequences for Survival." In Clements and Read, *Disabled People and the Right to Life*, 249–64.

Elliot, Carl. "The Drug Pushers." *Atlantic Monthly* 297, no. 3 (2006): 82–93.

Ellul, Jacques. *Perspectives on our Age: Jacques Ellul Speaks on His Life and Work*. Rev. ed. Edited by Willem H. Vanderburg. Toronto: Anansi, 2004.

———. *The Technological Society*. Translated by John Wilkinson. London: Jonathan Cape, 1964.

Errington, Andrew. "Every Good Path: Wisdom and Practical Reason in Christian Ethics and the Book of Proverbs." PhD diss., University of Aberdeen, 2017.

Eubanks Higgins, Sonja, Patricia McCarthy Veach, Ian M. McFarlane, L. DiAnne Borders, Bonnie LeRoy, and Nancy Callanan. "Genetic Counselling Supervisor Competencies: Results of a Delphi Study." *Journal of Genetic Counselling* 22 (2013): 39–57.

Evans, John H. *Playing God: Human Genetic Engineering and the Rationalization of Public Bioethical Debate*. Chicago: University of Chicago Press, 2002.

Evans, R. J. W. and Alexander Marr. *Curiosity and Wonder from the Renaissance to the Enlightenment*. Aldershot, U.K.: Ashgate, 2006.

Fayers, Peter M., and David Machin. *Quality of Life: Assessment, Analysis, and Interpretation*. Chichester, U.K.: Wiley and Sons, 2000.

Ferngren, Gary B. *Medicine and Health Care in Early Christianity*. Baltimore: John Hopkins University Press, 2009.

———. *Medicine and Religion: A Historical Introduction*. Baltimore: Johns Hopkins University Press, 2014.

Fine, Michael. "Eva Feder Kittay: Dependency Work and the Social Division of Care." In *The Palgrave Handbook of Social Theory in Health, Illness and Medicine*, edited by Fran Collyer, 628–43. New York: Palgrave Macmillan, 2015.

Finley, M. I. *Ancient Slavery and Modern Ideology*. New York: Viking, 1980.

Fitzgerald, Timothy. *Discourse on Civility and Barbarity: A Critical History of Religion and Related Categories*. Oxford: Oxford University Press, 2007.

Flexner, Stuart Berg, ed. *The Random House Dictionary of the English Language*. 2nd ed. New York: Random House, 1987.

Foucault, Michel. *Abnormal: Lectures at the Collège de France, 1974–1975*. Edited by Valerio Marchetti and Vanonela Salomoni. Translated by Graham Burchell. London: Verso, 2016.

———. *The Birth of the Clinic: An Archaeology of Medical Perception*. Translated by A. M. Sheridan Smith. New York: Vintage Books, 1994.

———. *Discipline and Punish: The Birth of the Prison*. Translated by Alan Sheridan. New York: Vintage Books, 1995.

———. *Madness and Civilization: A History of Insanity in the Age of Reason*. Translated by Richard Howard. New York: Random House, 1965.

———. *Society Must Be Defended: Lectures at the Collège de France, 1975–1976*. Translated by David Macey. London: Penguin, 1997.

Fox, Allison. "Why Autism Speaks Dropped the Word 'Cure' From Its Mission Statement." *Huffington Post*, October 18, 2016.

Fox, Renee C., and Judith P. Swazey. *Observing Bioethics*. New York: Oxford University Press, 2008.

Frankena, William. *Ethics*. 2nd ed. Englewood Cliffs, N.J.: Prentice-Hall, 1973.

Friedrich, Gerhard, ed. *Theological Dictionary of the New Testament*. Vol. 9. Edited and translated by Geoffrey W. Bromiley. Grand Rapids: Eerdmans, 1974.

Frison, Arne, and Samuel Kabue. *Interpreting Disability: A Church of All and for All*. Geneva, Switzerland: World Council of Churches, 2004.

Führer, Christian. *Und wir sind dabei gewesen: Die Revolution, die aus der Kirche kam*. Berlin: Ullstein, 2009.

Furnish, Victor Paul. *The Theology of the First Letter to the Corinthians*. Cambridge: Cambridge University Press, 1999.

Gallagher, Stephen, Anna C. Phillips, and Douglas Carroll. "Parental Stress Is Associated with Poor Sleep Quality in Parents Caring for Children with Developmental Disabilities." *Journal of Pediatric Psychology* 35, no. 7 (2010): 728–37.

Gardiner, Dan. *Risk: The Science and Politics of Fear*. London: Virgin Books, 2008.

Garland-Thomson, Rosemarie. *Extraordinary Bodies: Figuring Physical Disability in America*. New York: Columbia University Press, 1996.

———, ed. *Freakery: Cultural Spectacles of the Extraordinary Body*. New York: New York University Press, 1996.

Gaventa, Bill, and Erik de Jongh, eds. *Knowing, Being Known, and the Mystery of God: Essays in Honor of Professor Hans Reinders: Teacher, Friend, and Disciple*. Amsterdam: VU University Press, 2016.

Gayle, Damien. "Family Seek to Replace 'Sarcastic' Coroner after Autistic Daughter Died." *The Guardian*, May 5, 2018. https://www.theguardian.com/society/2018/may/10/family-seek-to-replace-sarcastic-coroner-after-autistic-daughter-died.

Gibbs, Robert. *Correlations in Rosenzweig and Levinas*. Princeton: Princeton University Press, 1992.

Gibson, Anne. "Entertaining Angels—A Faith and Light Experience." In Kearney, *Prophetic Cry*, 47–59.

Gillespie, Michael Allen. *The Theological Origins of Modernity*. Chicago: University of Chicago Press, 2008.

Glatzer, Nahum N., ed. *Franz Rosenzweig: His Life and Thought*. 2nd ed. New York: Schocken, 1961.

Gillibrand, John. *Disabled Church, Disabled Society: The Implications of Autism for Philosophy, Theology and Politics*. Foreword by Rowan Williams. London: Jessica Kingsley, 2010.

Goldingay, John. *Remembering Ann*. Carlisle: Piquant, 2011.

Govig, Stewart D. *Strong at the Broken Places: Persons with Disabilities and the Church*. Louisville: Westminster John Knox, 1989.

Graeber, David. *Debt: The First 5,000 Years*. Brooklyn: Melville House, 2011.

Grant, George. *Lament for a Nation*. Ottawa: Carleton University Press, 1995.

———. *Technology and Empire*. Concord, Ontario: Anansi, 1969.

Gray, Michelle, Haley Cripps, and Avneet Johal. *British Social Attitudes Survey: Attitudes toward the Rights of Disabled People*. Research Report 588. Norwich: Department of Work and Pensions, 2009.

Green, Bernard. *Christianity in Ancient Rome: The First Three Centuries*. London: T&T Clark, 2010.

Greig, Jason Reimer. *Reconsidering Intellectual Disability: L'Arche, Medical Ethics, and Christian Friendship*. Washington, D.C.: Georgetown University Press, 2015.

Greggs, Tom. *Theology against Religion: Constructive Dialogues with Bonhoeffer and Barth*. New York: T&T Clark, 2011.

Gregori , Pavel. "Plato's and Aristotle's Explanation of Human Posture." *Rhizai: A Journal for Ancient Philosophy and Science* 2 (2005): 183–96.

Gregory, Brad S. *Salvation at Stake: Christian Martyrdom in Early Modern Europe*. Cambridge, Mass.: Harvard University Press, 1999.

Gunton, Colin E. *A Brief Theology of Revelation*. Edinburgh: T&T Clark, 1995.

Hacking, Ian. *The Taming of Chance*. Cambridge: Cambridge University Press, 1990.

Hakimjune, Danny. "A Disabled Boy's Death, and a Troubled System." *New York Times*, June 6, 2011, A1.

Hall, Amy Laura. *Conceiving Parenthood: American Protestantism and the Spirit of Reproduction*. Grand Rapids: Eerdmans, 2008.

———. *Kierkegaard and the Treachery of Love*. Cambridge: Cambridge University Press, 2002.

———. "A Ravishing and Restful Sight: Seeing with Julian of Norwich." In Brock and Swinton, *Disability in the Christian Tradition*, 152–64.

Hamilton, Ross. *Accident: A Philosophical and Literary History*. Chicago: University of Chicago Press, 2008.

Hammond, Victoria. *The Dome in European Architecture*. Princeton: Princeton Architectural Press, 2005.

Handelman, Susan. *Fragments of Redemption: Jewish Thought and Literary Theory in Benjamin, Scholem, and Levinas*. Bloomington: Indiana University Press, 1991.

Harmon, Shawn H. E. "Abortion and Conscientious Objection: Doogan—A Missed Opportunity for an Instructive Rights-Based Analysis." *Medical Law International* 16, nos. 3–4 (2016): 143–73.

Harrill, James Albert. *The Manumission of Slaves in Early Christianity*. Tübigen, Germany: Mohr, 1995.

Harrison, Carol. *Augustine: Christian Truth and Fractured Humanity*. Oxford: Oxford University Press, 2000.

Harry, Beth, and Janette K. Klingner. *Why Are So Many Minority Students in Special Education? Understanding Race and Disability in Schools*. New York: Teacher's College Press, 2006.

Hartley, Sigan L., Marsha Mailick Seltzer, Lara Head, and Leonard Abbeduto. "Psychological Well-Being in Fathers of Adolescents and Young Adults with Down Syndrome, Fragile X Syndrome, and Autism." *Family Relations* 61, no. 2 (2012): 327–42.

Hassall, R., J. Rose, and J. McDonald. "Parenting Stress in Mothers of Children with an Intellectual Disability: The Effects of Parental Cognitions in Relation to Child Characteristics and Family Support." *Journal of Intellectual Disability Research* 49, no. 6 (2005): 405–18.

Hauerwas, Stanley. *After Christendom: How the Church Is to Behave if Freedom, Justice, and a Christian Nation Are Bad Ideas*. Nashville: Abingdon, 1999.

———. *Dispatches from the Front: Theological Engagements with the Secular*. Durham: Duke University Press, 1994.

———. "How Christian Ethics Became Medical Ethics: The Case of Paul Ramsey." In *Wilderness Wanderings: Probing Twentieth Century Theology and Philosophy*, 124–40. Boulder, Colo.: Westview, 1997.

———. *Performing the Faith: Bonhoeffer and the Practice of Nonviolence*. Grand Rapids: Brazos, 2004.

———. *Sanctify Them in the Truth: Holiness Exemplified*. Nashville: Abingdon, 1999.

———. *Suffering Presence: Theological Reflections on Medicine, the Mentally Handicapped, and the Church*. Edinburgh: T&T Clark, 1986.

———. "Timeful Friends: Living with the Handicapped." In Swinton, *Critical Reflections on Stanley Hauerwas' Theology of Disability*, 11–26.

———. "Why Jean Vanier Matters: An Exemplary Exploration." In Gaventa and de Jongh, *Knowing, Being Known, and the Mystery of God*, 229–39.

———. *The Work of Theology*. Grand Rapids: Eerdmans, 2015.

Hauerwas, Stanley, and Charles Pinches. *Christians among the Virtues: Theological Conversations with Ancient and Modern Ethics*. South Bend, Ind.: University of Notre Dame Press, 1997.

Hauerwas, Stanley, and Jean Vanier. *Living Gently in a Violent World: The Prophetic Witness of Weakness*. Downers Grove, Ill.: InterVarsity, 2008.

Hauerwas, Stanley, and Sam Wells, eds. *The Blackwell Companion to Christian Ethics*. 2nd ed. Oxford: Wiley-Blackwell, 2011.

Henriksen, Jan-Olav, and Karl Olav Sandnes. *Jesus as Healer: A Gospel for the Body*. Grand Rapids: Eerdmans, 2016.

Heslop, Pauline, Peter Blair, Peter Fleming, Mat Hoghton, Anna Marriott, and Lesley Russ. *Confidential Inquiry into Premature Deaths of People with Learning Disabilities (CIPOLD)*. Final report. Bristol: Norah Fry Research Centre, 2013.

Heuser, Stefan. "Bonhoeffer and Bioscience: Dialogues on the Hermeneutics of Life." In Wüstenberg, Heuser, and Hornung, *Bonhoeffer and the Biosciences*, 13–26.

———. "The Cost of Citizenship: Disciple and Citizen in Bonhoeffer's Political Ethics." *Studies in Christian Ethics* 18, no. 3 (2005): 49–69.

———. "The Human Condition as Seen from the Cross: Luther and Disability." In Brock and Swinton, *Disability in the Christian Tradition*, 184–99.

Hubach, Stephanie O. *Same Lake, Different Boat: Coming alongside People Touched by Disability*. Philipsburg: P&R Publishing, 2006.

Hughes, Bettany. *The Hemlock Cup: Socrates, Athens and the Search for the Good Life*. London: Vintage, 2011.

Hughes, Karen, Mark A. Bellis, Lisa Jones, Sara Wood, Geoff Bates, Lindsay Eckley, Ellie McCoy, Christopher Mikton, Tom Shakespeare, and Alana Officer. "Prevalence and Risk of Violence against Adults with Disabilities: A Systematic Review and Meta-analysis of Observational Studies." *The Lancet* 379 (2012): 1621–29.

Illich, Ivan. *Rivers North of the Future: The Testament of Ivan Illich as told to David Cayley*. Toronto: Anansi, 2005.

Ingold, Tim. *The Life of Lines*. New York: Routledge, 2015.

Iozzio, Mary Jo. "Genetic Anomaly or Genetic Diversity: Thinking in the Key of Disability on the Human Genome." *Theological Studies* 66 (2005): 862–81.

———. "Radical Dependence and the *Imago Dei*: Bioethical Implications of Access to Healthcare for People with Disabilities." *Christian Bioethics* 23, no. 3 (2017): 234–60.

———. "Solidarity: Restoring Communion with Those Who are Disabled." *Journal of Religion, Disability and Health* 25, no. 2 (2011): 139–52.

Iwand, Hans Joachim. "Wider den Mißbrauch des *pro me* as methodisches Princip in der Theologie." In *Briefe, Forträge, Predigtmeditationen*, edited by Peter-Paul Sänger, 225–30. Berlin: Evanglisiche Verlagsanstalt, 1979.

Jackson, Rebecca, Kimberly Gibson, Yvonne Wu, and Mary Croughan. "Perinatal Outcomes in Singletons Following In Vitro Fertilization: A Meta-analysis." *Obstetrics & Gynecology* 103 (2004): 551–63.

Jenkins, Timothy. *Of Flying Saucers and Social Scientists: A Re-Reading of When Prophecy Fails and of Cognitive Dissonance*. New York: Palgrave MacMillan, 2013.

Jennings, Michael W., Howard Eiland, and Gary Smith, eds. *Walter Benjamin: Selected Writings*. Vol. 2, part 2: *1931–1934*. Translated by Rodney Livingstone. Cambridge, Mass.: Harvard University Press, 1999.

Jennings, Willie James. *The Christian Imagination: Theology and the Origins of Race*. New Haven, Conn.: Yale University Press, 2010.

———. "Disfigurations of Christian Identity: Performing Identity as Theological Method." In *Lived Theology: New Perspectives in Method, Style and Pedagogy*, edited by Marsh et al., 67–89. Oxford: Oxford University Press, 2017.

Jensen, Michael. *Martyrdom and Identity: The Self on Trial*. London: Bloomsbury, 2013.

Johnson, Kelly S. *The Fear of Beggars: Stewardship and Poverty in Christian Ethics*. Grand Rapids: Eerdmans, 2007.

———. "Interceding: Poverty and Prayer." In Hauerwas and Wells, *Blackwell Companion to Christian Ethics*, 239–50.

Jones, David Albert. "Apostles of Suicide: Theological Precedent for Christian Support of 'Assisted Dying.'" *Studies in Christian Ethics* 29, no. 3 (2016): 331–38.

Juengst, Eric T. "What *Does* Enhancement *Mean*?" In *Enhancing Human Traits: Ethical and Social Implications*, edited by Erik Parens, 29–47. Washington, D.C.: Georgetown University Press, 1998.

Junker-Kenny, Maureen. "Genes and the Self: Anthropological Questions to the Human Genome Project." In *Brave New World: Theology, Ethics and the Human Genome*, edited by Celia Deane-Drummond, 124–25. London: T&T Clark International, 2003.

Kaczor, Christopher. "Conscientious Objection and Health Care: A Reply to Bernard Dickens." *Christian Bioethics: Non-Ecumenical Studies in Medical Morality* 18, no. 1 (2012): 59–71.

Kafka, Franz. *Collected Stories*. Edited by Gabriel Josipovici. Translated by Willa and Edwin Muir. New York: Alfred A. Knopf, 1993.

Kaposy, Chris. *Choosing Down Syndrome: Ethics and New Prenatal Testing Technologies*. Cambridge, Mass.: MIT Press, 2018.

Karłowicz, Dariusz. *The Archparadox of Death: Martyrdom as a Philosophical Category*. Frankfurt am Main: Peter Lang, 2016.

Käsemann, Ernst. "The Theological Problem Presented by the Motif of the Body of Christ." In *Perspectives on Paul*, translated by Margaret Kohl, 102–21. London: SCM Press, 1971.

Kaufman, Eleanor. *The Delirium of Praise: Bataille, Blanchot, Deleuze, Foucault, Kosowski*. Baltimore: Johns Hopkins University Press, 2001.

Kearney, Tim, ed. *A Prophetic Cry: Stories of Spirituality and Healing Inspired by L'Arche*. Dublin: Veritas, 2000.

———. "The Upside-Down Kingdom." In Kearney, *Prophetic Cry*, 68–83.

Keen, Craig. *After Crucifixion: The Promise of Theology*. Eugene: Cascade, 2013.

Kelly, Brendan. "Priesthood and Handicap—Some Personal Reflections." In Kearney, *Prophetic Cry*, 86–96.

Kierkegaard, Søren. *Fear and Trembling, Repetition*. Edited and translated by Howard Hong and Edna Hong. Kierkegaard's Writings 6. Princeton: Princeton University Press, 1983.

———. *Practice in Christianity*. Edited and translated by Howard Hong and Edna Hong. Kierkegaard's Writings 20. Princeton: Princeton University Press, 1991.

Kim, Yung Suk. *Christ's Body in Corinth: The Politics of a Metaphor*. Minneapolis: Fortress, 2008.

Kittel, Gerhard, ed. *Theological Dictionary of the New Testament*. Vol. 2. Edited and translated by Geoffrey W. Bromiley. Grand Rapids: Eerdmans, 1964.

———, ed. *Theological Dictionary of the New Testament*. Vol. 4. Edited and translated by Geoffrey W. Bromiley. Grand Rapids: Eerdmans, 1967.

Knight, Douglas. *The Eschatological Economy: Time and the Hospitality of God*. Grand Rapids: Eerdmans, 2006.

Kolářova, Kateřina. "Death by Choice, Life by Privilege: Biopolitical Circuits of Vitality and Debility in the Times of Empire." In Tremain, *Foucault and the Government of Disability*, 396–423.

Kovacs, Judith, trans. and ed. *First Corinthians: Interpreted by Early Christian Commentators*. Grand Rapids: Eerdmans, 2005.

Krötke, Wolf. *Sin and Nothingness in the Theology of Karl Barth: With a New Foreword by the Author*. Studies in Reformed Theology and History. Edited and translated by Philip Ziegler and Christina-Maria Bammel. Princeton: Princeton Theological Seminary, 2005.

Lactantius. *The Divine Institutes*. In *Ante-Nicene Christian Library*, vol. 21: *The Works of Lactantius*, edited by Alexander Roberts and James Donaldson, translated by William Fletcher. Edinburgh: T&T Clark, 1881.

Latour, Bruno. "Body, Cyborgs, and the Politics of Incarnation." In Sweeney and Hodder, *The Body*, 127–41.

———. *Reassembling the Social: An Introduction to Actor, Network Theory*. Oxford: Oxford University Press, 2005.

Lazier, Benjamin. *God Interrupted: Heresy and the European Imagination between the World Wars*. Princeton: Princeton University Press, 2008.

Lee, Jefferson. "The Staff of Jesus in Early Christian Art." *Religion and the Arts* 14, no. 3 (2010): 221–51.

Lehman, Paul. *Ethics in a Christian Context*. New York: Harper & Row, 1963.

Lehrer, Jonah. "The Truth Wears Off." *New Yorker*, December 13, 2010, 52–57.

Leroi, Armand Maire. *Mutants: On the Form, Varieties and Errors of the Human Body*. London: Harper Perennial, 2005.

Lewis, John. "Student Attitudes Toward Impairment and Accessibility: An Evaluation of Awareness Training for Urban Planning Students." *Vocations and Learning* 2 (2009): 109–25.

Lindemann, Andreas. "Die Kirche als Leib: Beobachtungen zur 'demokratischen' Ekklesiologie bei Paulus." *Zeitschrift für Theologie und Kirche* 92 (1995): 140–65.

Linden, David J. *Touch: The Science of Hand, Heart, and Mind*. London: Viking, 2015.

Lindforsa, Sara, Christina Eintreib, and Kristina Alexanderson. "Stress Factors Affecting Academic Physicians at a University Hospital." *Work* 34 (2009): 305–13.

Link, Jürgen. *Versuch über den Normalismus: Wie Normalität produciert wird*. Opladen, Germany: Westdeutscher Verlag, 1996.

Lippman, Abby, and Benjamin S. Wilfond. "Twice-Told Tales: Stories about Genetic Disorders." *American Journal of Human Genetics* 51 (1992): 936–37.

Locke, John. *An Essay Concerning Human Understanding*. Edited by Peter H. Nidditch. Oxford: Oxford University Press, 1975.

Logue, Larry M. *Race, Ethnicity, and Disability: Veterans and Benefits in Post-Civil War America*. Cambridge: Cambridge University Press, 2013.

Luhmann, Niklas. *Risk: A Sociological Theory*. Translated by Rhodes Barrett. Berlin: Walter de Gruyter, 1993.

Luther, Martin. "Large Catechism." In *The Book of Concord: The Confessions of the Evangelical Lutheran Church*, edited by T. G. Tappert. Philadelphia: Fortress, 1959.

———. *Luther's Works*. 55 vols. Edited by Helmut Lehman and Jaroslav Pelikan. St. Louis and Philadelphia: Concordia and Fortress, 1955–1986.

Macaskill, Grant. "Autism Spectrum Disorders and the New Testament: Preliminary Reflections." *Journal of Disability & Religion* 22, no. 1 (2018): 15–41.

MacDonald, Michael. *Mystical Bedlam: Madness, Anxiety, and Healing in Seventeenth-Century England*. Cambridge: Cambridge University Press, 1981.

MacIntyre. Alasdair. *After Virtue*. 3rd ed. London: Duckworth, 2007.

———. *Dependent Rational Animals: Why Human Beings Need the Virtues*. Chicago: Open Court, 1999.

———. *Three Rival Versions of Moral Inquiry: Encyclopedia, Genealogy, and Tradition*. London: Gerald Duckworth, 1990.

Mardell, Danny. *Danny's Challenge: The True Story of a Father Learning to Love His Son*. Edited by Sally Weal. London: Short Books, 2005.

Marion, Jean-Luc. *Givenness and Revelation*. Translated by Stephen E. Lewis. Oxford: Oxford University Press, 2016.

Marsden, George M. *Reforming Fundamentalism: Fuller Seminary and the New Evangelicalism*. Grand Rapids: Eerdmans, 1987.

Martin, Ralph. "Gifts, Spiritual." In *The Anchor Bible Dictionary*, vol. 2, edited by David Freedman, 1015–18. New York: Doubleday, 1992.

Mata, Douglas A., Marco A. Ramos, Narinder Bansal, Rida Khan, Constance Guille, Emanuele Di Angelantonio, and Srijan Sen. "Prevalence of Depression and Depressive Symptoms among Resident Physicians: A Systematic Review and Meta-analysis." *Journal of the American Medical Association* 314, no. 22 (2015): 2373–83.

Mathewes, Charles T. "Book One: The Presumptuousness of Autobiographies and the Paradoxes of Beginning." In *A Reader's Companion to Augustine's "Confessions,"* edited by Kim Paffenroth and Robert Peter Kennedy, 7–24. Louisville: Westminster John Knox, 2003.

Mathews, Thomas F. *The Clash of the Gods: A Reinterpretation of Early Christian Art*. Rev. and exp. version. Princeton: Princeton University Press, 1993.

McCullagh, John. "The Prophetic Voice of the Poor." In Kearney, *Prophetic Cry*, 25–35.

McCullers, Carson. *The Heart Is a Lonely Hunter*. Introduction and notes by Kasia Boddy. 1940. London: Penguin, 2008.

McGuire, Anne. "'Life Worth Defending': Biopolitical Frames of Terror in the War on Autism." In Tremain, *Foucault and the Government of Disability*, 350–71.

McVeigh, Tracy. "Sally Phillips's Film on Down's Is 'Unhelpful' for Families, Warns Antenatal Specialist." *The Guardian*, October 2, 2016.

Merleau-Ponty, Maurice. *The Phenomenology of Perception*. Translated by Colin Smith. London: Routledge, 1962.

Meskus, Mianna. "Personalized Ethics: The Emergence and the Effects in Prenatal Testing." *Biosciences* 7, no. 4 (2012): 373–92.

Messer, Neil. *Flourishing: Health, Disease, and Bioethics in Theological Perspective*. Grand Rapids: Eerdmans, 2013.

Metzler, Irina. *Disability in Medieval Europe: Thinking about Physical Impairment during the High Middle Ages, c.1100–1400*. Abingdon, U.K.: Routledge, 2006.

———. *Fools and Idiots? Intellectual Disability in the Middle Ages*. Manchester: Manchester University Press, 2016.

Mikton, Christopher, and Tom Shakespeare. "Introduction to Special Issue on Violence against People with Disability." *Journal of Interpersonal Violence* 29, no. 17 (2014): 3055–62.

Milavec, Aaron, ed. *The Didache: Text, Translation, Analysis, and Commentary*. Collegeville, Penn.: Liturgical, 2003.

Milbank, John. "Can a Gift Be Given? Prolegomena to a Future Trinitarian Metaphysic." *Modern Theology* 11, no. 1 (1995): 119–61.

Miller, Timothy S. *The Birth of the Hospital in the Byzantine Empire*. Rev. ed. Baltimore: Johns Hopkins University Press, 1985.

Minkoff, Howard, and Richard Berkowitz. "The Myth of the Precious Baby." *Obstetrics and Gynecology* 106 (2005): 607–9.

Minkoff, Howard, Kathleen Powderly, Frank Chervenak, and Lawrence McCullough. "Ethical Dimensions of Elective Primary Cesarean Delivery." *Obstetrics and Gynecology* 103 (2004): 387–92.

Mitchell, Lisa M., and Eugenia Georges. "Cross-Cultural Cyborgs: Greek and Canadian Women's Discourses on Fetal Ultrasound." *Feminist Studies* 23, no. 2 (1997): 373–401.

Monteith, W. Graham. *Epistles of Inclusion: St. Paul's Inspired Attitudes*. Guildford, U.K.: Grovesnor House, 2010.

———. *Visibly Invisible: A Pilgrimage as a Disabled Minister*. Guildford, U.K.: Grovesnor House, 2010.

Moyne, Samuel. *Origins of the Other: Emmanuel Levinas between Revelation and Ethics*. Ithaca, N.Y.: Cornell University Press, 2005.

Mumford, James. *Ethics at the Beginning of Life: A Phenomenological Critique*. Oxford: Oxford University Press, 2013.

Murgatroyd, Paul. *Mythical Monsters in Classical Literature*. London: Duckworth, 2007.

Murphy-O'Connor, Jerome. *Keys to First Corinthians: Revisiting the Major Issues*. Oxford: Oxford University Press, 2009.

Nausner, Michael. "Participating in Christ: Therapeutic Dimensions in Christian Discipleship from a Wesleyan Perspective." In Wendte, *Jesus der Heiler*, 99–116.

Niebuhr, Reinhold. *Moral Man and Immoral Society: A Study in Ethics and Politics*. New York: Scribner's, 1932.

Novatian, *De spectaculis: A Translation with an Introduction and Notes*. Translated by Jacoby Matthew Henry. Washington, D.C.: Catholic University of America Press, 1957.

Nussbaum, Martha. *Frontiers of Justice: Disability, Nationality, Species Membership*. Cambridge: Belknap Press, 2006.

O'Donovan, Oliver. *The Desire of the Nations: Rediscovering the Roots of Political Theology*. Cambridge: Cambridge University Press, 1996.

———. *Resurrection and Moral Order: An Outline for Evangelical Ethics*. 2nd ed. Leicester, U.K.: Apollos, 1994.

O'Donovan, Oliver, and Joan Lockwood O'Donovan, eds. *Irenaeus to Grotius: A Sourcebook in Christian Political Thought, 100–1625*. Grand Rapids: Eerdmans, 1999.

Öhman, Björn Nalle. *Kropp, handling och ritual: hur förstå religion och personer med grava funktionshinder?* Åbo, Finland: Åbo Akademis förlag, 2008.

O'Sullivan, Anne. "The White Stone." In Kearney, *Prophetic Cry*, 98–104.

Ouellette, Alicia. *Bioethics and Disability: Toward a Disability-Conscious Bioethics*. Cambridge: Cambridge University Press, 2011.

Parens, Erik. "Respecting Children with Disabilities—and Their Parents." *Hastings Center Report* 39, no. 1 (2009): 22–23.

Parvaz, D. "In Cringe-Worthy Speech, Trump Tells Paralympians They Were 'Tough to Watch,'" *Think Progress*, April 28, 2018.

Patterson, David, and Alberto C. S. Costa. "History of Genetic Disease: Down Syndrome and Genetics—a Case of Linked Histories." *Nature Reviews Genetics* 6 (2005): 137–47.

Peterson, James C. *Genetic Turning Points: The Ethics of Human Genetic Intervention*. Grand Rapids: Eerdmans, 2001.

Pick, Anat. *Creaturely Poetics: Animality and Vulnerability in Literature and Film*. New York: Columbia University Press, 2011.

Pistorius, Martin, with Megan Lloyd Davies. *Ghost Boy*. London: Simon & Schuster, 2011.

Plato. *Apology*. In *The Trials of Socrates: Six Classic Texts*, edited by C. D. C. Reeve, 26–61. Indianapolis: Hackett, 2002.

———. *Crito*. In *The Trials of Socrates: Six Classic Texts*, edited by C. D. C. Reeve, 62–78. Indianapolis: Hackett, 2002.

———. *The Republic*. Edited and translated by Chris Emlyn-Jones and William Preddy. Cambridge, Mass.: Harvard University Press, 2013.

———. *Timaeus*. In *Timaeus and Critias*, translated by Desmond Lee, 27–124. London: Penguin, 1977.

Poerksen. Uwe. *Plastic Words: The Tyranny of a Modular Language*. Translated by Jutta Mason and David Cayley. University Park: Pennsylvania State University Press, 1995.

Porterfield, Amanda. *Healing in the History of Christianity*. Oxford: Oxford University Press, 2005.

Proctor, Robert N. "The Destruction of 'Lives Not Worth Living.'" In *Deviant Bodies: Critical Perspectives on Difference in Science and Popular Culture*, edited by Jennifer Terry and Jacqueline Urla, 170–96. Bloomington: Indiana University Press, 1995.

Proust, Marcel. *Swann's Way*. Translated by Lydia Davis. London: Penguin, 2003.

Putnam, Hilary. "Introduction" to *Understanding the Sick and the Healthy: A View of World, Man, and God*, by Franz Rosenzweig. Translated and edited by Nahum Glatzer. Cambridge, Mass.: Harvard University Press, 1999.

Quinn, Dennis. *Iris Exiled: A Synoptic History of Wonder*. Lanham, Md.: University Press of America, 2002.

Quinones, Julian, and Arijeta Lajka. "'What Kind of Society Do You Want to Live in?': Inside the Country Where Down Syndrome Is Disappearing." *CBS News*, August 14, 2017.

Ramey, Joshua. *Politics of Divination: Neoliberal Endgame and the Religion of Contingency*. London: Rowan & Littlefield, 2016.

Ramsey, Paul. *Basic Christian Ethics*. Louisville: Westminster John Knox, 1993.

———. *The Patient as Person*. New Haven: Yale University Press, 1970.

Rapp, Rayna. *Testing Women, Testing the Fetus: The Social Impact of Amniocentesis in America*. New York: Routledge, 2000.

Rashkover, Randi. *Revelation and Theopolitics: Barth, Rosenzweig, and the Politics of Praise*. London: T&T Clark, 2005.

Ravaud, Jean-Francois, and Henri-Jacques Stiker. "Inclusion/Exclusion: An Analysis of Historical and Cultural Meanings." In Albrecht, Seelman, and Bury, *Handbook of Disability Studies*, 490–515.

Read, Janet, and Luke Clements. "Demonstrably Awful: The Right to Life and the Selective Non-treatment of Disabled Babies and Young Children." In Clements and Read, *Disabled People and the Right to Life*, 148–75.

Rees, Geoffrey. *The Romance of Innocent Sexuality*. Eugene, Ore.: Cascade, 2011.

Reeve, C. D. C., ed. *The Trials of Socrates: Six Classic Texts*. Indianapolis: Hackett, 2002.

Reinders, Hans S. "Being with the Disabled: Jean Vanier's Theological Realism." In Brock and Swinton, *Disability in the Christian Tradition*, 467–82.

———. *Disability, Providence, and Ethics: Bridging Gaps, Transforming Lives*. Waco, Tex.: Baylor University Press, 2014.

———. *The Future of the Disabled in Liberal Society: An Ethical Analysis*. South Bend, Ind.: University of Notre Dame Press, 2000.

———. "Life's Goodness: On Disability, Genetics, and 'Choice.'" In Swinton and Brock, *Theology, Disability and the New Genetics*, 29–43.

———. *Receiving the Gift of Friendship: Profound Disability, Theological Anthropology, and Ethics*. Grand Rapids: Eerdmans, 2008.

Reinders, Hans S., and Lydia Helwig Nazarowa. *Looking for Quality: Assessing Quality of Care in Long Term Services, toward a Narrative Approach*. Unpublished conference paper.

Reist, Melinda Tankard. *Defiant Birth: Women Who Resist Medical Eugenics*. North Melbourne: Spinifex, 2006.

Reynolds, Thomas E. "Love without Boundaries: Theological Reflections on Parenting a Child with Disabilities." *Theology Today* 62 (2005): 193–209.

———. "Theology and Disability: Changing the Conversation." *Journal of Religion, Disability and Health* 16 (2012): 33–48.

———. *Vulnerable Communion: A Theology of Disability and Hospitality*. Grand Rapids: Brazos, 2008.

Richards, Martin. "Annotation: Genetic Research, Family Life, and Clinical Practice." *Journal of Child Psychology* 39, no. 3 (1998): 291–305.

Richardson, Evin Winkelman, and Zolinda Stoneman. "The Road to Membership: The Role of Resilience in Seeking and Maintaining Membership in a Faith Community for Families of Children with Disabilities." *Journal of Disability and Religion* 19, no. 4 (2015): 312–39.

Rodowick, D. N. *Philosophy's Artful Conversation*. Cambridge, Mass.: Harvard University Press, 2015.

Romero, Miguel J. "The Goodness and Beauty of Our Fragile Flesh: Moral Theologians and Our Engagement With 'Disability.'" *The Journal of Moral Theology* 6, Special Issue no. 2 (2017): 206–53.

Rose, Beth. "Archbishop Justin Welby: I Don't Pray for My Daughter's Disability." BBC News, July 6, 2018.

Rose, Martha L. *The Staff of Oedipus: Transforming Disability in Ancient Greece*. Ann Arbor: University of Michigan Press, 2003.

Rosenzweig, Franz. *Star of Redemption*. Translated by Barbara E. Galli. Madison: University of Wisconsin Press, 2005.

———. *Understanding the Sick and the Healthy: A View of World, Man, and God*. Edited and translated by Nahum Glatzer. Cambridge, Mass.: Harvard University Press, 1999.

Rotenstein, Lisa S., Marco A. Ramos, Matthew Torre, J. Bradley Segal, Michael J. Peluso, Constance Guille, Srijan Sen, and Douglas A. Mata. "Prevalence of Depression, Depressive

Symptoms, and Suicidal Ideation among Medical Students: A Systematic Review and Meta-analysis." *Journal of the American Medical Association* 316, no. 21 (2016): 2214–36.

Rothman, Barbara Katz. "Spoiling the Pregnancy: Prenatal Diagnosis in the Netherlands." In *Birth by Design: Pregnancy, Maternity Care and Midwifery in North America and Europe*, edited by Raymond De Vries, Cecilia Benoit, Edwin van Teijlingen, and Sirpa Wrede, 180–98. New York: Routledge, 2001.

———. *The Tentative Pregnancy: Prenatal Diagnosis and the Future of Motherhood*. New York: Penguin Books, 1987.

Rowe, C. Kavin. *World Upside Down: Reading Acts in the Graeco-Roman Age*. Oxford: Oxford University Press, 2010.

Ryan, Sara. *Justice for Laughing Boy: A Death by Indifference*. London: Jessica Kingsley, 2018.

Sacks, Jonathan. *Not in My Name: Confronting Religious Violence*. London: Hodder & Stoughton, 2015.

Santner, Eric. *On the Psychotheology of Everyday Life: Reflections of Freud and Rosenzweig*. Chicago: University of Chicago Press, 2001.

Satz, Debra. *Why Some Things Should Not Be for Sale: The Moral Limits of Markets*. Oxford: Oxford University Press, 2010.

Savulescu, Julian, and Udo Schuklenk. "Doctors Have No Right to Refuse Medical Assistance in Dying, Abortion or Contraception." *Bioethics* 31, no. 3 (2017): 162–70.

Schaeffer, Hans, Gerard den Hertog, and Stefan Paas, eds. *Mercy: Theories, Concepts, Practices*. Zürich: Lit Verlag, 2018.

Schmidt, Leigh Eric. *Hearing Things: Religion, Illusion, and the American Enlightenment*. Cambridge, Mass.: Harvard University Press, 2000.

Schroeder, C. Paul. *On Social Justice: Basil the Great*. Crestwood, N.Y.: St. Vladimir's Seminary, 2009.

Schweik, Susan. *The Ugly Laws: Disability in Public*. New York: New York University Press, 2009.

Screech, M. A. *Laughter at the Foot of the Cross*. Boulder, Colo.: Westview, 1999.

Serres, Michel. *The Five Senses: A Philosophy of Mingled Bodies (I)*. Translated by Margaret Sankey and Peter Cowley. London: Continuum International, 2008.

Shakespeare, Tom. "Just What Is the Disability Perspective on Disability?" *Hastings Center Report* 46, no. 3 (2016): 31–32.

———. "'Losing the Plot'? Medical and Activist Discourses of Contemporary Genetics and Disability." *Sociology of Health and Illness* 21, no. 5 (1999): 669–88.

———. "Still a Health Issue." *Disability and Health Journal* 5 (2012): 129–31.

Shaw, Brent D. "The Passion of Perpetua." *Past and Present* 139 (May 1993): 3–45.

Shea, Sarah. "Theological Reflection on Inter-country Adoptions of Special Needs Children from Mainland China." In Swinton and Brock, *Graceful Embrace*, 161–82.

Shrier, Paul. "Messengers of Hope: A Boy with Autism, His Church, and the Special Olympics." *Journal of Disability & Religion* 21, no. 2 (2017): 230–44.

Sigurdson, Ola. *Heavenly Bodies: Incarnation, the Gaze, and Embodiment in Christian Theology*. Translated by Carl Olson. Grand Rapids: Eerdmans, 2016.

Silberman, Steve. *Neurotribes: The Legacy of Autism and How to Think Smarter about People Who Think Differently*. London: Allen and Unwin, 2015.

Simons, Maarten, and Jan Masschelein. "Inclusive Education." In Tremain, *Foucault and the Government of Disability*, 208–28.

Simplican, Stacy Clifford. *The Capacity Contract: Intellectual Disability and the Question of Citizenship*. Minneapolis: University of Minnesota Press, 2015.

Simplican, Stacy Clifford, Geraldine Leader, John Kosciulek, and Michael Leahy. "Defining Social Inclusion of People with Intellectual and Developmental Disabilities: An Ecological Model of Social Networks and Community Participation." *Research in Developmental Disabilities* 38 (2015): 18–29.

Simpson, J. A., and E. S. C. Weiner, eds. *The Oxford English Dictionary*. 2nd ed. Vol. 12: *Poise–Quelt*. Oxford: Clarendon, 1989.

Sivberg, Bengt. "Coping Strategies and Parental Attitudes, a Comparison of Parents with Children with Autistic Spectrum Disorders and Parents with Non-autistic Children." *International Journal of Circumpolar Health* 61, no. 2 (2002): 36–50.

Skidelsky, Robert. *Keynes: The Return of the Master*. New York: Public Affairs, 2010.

Sklansky, Mark. "Neonatal Euthanasia: Moral Considerations and Criminal Liability." *Journal of Medical Ethics* 27 (2001): 5–11.

Slavin, Stuart J. "Medical Student Mental Health: Culture, Environment, and the Need for Change." *Journal of the American Medical Association* 316, no. 21 (2016): 2195–96.

Smietana, Bob. "Few Churches Are Autism Friendly." *Facts & Trends.net*. July 30, 2018.

Smith, Mitch, and Richard Pérez-Penajan. "Beating of a Disabled Teenager Highlights a Crime That's Often Unseen." *New York Times*, January 6, 2017, A8.

Smith, Ted A. *The New Measures: A Theological History of Democratic Practice*. Cambridge: Cambridge University Press, 2007.

Soskice, Janet Martin. *The Kindness of God: Metaphor, Gender, and Religious Language*. Oxford: Oxford University Press, 2007.

Soukhanov, Anne, ed. *The American Heritage Dictionary of the English Language*. 3rd ed. Boston: Houghton Mifflin, 1992.

Sowell, Thomas. "Autism Crusade Will Backfire on Children." *Redding.com*, November 14, 2007.

Stach, Reiner. *Kafka: The Decisive Years*. Translated by Shelley Frisch. Princeton: Princeton University Press, 2005.

———. *Kafka: The Years of Insight*. Translated by Shelley Frisch. Princeton: Princeton University Press, 2013.

Stainton, Tim. "Reason, Grace and Charity: Augustine and the Impact of Church Doctrine on the Construction of Intellectual Disability." *Disability and Society* 23, no. 5 (2008): 485–96.

Stegenga, Jacob. *Medical Nihilism*. Oxford: Oxford University Press, 2018.

Stevens, Katherine J. "Working with Children to Develop Dimensions for a Preference-Based, Generic, Pediatric, Health-Related Quality-of-Life Measure." *Qualitative Health Research* 20, no. 3 (2010): 340–51.

Stiker, Henri-Jacques. *A History of Disability*. Translated by William Sayers with a foreword by David T. Mitchell. Ann Arbor: University of Michigan Press, 1999.

Stout, Jeffrey. *Democracy and Tradition*. Princeton: Princeton University Press, 2004.

Sweeney, Sean T., and Ian Hodder, eds. *The Body*. Cambridge: Cambridge University Press, 2002.

Sweet, Victoria. *God's Hotel: A Doctor, A Hospital, and a Pilgrimage to the Heart of Medicine*. New York: Riverhead Books, 2012.

Swinger, Maureen. "The Teacher Who Never Spoke: How My Brother Who Could Never Walk or Talk Coached Dozens of His Peers into Manhood." *Plough Quarterly* 12 (2017): 18–27.

Swinton, John, ed. *Critical Reflections on Stanley Hauerwas' Theology of Disability: Disabling Society, Enabling Theology*. Binghamton, N.Y.: Hayworth Pastoral, 2004.

———. *Becoming Friends of Time: Disability, Timefullness, and Gentle Discipleship*. Waco, Tex.: Baylor University Press, 2016.

———. *Dementia: Living in the Memories of God*. Grand Rapids: Eerdmans, 2012.

———. *From Bedlam to Shalom*. New York: Peter Lang, 2000.

———. "How Do We Know That Kelly Doesn't Know? Some Reflections on the Experiences of People with Profound Intellectual Disabilities." In Gaventa and de Jongh, *Knowing, Being Known, and the Mystery of God*, 175–82.

———. *Raging with Compassion: Pastoral Responses to the Problem of Evil*. Grand Rapids: Eerdmans, 2007.

———. "What's in a Name? Why People with Dementia Might Be Better Off without the Language of Personhood." *International Journal of Practical Theology* 18, no. 2 (2014): 1–14.

Swinton, John, and Brian Brock, eds. *A Graceful Embrace: Theological Reflections on Adopting Children*. Leiden: Brill, 2018.

———, eds. *Theology, Disability and the New Genetics: Why Science Needs the Church*. London: T&T Clark, 2007.

Swinton, John, and Stephen Pattison. "Moving Beyond Clarity: Towards a Thin, Vague, and Useful Understanding of Spirituality in Nursing Care." *Nursing Philosophy* (2010): 226–37.

Taylor, Ashley. "Expressions of 'Life Worth Living' and Their Foreclosure through Philosophical Theorizing on Moral Status and Intellectual Disability." In Tremain, *Foucault and the Government of Disability*, 372–95.

Taylor, Charles. *Sources of the Self: The Making of the Modern Identity*. Cambridge, Mass.: Harvard University Press, 1989.

Tertullian. *Apologetical Works*. Translated by R. Arbesmann, E. J. Daily, and E. A. Quain. Fathers of the Church 10. Washington, D.C.: Catholic University of America Press, 1950.

———. *On Fasting*. In *Ante-Nicene Fathers*, vol. 4: *Tertullian, Minucius Felix, Commodianus, Origen*, edited by Alexander Roberts and James Donaldson. Grand Rapids: Eerdmans, 1979.

———. *Tertullian: Apology, de Spectaculis, Minucius Felix*. Translated by T. R. Glover and Gerald Rendall. Loeb Classical Library 250. Cambridge, Mass.: Harvard University Press, 1931.

Thiselton, Anthony. *The First Epistle to the Corinthians: A Commentary on the Greek Text*. Grand Rapids: Eerdmans, 2000.

Thomas, Gareth M. *Down Syndrome Screening and Reproductive Politics: Care, Choice, and Disability in the Prenatal Clinic*. Abingdon: Routledge, 2017.

Thomas, Gareth M., and Barbara Katz Rothman. "Keeping the Backdoor to Eugenics Ajar? Disability and the Future of Prenatal Screening." *American Medical Association Journal of Ethics* 18, no. 4 (2016): 406–15.

Thompson, Samantha. "The *Confessions* of Saint Augustine: Accessory to Grace." In *Autobiography as Philosophy: The Philosophical Uses of Self-Presentation*, edited by Thomas Mathein and D. G. Wright, 31–63. Abingdon, U.K.: Routledge, 2006.

Thomson, Judith Jarvis. "A Defense of Abortion." *Philosophy and Public Affairs* 1, no. 1 (1971): 47–66.

Tremain, Shelley, ed. *Foucault and the Government of Disability*. Rev. ed. Ann Arbor: University of Michigan Press, 2015.

Trevett, Christine. "Asperger's Syndrome and the Holy Fool: The Case of Brother Juniper." *Journal of Religion, Disability and Health* 13, no. 2 (2009): 129–50.

Trigg, Joseph W. *Origen*. London: Routledge, 1998.

Troeltsch, Ernst. *The Social Teaching of the Christian Churches*. 2 vols. Translated by Olive Wyon. Foreword by James Luther Adams. Louisville: Westminster John Knox, 1992.

Tuffrey-Wijne, Irene, Leopold Curfs, Ilora Finlay, and Sheila Hollins. "Euthanasia and Assisted Suicide for People with an Intellectual Disability and/or Autism Spectrum Disorder: An Examination of Nine Relevant Euthanasia Cases in the Netherlands (2012–2016)." *BMC Medical Ethics* 19, no. 17 (2018). Published online March 5, 2018.

Tyson, Paul G. "The Wounds of Faith and Medicine, and the Balm of Paradox." *Christian Bioethics* 20, no. 3 (2014): 330–58.

UK Department of Health. *Transforming Care: A National Response to Winterbourne View Hospital*. https://www.gov.uk.

Ulrich, Hans G. "Bonhoeffer's Work—Challenging the Ethical Approach in the Field of Bioethics for a Critical Hermeneutics of Life: Shared Insights from a Multiple Dialogue." In Wüstenberg, Heuser, and Hornung, *Bonhoeffer and the Biosciences*, 169–74.

———. *Eschatologie und Ethik: Die Theologische Theorie der Ethik in ihrer Beziehung auf die Rede von Gott seit Freidrich Schliermacher*. Munich: Chr. Kaier Verlag, 1988.

———. *Wie Geschöpfe leben: Konturen evangelischer Ethik*. Münster: Lit Verlag, 2005.

———. "The Messianic Contours of Evangelical Ethics." In *The Freedom of a Christian Ethicist*, edited by Brian Brock and Mike Mawson, 39–64. London: Continuum, 2015.

van Hooff, Anton J. L. "Ancient Euthanasia: 'Good Death' and the Doctor in the Graeco-Roman World." *Social Science & Medicine* 58, no. 5 (2004): 975–85.

Vanier, Jean. *Becoming Human*. New York: Paulist, 1998.

———. *Community and Growth*. 2nd rev. ed. London: Darton, Longman and Todd, 1989.

———. *Made for Happiness: Discovering the Meaning of Life with Aristotle*. Translated by Kathryn Spink. Toronto: Anansi, 2012.

Verhey, Allen. *Reading the Bible in the Strange World of Medicine*. Grand Rapids: Eerdmans, 2003.

Volpe, Medi Ann. "Irresponsible Love: Rethinking Intellectual Disability, Humanity, and the Church." *Modern Theology* 25, no. 3 (2009): 491–501.

Voorhoeve, Alex. *Conversations on Ethics*. Oxford: Oxford University Press, 2009.

Vosloo, Robert. "Body and Health in the Light of the Theology of Dietrich Bonhoeffer." *Religion and Theology* 13, no. 1 (2006): 23–37.

Waldschmidt, Anne. "Who Is Normal? Who Is Deviant? 'Normality' and 'Risk' in Genetic Diagnostics and Counselling." In Tremain, *Foucault and the Government of Disability*, 191–207.

Wall, Benjamin S. *Welcome as a Way of Life: A Practical Theology of Jean Vanier*. Eugene, Ore.: Cascade, 2016.

Wannenwetsch, Bernd. "Angels with Clipped Wings: The Disabled as Key to the Recognition of Personhood." In Swinton and Brock, *Theology, Disability and the New Genetics*, 182–200.

———. "But to *Do* Right . . . Why the Language of 'Rights' Does Not Do Justice to Justice." *Studies in Christian Ethics* 23, no. 2 (2010): 138–46.

———. "From *Ars Moriendi* to Assisted Suicide: Bonhoefferian Explorations into Cultures of Death and Dying." *Studies in Christian Ethics* 24, no. 4 (2011): 428–40.

———. "The Liturgical Origin of the Christian Politeia: Overcoming the 'Weberian' Temptation." In *Church as Politeia: The Political Self-Understanding of Christianity*, edited by Christoph Stumpf and Holger Zaborowski, 323–40. Berlin: Walter de Gruyter, 2004.

———. "Loving the Limit: Dietrich Bonhoeffer's Hermeneutics of Human Creatureliness and Its Challenge for an Ethics of Medical Care." In Wüstenberg, Heuser, and Hornung, *Bonhoeffer and the Biosciences*, 89–108.

———. "'Members of One Another': *Charis*, Ministry and Representation: A Politico-Ecclesial Reading of Romans 12." In *A Royal Priesthood? The Use of the Bible Ethically and Politically: A Dialogue with Oliver O'Donovan*, ed. Craig Bartholomew, Jonathan Chaplin, Robert Song, and Al Wolters, 196–220. Carlisle: Paternoster, 2002.

———. "'My Strength Is Made Perfect in Weakness': Bonhoeffer and the War over Disabled Life." In Brock and Swinton, *Disability in the Christian Tradition*, 353–69.

———. "Plurale Sinnlichkeit: Glaubenswahrnehmung im Zeitalter vitueller Realität." In *Neue Zeitschrift für Systematische Theologie und Religionsphilosphie* 42 (2000): 299–315.

———. *Political Worship: Ethics for Christian Citizens*. Translated by Margaret Kohl. Oxford: Oxford University Press, 2004.

———. "Der Profi: Mensch ohne Eigenschaften: Warum die Kirche Amageure braucht." In *Alles ist Nichts: Evangelium Hören II*, edited by Arbeitskreis Kirche in der Marketgesellschaft, 45–55. Nürnberg, 2001.

———. "Representing the Absent in the City: Prolegomena to a Negative Political Theology According to Revelation 21." In *God, Truth, and Witness: Engaging Stanley Hauerwas*, edited by L. G. Jones, R. Hütter, and C. R. Velloseo Ewell, 167–92. Grand Rapids: Brazos Press, 2005.

Warnock, Joanne. "Fyvie Parents' Joy at Health Board's U-Turn on Willow's Life-Saving Operation." *Aberdeen Press and Journal*, May 8, 2018, 3.

Warnock, Mary. "The Bioethics of Reproduction: Have the Problems Changed?" In Sweeney and Hodder, *The Body*, 39–56.

Wasserman, David, Adrienne Asch, and Jerome Bickenbach. "Mending, Not Ending: Cost-Effectiveness Analysis, Preferences and the Right to a Life with Disabilities." In Clements and Read, *Disabled People and the Right to Life*, 30–56.

Wasserman, David, Jerome Bickenbach, and Robert Wachbroit, eds. *Quality of Life and Human Difference: Genetic Testing, Health Care, and Disability*. Cambridge: Cambridge University Press, 2005.

Webb-Mitchell, Brent. *Beyond Accessibility: Toward Full Inclusion of People with Disabilities in Faith Communities*. New York: Church Publishing, 2010.

———. "Crafting Christians into the Gestures of the Body of Christ." In Eiesland and Saliers, *Human Disability and the Service of God*, 267–80.

Weir, Lorna. "Recent Developments in the Government of Pregnancy." *Economy and Society* 25 (1996): 372–92.

Wen, Leana, and Joshua Kosowsky. *When Doctors Don't Listen: How to Avoid Misdiagnoses and Unnecessary Tests*. New York: St. Martin's, 2012.

Wendte, Martin, ed. *Jesus der Heiler und die Gesundheitsgesellschaft: Interdisziplinäre und Internationale Perspectiven*. Leipzig: Evangelishe Verlagsanstalt, 2018.

———. "Mystical Foundations of Politics? Luther on God's Presence and the Place of Human Beings." *Studies in Christian Ethics* 31, no. 4 (2018): 1–13.

———. "On Hegel's View of People with Disabilities." In Brock and Swinton, *Disability in the Christian Tradition*, 251–85.

Williams, Bernard. "Introductory Essay." In *Meditations on First Philosophy with Selections from the Objections and Replies*. By René Descartes. Rev. ed. Cambridge: Cambridge University Press, 1996.

Williams, Clare. "Framing the Fetus in Medical Work: Rituals and Practices." *Social Science and Medicine* 60 (2005): 2085–95.

Williams, Rowan. "The Body's Grace." In *Theology and Sexuality: Classic and Contemporary Readings*, edited by Eugene F. Rogers, Jr., 309–21. Oxford: Blackwell, 2002.

Williams, Sarah. *The Shaming of the Strong: The Challenge of an Unborn Life*. Lottbridge Drove, U.K.: Life Journey/Kingsway Communications, 2005.

Wood, Don. "Barth on the Concrete Freedom of Human Life." In Brock and Swinton, *Disability in the Christian Tradition*, 391–426.

Wüstenberg, Ralf K., Stefan Heuser, and Esther Hornung, eds. *Bonhoeffer and the Biosciences: An Initial Exploration*. Frankfurt am Main: Peter Lang, 2010.

Wyatt, John. *Matters of Life and Death: Human Dilemmas in the Light of the Christian Faith*. Rev. ed. Foreword by John Stott. Nottingham, U.K.: InterVarsity, 2009.

Yong, Amos. *The Bible, Disability, and the Church: A New Vision of the People of God*. Grand Rapids: Eerdmans, 2011.

———. "Disability and the Gifts of the Spirit: Pentecost and the Renewal of the Church." *Journal of Pentecostal Theology* 19, no. 1 (2010): 76–93.

———. *Theology and Down Syndrome: Reimagining Disability in Late Modernity*. Waco, Tex.: Baylor University Press, 2007.

Young, Frances M. *Brokenness and Blessing: Towards a Biblical Spirituality*. London: Darton, Longman and Todd, 2007.

———. *Face to Face: A Narrative Essay in the Theology of Suffering*. Edinburgh: T&T Clark, 1990.

Zablotsky, Benjamin, Catherine P. Bradshaw, and Elizabeth A. Stuart. "The Association between Mental Health, Stress, and Coping Supports in Mothers of Children with Autistic Spectrum Disorders." *Journal of Autism and Developmental Disorders* 43 (2013): 1380–93.

Ziegler, Philip. *Militant Grace: The Apocalyptic Turn and the Future of Christian Theology*. Grand Rapids: Baker Academic, 2018.

Zuckoff, Mitchell. *Choosing Naia: A Family's Journey*. Boston: Beacon, 2002.

Zuger, Abigail. "A Prescription for Frustration." *New York Times*, April 1, 2013.

Scripture Index

Ancient Sources and Church Fathers Index

Author Index

Subject Index

Also Available in the SRTD Series

Disability and Spirituality: Recovering Wholeness
William C. Gaventa

Crippled Grace: Disability, Virtue Ethics, and the Good Life
Shane Clifton

The Bible and Disability: A Commentary
Edited by Sarah J. Melcher, Mikeal C. Parsons, and Amos Yong

Pastoral Care and Intellectual Disability: A Person-Centered Approach
Anna Katherine Shurley

Becoming Friends of Time: Disability, Timefullness, and Gentle Discipleship
John Swinton

Disability and World Religions: An Introduction
Edited by Darla Y. Schumm and Michael Stoltzfus

Madness: American Protestant Responses to Mental Illness
Heather H. Vacek

Disability, Providence, and Ethics: Bridging Gaps, Transforming Lives
Hans S. Reinders

Flannery O'Connor: Writing a Theology of Disabled Humanity
Timothy J. Basselin

Theology and Down Syndrome: Reimagining Disability in Late Modernity
Amos Yong